This book, from one of the world's most prestigious heart centers, is a veritable treasure chest of information concerning the diagnosis, treatment, and—especially—the prevention of cardiovascular diseases. I enthusiastically recommend it to anyone interested in staying "heart healthy."

Roman W. DeSanctis, M.D.
Professor of Medicine, Harvard Medical School
Director, Clinical Cardiology
Massachusetts General Hospital

A great owner's manual for the heart—comprehensive, coherent, and caring—from the institute founded by Denton Cooley, the best of the best.

Albert Starr, M.D.
Professor of Surgery, Oregon Health Sciences University
Director of Heart Institute, St. Vincent Hospital, Portland, Oregon

Provides concise, easy-to-understand, and up-to-date information on heart disease, from the staff at the acclaimed Texas Heart Institute. It will undoubtedly serve as a practical guide for preventing heart attacks, and helping reduce risks and complications of heart disease.

Valentin Foster, M.D., Ph.D.
Director, Cardiovascular Institute
Dean of Academic Affairs
Mt. Sinai Medical Center

Dr. Cooley and his colleagues have made available a very comprehensive yet understandable commonsense guide to assist each of us as we pursue the goal of maximizing our health.

Dr. James "Red" Duke
Professor of Surgery
University of Texas Medical School, Houston

Dr. Cooley and his team at Texas Heart Institute bring you an outstanding source of information about the heart, providing complete, understandable answers to all your questions.

Mortimer J. Buckley, M.D.
Professor of Surgery, Harvard Medical School
Chief, Cardiac Surgical Unit, Massachusetts General Hospital

This book, written by a knowledgable group, describes various methods to diagnose and treat problems of the heart, but more important, it conveys methods to keep you from needing their expertise.

John Ochsner, M.D.
Chairman Emeritus, Ochsner Clinic

This comprehensive handbook provides people with the insight necessary to understand some of the complexities of heart disease so they can rationally adjust their lifestyles to reduce their risk.

Jay N. Cohn, M.D.
Professor of Medicine
Head, Cardiovascular Division
University of Minnesota Medical School

An excellent handbook that fills a great need. Provides up-to-date information for anyone interested in prevention of heart disease, for heart patients and their families, and even for medical personnel.

W. Proctor Harvey, M.D.
Professor of Medicine, Division of Cardiology
Georgetown University Medical Center

Dr. Cooley and the Texas Heart Institute are the team whose advice is constantly sought on the management of patients with cardiovascular disease. This book clearly exemplifies their expertise, and I heartily endorse it. A significant contribution to the literature to help you understand, care for, and protect this most precious possession—the cardiovascular system.

George J. Magovern, M.D.
Professor of Surgery, Medical College of Pennsylvania and Hahnemann University
Executive Vice President, Health Services Delivery, Allegheny Health, Education and
Research Foundation

You should take the Texas Heart Institute "Heart Health Test." If you score above 12 you must read this book and take its messages seriously. It was expertly and sensibly crafted by health care workers from one of the world's leading heart centers—the Texas Heart Institute.

Tirone E. David, M.D.
Professor of Surgery, University of Toronto
Chief, Division of Cardiovascular Surgery, The Toronto Hospital

The most comprehensive self-help guide available in the area of heart disease. Presented for the nonmedical reader, but a fund of information for health professionals, too. As applicable to international readers as to those in the United States. Everyone who has concerns about their health would benefit from the wealth of knowledge and advice presented.

Stephan Westaby, Consultant Cardiothoracic Surgeon
Oxford Heart Centre
John Radcliffe Hospital
Oxford, England

TEXAS HEART INSTITUTE
HEART OWNER'S HANDBOOK

Foreword by Denton A. Cooley, M.D.
Founder and Surgeon-in-Chief,
Texas Heart Institute

John Wiley & Sons
New York ■ Chichester ■ Brisbane ■ Toronto ■ Singapore

Copyright © 1996 by Texas Heart Institute
Published by John Wiley & Sons, Inc.

Library of Congress Cataloging-in-Publication Data
The Texas Heart Institute heart owner's handbook / Texas Heart
  Institute.
        p. cm.
    Includes bibliographical references and index.
      ISBN 0-471-05982-X (alk. paper). — ISBN 0-471-04420-2 (pbk. :
  alk. paper)
      1. Heart—Diseases—Prevention. 2. Cardiology—Popular works.
  3. Consumer education.   I. Texas Heart Institute.
  RC672.T49 1995
  616.1'2—dc20   95-33694

Printed in the United States of America

10 9 8 7 6 5 4 3 2 1

Contents

PART SEVEN   WHEN SOMETHING GOES WRONG

Foreword

Suppose that you could look 5 years into the future. You see yourself in an intensive care unit, having just suffered a heart attack or stroke, when a doctor walks in the room and tells your family that your chances of dying are one in three. If you knew that you might avoid this fate by making changes in your lifestyle, would you make those changes? More than likely, you would. If you knew that if you didn't make those changes, you could become so ill from heart disease that you could no longer work and support your family, would you make them? Most likely, you would.

Unfortunately, we cannot see into the future. And as a result, many of us don't think about the possibility of heart disease until it's too late. Each year, at least 1.7 million years of potential life are lost to cardiovascular disease by persons 65 or younger. In the United States alone, this disease claims a life every 34 seconds. New diagnostic and treatment methods have helped decrease the death rate due to heart disease, but they have not decreased its prevalence. As of 1992, approximately 59 million Americans were afflicted with some form of cardiovascular disease; and heart disease is prevalent in many other parts of the world also.

Such statistics are frightening, but the news is not all bad. We have learned much about heart disease. Although a few risk factors (mainly, gender and heredity) cannot be controlled, dying from cardiovascular disease is no longer inevitable. In many cases, cardiovascular disease can be treated or even prevented. New technologies and surgical techniques—including pacemakers, balloon angioplasty, and heart transplants—have given years of extra life to patients who would have died from their illnesses. Most babies with congenital heart defects, who once died within days of birth, can now live normal lives. New diagnostic techniques allow us to identify and treat heart disease in its early stages. In addition, we've learned much about what causes heart disease and what measures must be taken to prevent it.

Somehow, however, the warnings about heart disease seem to be falling on deaf ears. Even though more people today are aware that lifestyle changes can make a difference, cardiovascular disease remains a major health and economic problem. Too few people are making the changes they need to make. We know we should:

- Eat less fat. Yet high-fat, fast-food restaurants continue to be our cities' most popular eateries. (Today, even Russians eat Big Macs.)
- Exercise regularly. Yet television remains our national pastime.
- Quit smoking. Yet tobacco companies continue to prosper, here and overseas.
- Lose weight. Yet 25 to 30 percent of Americans are overweight, including our children. The average American gains almost a pound a year between the ages of 20 and 50.
- Decrease our blood pressure. Yet many of us still salt our food without tasting it.

All the medical advances in the world won't eradicate heart disease if people don't alter these patterns of behavior. As I once read, "If you do not think about the future, you cannot have one."

At the Texas Heart Institute, we want to encourage you to look toward your future and to take the steps necessary to prevent heart disease. We hope you find the *Heart Owner's Handbook* to be a useful guide. Used properly, this handbook may help you avoid becoming part of a statistic—one of the almost 59 million people in the United States who suffer from cardiovascular disease. If you already have cardiovascular disease, you and your family can use this handbook to learn about your disease. By making some lifestyle changes, you may be able to prevent or delay the disease from recurring. The *Heart Owner's Handbook* will even give you tips on how to be assertive health care consumers, which is becoming more important as managed care changes the traditional patient-physician relationship.

In this handbook, you'll learn how to assess your risk of cardiovascular disease, how to reduce that risk, and what to do if you have or develop the disease. For those of you who know someone with heart disease (either congenital or acquired), we hope the *Heart Owner's Handbook* will answer your questions as well. However, because we've seen thousands of patients since the Institute was chartered in 1962 (approximately 90,000 open-heart surgery patients and 160,000 heart catheterization patients alone), we know that you'll probably have more questions. If you do, you may call our Heart Information Service at 800–292–2221(outside the United

States, call 713–794–6536. You will be charged the normal rate for international calls). This free service was started for people just like you. Someone will be happy to answer your questions.

In most cases, success must be earned. Although a few achieve success through luck, I believe that the harder you work, the luckier you become. The same philosophy applies to health. As a nation, we must work harder to become healthier. At the Texas Heart Institute, we emphasize the importance of individual responsibility in preventing heart disease. However, until heart disease is conquered, we will continue to generate new knowledge and perform more research to ensure that patients receive the newest, safest, and most effective treatments available. We will also continue to educate, because we will only conquer heart disease if we work together. In the words of former President Dwight Eisenhower, "Together we shall achieve victory."

Denton A. Cooley, M.D.
Founder and Surgeon-in-Chief,
Texas Heart Institute

Acknowledgments

The Board of Trustees and the officers of the Texas Heart Institute appreciate the efforts and assistance of all who have contributed to the making of this book.

Medical Reviewers
> Patrick J. Hogan, M.D., Chairman
> Camilo Barcenas, M.D.
> Denton A. Cooley, M.D.
> Susan Denfield, M.D.
> O. H. Frazier, M.D.
> Alan Hoffman, M.D.
> Ali Massumi, M.D.
> Charles E. Mullins, M.D.
> James T. Willerson, M.D.

Illustrations (except Figures 11–19)
> Carol J. Latta

Editorial/Research
> Jerry Eastman
> Marianne Mallia
> Brook Watts

John Wiley & Sons, Inc. Staff
> Judith N. McCarthy
> Nana D. Prior

Professional Book Center
> Jennifer Ballentine
> Lee Ballentine
> Brian Jones

Introduction

The Texas Heart Institute exists to help you, your family, your community, and your physician. The collective knowledge and experience of the entire Texas Heart Institute staff is at your service through this handbook.

We are a nonprofit organization dedicated to the study and treatment of cardiovascular disease. The Institute was founded in 1962 by Denton A. Cooley, M.D., and is now the largest center in the world devoted to heart disease research and treatment.

More than 160 medical doctors and scientists combine their talents to conduct research, teach physicians and other health professionals, diagnose disease, and deliver comprehensive patient care. Physicians at the Texas Heart Institute have performed more than 160,000 cardiac catheterization diagnostic procedures, 90,000 open-heart surgeries, 600 heart transplants, and 80,000 other heart, chest, and blood vessel operations. The pioneering research they have done has resulted in findings, equipment, treatment techniques, and prevention regimens that have become the standard by which progress is measured.

The Texas Heart Institute's Heart-Health Message

Our primary message is simple: Take care of your heart.

Your heart works hard for you. It circulates the approximately 10½ pints of blood in your body through a progression of arteries and veins that finally become so small that a dozen of them together are the thickness of one human hair. Your heart—the power unit for this intricate cardiovascular network—should last you for many years. However, to a great extent, how you treat your heart controls how long and how well it will continue to work for you.

This handbook contains all the information you need to make the life of your heart as long and as healthy as possible. We have an urgent need to share this lifesaving information with you. Heart disease is the number-one cause of death in the United States and in many other nations. Over 150,000 Americans under 65 died from diseases of the heart in 1992.

An estimated 11.2 million people in the United States alone have been diagnosed with disease of the coronary arteries, the tiny vessels that supply blood to the heart muscle. Millions more have heart problems that go undiagnosed because their illness has not yet progressed to the point where symptoms appear. That's the bad news.

The good news, as recent statistics from the Centers for Disease Control and Prevention indicate, is that the death rate for heart disease in the United States has fallen by about 50 percent since 1970. This improvement is largely due to better diagnostic procedures, more effective treatment, and the acceptance by a growing number of people of their own role in living healthier lives.

By choosing this handbook, you have shown that you're part of that growing number. Congratulations on your decision to take control of your own heart health.

What Good Health Really Means

Most of us tend to consider ourselves in "good health" when we're not experiencing actual signs of illness. True health, though, is much more than the absence of symptoms. Indeed, the first symptoms of many heart disorders are actually indications that serious harm has already been done. Coronary artery disease is a good example. Slowly, one or more arteries supplying oxygen-rich blood to the heart have become blocked. Although this might take years, the very first symptoms of this blockage could well be chest pain or a sudden, fatal heart attack.

Taking direct actions to improve your chances of avoiding future illness is the key to longevity and true health. People in ancient China understood this concept of prevention perfectly. They paid their physicians a monthly fee to keep them well. If a person became ill, the fee was not paid, because the doctor was clearly not doing a good job.

The Good-Health Triangle

Good health, then, goes beyond just feeling well today. Achieving or maintaining good health requires your commitment to take three vital steps. The first is to get the best available information on how your life-style affects your heart. The second step is to resolve to act in your own best interest and to follow through on an informed program of heart-health risk control. And the third is to ensure that you have sound medical care as soon and as often as you need it. Together, these three mutually supportive elements form a triangle that defines the basic requirements for good health—and that also provides the basic organizing framework for this book.

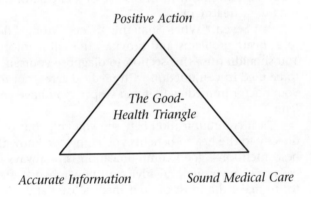

Positive Action

*The Good-
Health Triangle*

Accurate Information   *Sound Medical Care*

Accurate Information

Reliable, up-to-date information allows you to take effective steps to improve your health habits. This means first knowing what affects your heart health. Part One, "Your Personal Heart-Health Profile," provides our test to help you determine your overall heart health and pinpoint your individual risk factors.

You can then personalize the book by looking up your risk factors in Part Two, "Healthy Heart Habits," Part Three, "Controllable Health Factors," and Part Four, "Risk Factors You Can't Change But Need to Assess." In these sections, you'll find what you need to know about your personal risk factors and what you can do about each one.

Positive Action

Once you have the information you need, your good health depends largely on your taking positive action based on that information.

Part Five, "Your Personal Heart-Smart Programs," shows you how with easy-to-follow, proven programs that work whether you're trying to prevent or recover from heart disease, are a woman or a man, young or old, on your own or with a family of eight.

Part Six, "Heart-Smart Cooking," is especially valuable because proper nutrition is key to good heart health even if you have no other obvious risk factors. It provides more than 30 delicious, heart-healthy recipes to help make your transition to good eating much easier.

Sound Medical Care

Periodic examination, testing, and evaluation by a trained physician are crucial to your overall heart health and are important for people of all ages and physical conditions. Regular checkups are especially vital if you're already suffering from heart disease or a circulatory condition that requires long-term treatment.

Part Seven, "When Something Goes Wrong," describes the most common heart problems and provides the latest information on treatments. You shouldn't use this section to diagnose yourself, however. This book is to be used in conjunction with medical care—not to replace it. Always see your doctor immediately if you suspect you have any kind of health problem.

Clear communication between you and your physician will contribute directly to the health benefits you enjoy. We know that, despite everyone's best intentions, good communication isn't always easy. So in Part Seven, we also give you helpful advice on how to work effectively with your doctor to make the most of your medical care and how to achieve your best possible heart health.

Heart Doctors

If you are feeling ill or just having a regular check-up, most likely the physician you visit will be a doctor of internal medicine (internist) or of family medicine. If your condition requires it, these "gatekeepers" of the medical system will refer you to other physician specialists. If your doctor suspects that you have problem with your heart or blood vessels, he or she will refer you to a *cardiologist,* who specializes in diseases of the cardiovascular system. (If your child has heart problems, your pediatrician will refer you to a *pediatric cardiologist.*) Cardiologists may treat your heart or vascular condition with diet, drugs, or invasive but nonsurgical procedures such as balloon angioplasty. If your cardiologist thinks that surgery is required, he or she will refer you to a *cardiovascular surgeon,* who operates to repair, replace, or bypass diseased parts of the heart and vascular system.

Who This Book Is For

This book is for everyone who is concerned about his or her heart health. It is for the young and the old, for men and women, for those who have had heart trouble in the past and those who have never felt sick in their lives, for adults and whole families. In short, it is for you.

Here's some advice on how best to use this book for those with special concerns:

- If you're recovering from heart disease, anything you can do to alleviate your condition and prevent further complications will greatly improve your quality of life. But it's especially important that you act under a doctor's care. We have outlined programs that work well for recovery, but every person is slightly different, so be sure your doctor approves it before you begin any kind of program.

- If you're a woman, you'll notice that we address the special concerns that women may have about heart disease throughout this handbook, but that we have not set this discussion apart (in a separate chapter, for example) because we feel that women's health is *not* a separate issue to be addressed in a segregated, marginalized manner. Where there are differences based on gender, these will be noted in the appropriate section so that complete information is provided throughout the book for *all* readers.

- If you're older, don't underestimate your ability to change your lifestyle for the better. We give special attention to the concerns of seniors regarding safe ways to exercise and achieve fitness.

- If you're young and have never worried seriously about your heart, bear in mind that everything you do now sets the course for your health in later life. Take the self-test in Part One—you may be surprised at how much more you can do for your heart.

- If you have a family, it's never too soon to get your children interested in a heart-healthy lifestyle. You'll find guidelines and advice on healthy weight and nutrition for children that can set positive patterns for their future. And we're sure your family will like the heart-healthy recipes in Part Six.

- If you're already a convert to heart-healthy living or find that this book helps you, share it with your family members, friends, and colleagues. You'll be doing them a favor.

The Texas Heart Institute Free Heart Information Service

While we've tried to bring you the most complete, up-to-date information about your heart health, no book can answer every person's concerns. So, if you have further questions about your heart, your cardiovascular system, good health habits, or any medical treatment for a heart condition, you're invited to call 800–292–2221, to speak with a member of our staff of Information Specialists, who will be happy to help you.

This service is offered throughout the United States at no cost, as part of our commitment to heart-health awareness. Our Information Specialists are on duty Monday through Friday, between 8:00 A.M. and 5:00 P.M., Central Time. Calls made during other hours will be recorded on an answering machine, so you can leave your name, phone number, and question(s), and one of our Information Specialists will call you back with a reply.

Texas Heart Institute's Heart Information Service
800–292–2221

Outside the United States, call 713–794–6536.
You will be charged the normal rate for international calls.

PART ONE

Your Personal Heart-Health Profile

How Healthy Is Your Heart?

CHAPTER 1

How Healthy Is Your Heart?

The world's leading scientific and medical experts all agree: A healthier heart can add years to your life and dramatically increase your vitality. If this sounds good to you, you've picked up the right book.

At the Texas Heart Institute, we believe that a healthier heart is within everyone's reach. But first, you must be willing to take a very close look at how healthy your heart is today. To help you, we've designed a simple test that will give you an accurate estimate of your heart's health almost instantly.

About the Test

Everyone should take this test. You can't fail it; you can only come out ahead. It's based on numerous scientific studies of nine factors that affect the average person's heart. These factors are your personal health history, how much you exercise, your weight, whether you smoke or use tobacco in any form, your blood pressure, your total cholesterol, whether you have diabetes, your gender, and your age.

You may be wondering why we haven't included diet, alcohol, stress, or genetic factors such as race and family health history on this list. It is, after all, well known that these factors also affect your heart, and we will help you assess them thoroughly later on, in chapters 3, 6, 7, and 13. But for a quick rating of your heart health, the nine factors we've identified provide the most reliable measurement based on current scientific data.

Please be aware, though, that these data come from large groups of people. Because individuals are affected differently, this test is *not* intended to be a personal medical assessment. It is intended to do two other important things: (1) heighten your awareness of how much you can improve your heart's health, and (2) point the way to a smarter, happier, healthier lifestyle.

Answer each question, giving yourself the number of points shown next to your answer. When you've finished, add up your points for your total score, and check your results. Answer the questions as honestly as you can. The only way you can blow this test is to fudge the truth.

THE TEXAS HEART INSTITUTE HEART-HEALTH TEST

▶ Personal Health History

I have a diagnosed heart or blood vessel disease.

Yes **4**

No **0**

▶ Exercise

I perform aerobic exercise (such as walking, jogging, cycling, swimming, step-training, or dance) for a daily total of 30 minutes four or more times each week.

No **4**

Yes **0**

▶ Weight

Use Table 1 to find your healthy weight range. Using the appropriate table for your gender, look up your height (without shoes) and body frame size to find your healthy weight range (ranges include 3 pounds (1.3 kg) of clothing for women, 5 (2.3 kg) pounds for men). To determine your body frame size, place your left thumb and middle finger around your right wrist and squeeze tightly. If your thumb and finger overlap, you have a small frame; if they just touch, you have a medium frame; if they do not touch, you have a large frame.

My weight is

20 pounds (9 kg) or more
above my healthy range **3**

10 to 20 pounds (4.5 to 9 kg)
above my healthy range **2**

5 to 10 pounds (2.3 to 4.5 kg)
above my healthy range **1**

Within 5 pounds (2.3 kg) of
my healthy range **0**

TABLE 1   Weight Guideline for Adults

	Women			Men			
Height (in ft & in)	Small Frame (in lb)	Medium Frame (in lb)	Large Frame (in lb)	Height (in ft & in)	Small Frame (in lb)	Medium Frame (in lb)	Large Frame (in lb)
4' 9"	102–111	109–121	118–131	5' 1"	128–134	131–141	138–150
4' 10"	103–113	111–123	120–134	5' 2"	130–136	133–143	140–153
4' 11"	104–115	113–126	122–137	5' 3"	132–138	135–145	142–156
5' 0"	106–118	115–129	125–140	5' 4"	134–140	137–148	144–160
5' 1"	108–121	118–132	128–143	5' 5"	136–142	139–151	146–164
5' 2"	111–124	121–135	131–147	5' 6"	138–145	142–154	149–168
5' 3"	114–127	124–138	134–151	5' 7"	140–148	145–157	152–172
5' 4"	117–130	127–141	137–155	5' 8"	142–151	148–160	155–176
5' 5"	120–133	130–144	140–159	5' 9"	144–154	151–163	158–180
5' 6"	123–136	133–147	143–163	5' 10"	146–157	154–166	161–184
5' 7"	126–139	136–150	146–167	5' 11"	149–160	157–170	164–188
5' 8"	129–142	139–153	149–170	6' 0"	152–164	160–174	168–192
5' 9"	132–145	142–156	152–173	6' 1"	155–168	164–178	172–197
5' 10"	135–148	145–159	155–176	6' 2"	158–172	167–182	176–202
5' 11"	138–151	148–162	158–179	6' 3"	162–176	171–187	181–207
6' 0"	141–154	151–165	161–182	6' 4"	166–180	175–191	186–212
6' 1"	144–157	154–168	164–185	6' 5"	169–183	179–195	191–217
6' 2"	147–160	157–171	167–188	6' 6"	172–186	183–199	196–222

(continued next page)

TABLE 1   *Weight Guideline for Adults (continued)*

	Women				Men		
Height (in cm)	Small Frame (in kg)	Medium Frame (in kg)	Large Frame (in kg)	Height (in cm)	Small Frame (in kg)	Medium Frame (in kg)	Large Frame (in kg)
145–146	46–50	49–54	53–59	155–156	58–60	59–63	62–68
147–149	46–51	50–55	54–60	157–158	59–61	60–64	63–69
150–151	47–52	51–57	55–62	159–160	59–62	61–65	64–70
152–154	48–53	52–58	56–63	161–163	60–63	62–67	65–72
155–156	49–54	53–59	58–64	164–166	61–64	63–68	66–74
157–158	50–56	54–61	59–66	167–168	62–65	64–69	67–76
159–160	51–57	56–62	60–68	169–171	63–67	65–71	68–77
161–163	53–59	57–63	62–70	172–173	64–68	67–72	70–79
164–166	54–60	59–65	63–72	174–176	65–69	68–73	71–81
167–168	55–61	60–66	64–73	177–178	66–71	69–75	72–83
169–171	57–63	61–68	66–75	179–181	67–72	71–77	74–85
172–173	58–64	63–69	67–77	182–183	68–74	72–78	76–86
174–176	59–65	64–70	68–78	184–186	70–76	74–80	77–89
177–178	61–67	65–72	70–79	187–188	71–77	75–82	79–91
179–181	62–68	67–73	71–81	189–191	73–79	77–84	81–93
182–183	63–69	68–74	72–82	192–194	75–81	79–86	84–95
184–186	65–71	69–76	74–83	195–196	76–82	81–88	86–98
187–188	66–72	71–77	75–85	197–199	77–84	82–90	88–100

Adapted from the Metropolitan Life Insurance Company, New York, 1983. Data from the 1979 Build Study, Society of Actuaries and Associates of Life Insurance Medical Directors of America, 1980. The weights presented are those associated with the lowest mortality between the ages of 25 and 59.

▶ Smoking and Tobacco

I smoke cigarettes every day . . . 4

I used to smoke, but I quit
less than 3 years ago 3

I don't smoke but I live or work
(or both) with people who do . . 2

I don't smoke cigarettes,
but I do smoke a pipe or cigars . . 2

I used to smoke, but I quit
more than 3 years ago 1

I don't smoke 0

▶ Blood Pressure
(for adults 18 or older)

My blood pressure is

Above 160/90 4

Between 140/90 and 160/90 . . . 2

Below 140/90 0

▶ Total Cholesterol

My cholesterol is

Above 240 mg/dL
(6.2 mmol/L) 3

200 to 240 mg/dL
(5.2 to 6.2 mmol/L) 2

I don't know my
cholesterol count 1

200 mg/dL
(5.2 mmol/L) or below 0

▶ Diabetes

I have high blood sugar or diabetes.

Yes 4

No 0

▶ Gender

I am

Male 4

Female, have gone through
menopause, and am not taking
hormone replacement therapy . . 3

Female, have gone through
menopause, and am taking
hormone replacement therapy . . 1

Female and have not gone through
menopause 0

▶ *Age*

I am male and

Over 60 4

45 to 60 3

30 to 44 2

Under 30 0

I am female and

Over 60 3

45 to 60 2

30 to 44 1

Under 30 0

▶ *Add up your points for all the questions to get your total score:*

Personal Health History _____

Exercise _____

Weight _____

Smoking and Tobacco _____

Blood Pressure _____

Total Cholesterol _____

Diabetes _____

Gender _____

Age _____

What Your Score Means

Check your total score against the categories described below. This will give you an indication of your overall heart health.

0–12

You are at *low risk*. Congratulations! Chances are good that your current lifestyle will keep your heart healthy for many years. This book will help you understand what you're doing right and provide information that could make your heart even healthier in the years to come. If your score was relatively high on any item(s), be sure to read the relevant chapter(s) of this book carefully. Also take note of the chapters on diet, alcohol, stress, and genetic factors.

13–24

You are at *medium risk*. You should modify your lifestyle to lower your risk of heart disease. If you have not yet discussed your heart risks with your doctor, make an appointment for a complete checkup.

Carefully read the chapters in this book on each of the factors that increased your score, as well as the chapters on diet, alcohol, stress, and genetic factors. As you begin the recommended programs to make the necessary adjustments to your lifestyle, discuss your plans and progress with your doctor.

25–34   You are at *high risk*. If you are not already being treated for heart disease, *see your doctor immediately*. It is important that you begin to reduce your risk as soon as possible. And if you already have a heart problem, you can do much to prevent your condition from becoming worse.

Once you have talked with your doctor, read the chapters in this book on each of the factors that increased your score, as well as the chapters on diet, alcohol, stress, and genetic factors. With your doctor's okay, begin living a healthier lifestyle by following the programs described in Part Five of this handbook. Also, begin eating a more healthy diet right away by using the recipes provided in Part Six.

If, after reading the information here, you have further questions about anything related to your heart health, you are invited to call our free Heart Information Service. Our staff of Information Specialists will be happy to help you at no charge.

Texas Heart Institute's Heart Information Service
800–292–2221

Outside the United States, call 713–794–6536.
You will be charged the normal rate for international calls.

You Can Improve Your Score

Almost everyone can improve their heart health in some way. Don't be content with a score of "medium risk" or even "low risk." Your health—and your life—are too important. Remember, a healthier heart is the key to longer life. Research shows that the average American over 35 can expect to live several months or even years longer—simply by controlling one or more heart-health risk factors. The most conclusive studies demonstrating the correlation between risk factor modification and increased life expec-

TABLE 2   *Years You May Gain by Caring for Your Heart*
(for Americans 35 years old who have one or more risk factors)

Risk Factor Controlled	Potential Added Years	
	Men	*Women*
Weight	0.7–1.7	0.5–1.1
Smoking and tobacco use	1.2–2.3	1.5–2.8
Blood pressure	1.1–5.3	0.9–5.7
Total cholesterol	0.5–4.2	0.4–6.3

Adapted from Tsevat, J., Weinstein, M.C., Williams, L.W., Tosteson, A.N., Goldman, L. Expected gains in life expectancy from various coronary heart disease risk factor modifications. *Circulation* 83, no. 4 (1991), pp. 1194–201. Reproduced with permission. Copyright © 1991 American Heart Association.

tancy have focused on four risk factors in particular: weight, smoking and tobacco use, blood pressure, and total cholesterol. The average number of years you could expect to gain by controlling these risk factors are shown in Table 2.

Perhaps even more important than extending your life, reducing risk factors can increase your *quality* of life. You are likely to feel more vigorous and alive if you take steps to improve your heart health.

PART TWO

Healthy Heart Habits

Exercise and Physical Fitness

Good Nutrition

Weight Control

No More Smoking and Tobacco

*Moderate or No Drinking
and No Illegal Drugs*

CHAPTER 2

Exercise and Physical Fitness

WHAT YOU NEED TO KNOW

If your self-test showed that you don't exercise enough to keep your heart healthy, read on, because exercise plays a fundamental role in reducing your risk of cardiovascular disease.

What Exercise Can Do for You

Aerobic exercise has been associated with lower blood pressure, is an effective component of weight-control programs, can decrease the insulin dosages needed to control diabetes, and produces increased levels of HDL ("good") cholesterol in the blood. (High blood levels of HDL cholesterol have been linked to a lowered risk of heart disease.) Also, people who exercise are more likely to stop or reduce smoking. Exercise may also keep blood vessels more flexible, which has significant potential benefit for all of us, but particularly for men and women over 50. Finally, physical activity generates greater psychological well-being for many people.

At the Texas Heart Institute, we recommend adequate exercise for most patients who are recovering from heart disease or other cardiovascular problems. And we're not alone. Both the American Heart Association and the National Heart, Lung and Blood Institute recognize physical inactivity as an important risk factor for developing coronary artery disease. And data gathered by the U.S. Centers for Disease Control and Prevention have indicated that people with a sedentary lifestyle are at higher risk for death from heart disease than those who exercise regularly. Indeed, several reputable studies have demonstrated that physical activity seems to reduce death not only from heart disease but from all causes.

What Kind of Exercise Should You Do?

There are two broad categories of exercise:

▶ 1. *Aerobic exercise* uses large groups of muscles and can be continued for long periods of time. Examples include walking, jogging, and cycling. Aerobic exercise drives the body to use oxygen more efficiently and delivers maximum benefits to the heart, lungs, and circulatory system.

▶ 2. *Anaerobic exercise*, experienced during short, high-effort activities, builds muscle strength, muscle endurance, and bone density. Examples include weight lifting and sprinting. Since the activity is intense and quickly over, the body receives less training in efficient oxygen use.

Anaerobic exercise does little to develop cardiovascular fitness and may, in certain cases, be harmful for those with high blood pressure. Even so, most well-balanced exercise programs involve some degree of anaerobic training because certain muscle groups, including those in the waist, back, and stomach, respond best to anaerobic conditioning. However, it is aerobic exercise that best conditions the heart.

How Much Is Enough?

A good general guideline (recently established by the Centers for Disease Control and Prevention and the American College of Sports Medicine) is to perform about 30 minutes of moderate to intense physical activity most days of the week. Such exercise can include active gardening, climbing stairs instead of using an elevator, or brisk housework. And it is not necessary to perform the same exercise each day. In fact, varying the type of exercise will probably lead to higher levels of overall fitness because you will use different muscle groups.

If you cannot arrange your schedule to accommodate a 30-minute block of exercise time, three 10-minute exercise periods per day will still produce positive effects.

To help you determine how much exercise you should do, remember the words "brisk," "sustained," and "regular":

■ A *brisk* workout raises your heart and breathing rates.

■ A *sustained* workout lasts 30 minutes (or longer).

■ A *regular* workout takes place four or more times per week.

Your Heart Rate during Exercise

Your heart rate is your best guide to the intensity of your workout. For optimum cardiovascular conditioning, you want to be in your "Fitness Zone," which is defined as 50 to 75 percent of your maximum heart rate. (This range is also referred to as your target heart rate.) The maximum heart rate declines as you grow older, so the exact parameters of your Fitness Zone depend on your age.

To determine your individual Fitness Zone, first calculate your maximum heart rate (in beats per minute) by subtracting your age from 220. Then multiply that number by 50 percent and 75 percent to determine the lower and upper boundaries, respectively, of your target heart rate. For example, if you are 50, your Fitness Zone would be a heart rate of 85 to 128 beats per minute (220 − 50 = 170; 170 × 0.50 = 85; 170 × 0.75 = 127.5). Table 3 shows the target heart rates for various ages.

Stay within your Fitness Zone when you exercise. Increasing your heart rate above the upper boundary does not appreciably improve cardiovascular conditioning and could be dangerous; and failing to maintain your heart rate above the lower boundary decreases the benefits of exercise.

You can check your heart rate, or pulse, at your neck or wrist, as shown in Figure 1. To do this, stop your exercise and place two fingers *either* between your wrist bone and the tendon on the thumb side of your wrist *or* along the left side of your neck. You should feel the pulsing of the artery with gentle pressure (pressing too hard, however, will block the flow of blood, and you won't feel anything). Count the number of beats you feel in 10 seconds, then multiply that by 6 to determine your heart rate in beats per minute.

TABLE 3   *Healthy Heart Rates*

Age (in years)	Fitness Zone (in beats per minute)
20	100–150
25	98–146
30	95–143
35	93–139
40	90–135
45	88–131
50	85–128
55	83–124
60	80–120
65	78–116
70	75–113

Source: National Heart, Lung, and Blood Institute and the
American Heart Association, *Exercise and Your Heart: A Guide to
Physical Activity,* 1993.

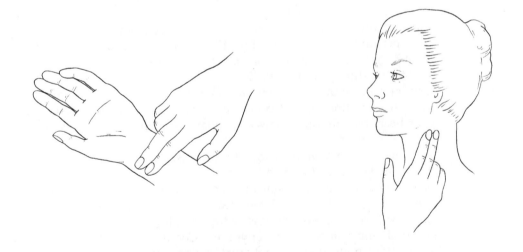

FIGURE 1   *Using two fingers, check your pulse at either your wrist or your neck.*

The Importance of Exercising Properly

When exercise is done properly, the benefits are quite amazing. But exercise can pose health risks if not done properly. The most common harmful effect associated with exercise is injury from placing too great a strain on muscles and joints. Too much effort too soon or for too long will harm even highly trained professional athletes. The wrong kind of exercise can also trigger existing heart problems. An especially dangerous situation arises when someone who exercises only occasionally suddenly engages in a physically challenging activity (sometimes referred to as the "weekend-warrior syndrome").

A study of 1,228 heart attack survivors at 45 U.S. hospitals showed that 4.4 percent of the heart attacks occurred within an hour of heavy exercise, and exercise probably precipitated 3.8 percent of them. The research also indicated that those who exercised less than once a week were more at risk for heart attack after performing an arduous task, such as pruning trees, shoveling snow, jogging, laying bricks, swimming, or climbing a ladder.

To make sure this doesn't happen to you, see your physician before undertaking any exercise regimen; but in any case, stop exercising the moment you feel weak, short of breath, or nauseated, and see your doctor as soon as possible.

Even though exercise can provide important health benefits, it is *vital* to manage your exertion level, work out properly on a regular basis, and be aware of how fit you are.

Preventing Exercise Injuries

The four most important ways to avoid exercise-related injuries follow.

▶ 1. *Start Your Program Slowly.* Begin your journey into fitness slowly. We crawl before we walk, and walk before we run. Each stage builds the body for the next step. Crawl and walk, figuratively speaking, before trying to run in the sport or activity you select. Expecting or trying too much too soon has ruined too many exercise programs and caused too many injuries. Start slowly, progress gradually, and you'll have a much better chance of staying with the activity. This rule is true for everyone, but if you're over 40, you should take special care to build your exercise program *gradually.*

▶ **2.** *Warm Up—Every Time.* Before attempting any strenuous physical activity, take 4 to 5 minutes to warm up. Walk leisurely, move about, or do any gentle movements that will slightly increase your heart rate and loosen and warm your joints and muscles. Shifting suddenly from a resting state to performing at or near your maximum physical capability places an enormous demand on your cardiovascular system. In many cases, the heart cannot meet the challenge.

Start slowly. Move smoothly. Give your body a chance to warm up gradually. Then increase the intensity of your exercise to your target heart rate.

▶ **3.** *Stretch Properly.* Professional athletes know the value of stretching before, during, and after exercise. Stretching should be part of your warm-up and cool-down routines; it is the great preventer of muscle and joint problems. Like exercise, stretching must be done properly to avoid injury. See chapter 15 for more information about stretching. Many of our patients at the Texas Heart Institute discover the benefits of gentle stretching during their recovery process.

▶ **4.** *Use Good Judgment.* Good judgment means staying within your physical limits. Light exercise, performed frequently, is much better for you than one gut-wrenching, muscle-quaking workout session per week. Even professional coaches and athletes counsel that physical conditioning is gained a little at a time.

Proper judgment also includes remembering that exercise is not limited to working out in a gym or jogging around a track. Pushing a lawn mower, putting up storm windows, and vacuuming a rug are all forms of exercise—although they may not qualify as aerobic exercise. Remember that the guidelines for warming up and stretching apply to these kinds of physical work as well.

Proper judgment can also help you avoid other exercise-related difficulties. Heat- or sunstroke, for example, may be prevented by being aware of the weather and taking simple precautions. These include drinking adequate amounts of water and avoiding overexertion or overexposure to the sun. (See also the discussions under "Paying Attention to Your Body" and "Using Common Sense," below.)

The Five-Step Aerobic Exercise Session

The four guidelines for avoiding exercise-related injuries also allow you to derive the most benefit from your exercise. Notice how they are incorporated into the basic five-step exercise session.

Please Note: These are general guidelines only. Part Five of this handbook details a complete exercise program.

▶ **Step 1.** *Stretch Thoroughly.* To begin, perform a few simple stretches that include all of your main muscle groups, not just the ones you are about to use. Stretch gently for at least 2 to 3 minutes.

The benefits derived from adequate stretching are hard to overstate. Many competitive athletes stretch as much or more than they practice their sport. Stretching is especially important as we age, to help maintain flexibility.

▶ **Step 2.** *Begin Slowly.* Start your exercise routine at a reduced level. You want a gradual effort that will slowly raise your heart rate. Never begin by calling suddenly on your body's maximum output. This places a severe strain on your entire circulatory system. Moreover, even after stretching, your muscles are not yet ready for a supreme effort.

▶ **Step 3.** *Intensify Gradually.* After gentle stretching and an easy beginning, you should slowly intensify your activity over a 5-minute period until you attain your target heart rate.

▶ **Step 4.** *Remain in Your Fitness Zone.* Once your heart rate is inside your Fitness Zone, try to keep it there. At first, even a minute or so at the lower end of your target heart rate might be uncomfortable. Then again, your heart rate might jump to the upper end fairly quickly. If this happens, slow down. Stay inside your Fitness Zone. After several sessions, you'll be able to maintain your heart rate at the desired level for longer periods.

For cardiovascular fitness, exercising in your Fitness Zone for 30 minutes at a time is enough. If you're also exercising as part of a weight-loss plan, longer periods are acceptable. Be sure, though, to keep your heart rate in the Fitness Zone.

▶ **Step 5.** *Ease Off Slowly and Stretch Again.* After exercising in your Fitness Zone for your desired length of time (duration), don't just stop. Teach yourself to slow down gradually, then stop and stretch some more. Take another 5 minutes to complete this cycle, allowing your body to ease off the effort of a full-intensity workout.

Remember that the routine of a 10-minute warm-up, 30 minutes inside your Fitness Zone, and 5 minutes of cool-down not only makes for an efficient, beneficial workout, but is also one of your best protections against exercise-related injury.

Keeping Realistic Goals

Another safeguard against exercise-related injury is to maintain realistic expectations and goals. Physical conditioning takes place at the rate set by the body, not imagined in the brain. Keeping realistic goals and objectives will help you avoid pushing yourself too hard too soon.

Paying Attention to Your Body

Your body is a reliable judge of exercise intensity—so pay attention. A sharp pain or a slowly building ache are warning signs. If discomfort occurs, discontinue the activity until you understand the cause. A sudden dizzy feeling, fainting, cold sweat, or pallor are other signs to stop. Pain or pressure in the middle or on the left side of your chest or in your left shoulder or arm, during or just after exercise, may be a *serious warning sign*. If any of these symptoms occurs, *see your physician immediately*.

Using Common Sense

Relying on common sense is one of the most important ways to prevent injury. Do not exercise right after eating; wait about an hour. Likewise, wait 20 minutes or so after exercise before eating. Drink lots of water before, during, and after exercise.

If you go outside, wear appropriate clothing. Protect your skin from the sun, either with clothing or sunscreen or both. Be extra careful on hot, humid days: Monitor your heart rate more frequently. On cold days, extend your warm-up routine because the blood vessels in your arms and legs tend to constrict when cold, which raises your blood pressure and causes your heart to work harder. And last, but far from least, when exercising on roads and streets, watch out for cars.

Exercise during Pregnancy

Conventional wisdom once held that women should not exercise during pregnancy. Most doctors now recommend regular, moderate exercise, with certain additional precautions.

If you're pregnant, you should be careful to select exercises appropriate to the stage of your pregnancy. While there is no difficulty in lying flat on your back during the first trimester, this position can interfere with your circulation and respiration during the later stages of pregnancy. So, you should avoid exercising in this position during the final 2 trimesters. Likewise, strenuous weight lifting and conventional abdominal exercises are not recommended in the later stages of pregnancy.

You must also avoid overheating your body as this could have adverse effects on fetal development. Stop your workout before you become fatigued, and be sure to drink plenty of water before, during, and after exercise.

The goal of exercise during pregnancy should be to maintain a sound level of cardiovascular and overall fitness. This will help you control your weight and will also ease the transition back to your normal exercise program after you give birth. However, be sure to allow ample recovery time after childbirth before attempting to resume your prepregnancy level of exercise activity.

Naturally, because pregnancies and physical fitness vary greatly among women, it is important to discuss any exercise plans with your obstetrician or other care provider. For more details about exercise and pregnancy, see the listing for the American College of Obstetricians and Gynecologists under "Exercise" in the "Resources" appendix of this book.

Fitness in Later Years

It is a medically accepted fact that as we age, our bodies lose some aerobic capacity. A variety of new studies, though, indicate that the decline in aerobic capacity might be less than previously thought and may begin later. The decline in fitness experienced by many seniors may therefore be due more to decreased activity levels than to physiological changes from aging.

In any case, the benefits of aerobic exercise—namely, improved cardiovascular health, increased physical strength, and improved psychological outlook—are available to anyone, regardless of age. Indeed, a person over 70 who follows a good fitness plan may well be in better shape than an inactive 40-year-old.

People in their 60s and older may find that a modified conditioning program is best (once again, see Part Five for your personal exercise program). Such a program includes longer warm-up and cool-down periods and requires slower movements during the actual activity. For many older adults, special attention should be paid to avoiding high-impact exercises, like jogging, which place undue strain on muscles and joints. Walking, swimming, and low-impact aerobics are good substitutes. In any case, older adults should significantly increase the time and emphasis devoted to stretching.

WHAT YOU CAN DO

Exercise is crucial to a healthy heart. Here are some things to consider as you get started.

See a Doctor before Beginning a Fitness Program

Seeing your doctor is especially important if you have any of the following health risks:

- You're taking a prescription medication.
- You've ever had any kind of heart problem, especially a heart attack.
- You have diabetes.
- You have bone or joint difficulties.
- You have uncontrolled high blood pressure.
- You have a family history of heart disease.
- You are a man over 45 or a woman over 50, if you are not accustomed to even moderate levels of exercise.
- You smoke.
- You're significantly overweight (10 percent to 20 percent above the maximum weight in your healthy weight range).

If you don't have any of these conditions but feel more comfortable having a doctor's okay before you begin, by all means contact your physician. One of the purposes of exercise is to enjoy yourself, and that's hard to do if you have any doubts about your physical condition and the risks of your activity.

Carefully Choose a Fitness Program

Most people who succeed in making exercise a part of their lives find some pleasure or enjoyment in the exercise they select. So first and foremost, try to find one or more activities you like or that give you satisfaction.

There are several other considerations you need to review when setting up your own exercise program.

Matching Benefits to Your Workout

Decide on the benefits you want from exercise, then match the exercise to those benefits. That sounds simple enough, yet many people fail to define their fitness program in terms of goals. Weight control, for instance, requires long-duration aerobic activity to burn maximum calories; while building muscle definition depends more on working specific muscles against resistance for brief periods.

Selecting Facilities and Equipment Necessary

No one needs to spend a great deal of money to exercise properly. In fact, there is no need to spend any money at all. Private health clubs may offer facilities and amenities that you prefer, such as a pool, sophisticated exercise machines, or exercise classes; however these may be expensive. Instead, you can walk aerobically through your neighborhood (or through the local mall if the weather is bad), you can buy a used stationary bicycle or treadmill, or you can buy and follow exercise videotapes. Perhaps your community has fitness facilities available at low or no cost. A growing number of communities also offer organized exercise programs, free or at reasonable rates. Use your imagination. There's no need to pay a lot of money to exercise.

Finding the Time to Exercise

Lack of time is often the downfall of well-intended exercise programs. It is easier to fit exercise into your life if you set aside the same time each day for the activity.

In a recent survey of 1,018 Americans, 64 percent said they would like to exercise but just didn't have enough hours in the day to fit it in. Most said they had fewer than 10 hours for leisure activity per week. Yet 84 percent watched television for at least 3 hours during a typical day.

Never let the excuse of insufficient time keep you from exercising. Even 30 minutes a day, broken into separate 5-, 10-, or 15-minute periods, will be enough to make a heart-healthy difference. Many people find that they can catch the TV news or keep up with their favorite programs while putting in some time on a stationary bike or treadmill.

Make Exercise a Regular Part of Your Life

Exercise is where we find it. Many physically undemanding occupations provide opportunity for brief periods of exercise. Climbing stairs instead of using the elevator, parking farther away from your office, or taking a brief, brisk walk at lunchtime are just a few ways to find fitness at the office.

If your job calls for a physically taxing effort, then you are exercising as you work. Stretching, a warm-up, and a cool-down are just as important to a painter or bricklayer as to a tennis pro.

Make exercise a part of your life and chances are your quality of life will improve. At the same time, you will be building cardiovascular fitness and lowering your risk of heart attack. For more information on how to do this, see Part Five of this handbook.

CHAPTER 3

Good Nutrition

WHAT YOU NEED TO KNOW

If you are currently not eating a healthy diet, you should know that the old adage "you are what you eat" is taking on new meaning as health experts learn more about the connections between the foods we eat and how our bodies process those foods. Good eating habits can significantly decrease our risk of heart disease, stroke, high blood pressure, diabetes, and some types of cancer.

Many organizations, professional associations, and federal agencies offer guidelines and recommendations for good nutrition. In this chapter, we'll try to translate all this government/institution–speak into readily understandable information you can use to improve your daily diet and overall heart health.

Consider what follows vital background material that will help you make sense of all the media noise telling you what to eat and why. We provide a framework—as well as the resources—for you to make sound decisions. We begin with the basics.

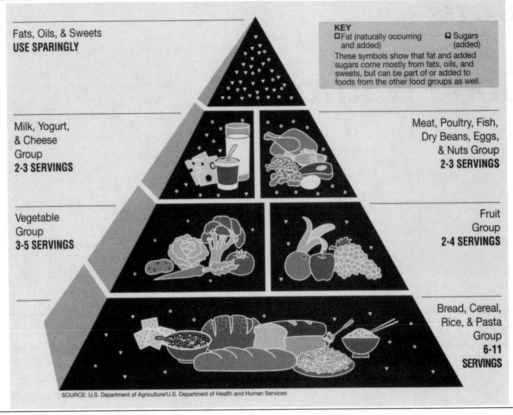

Fats, Oils, & Sweets
USE SPARINGLY

KEY
□ Fat (naturally occurring
and added)   ◩ Sugars
(added)
These symbols show that fat and added
sugars come mostly from fats, oils, and
sweets, but can be part of or added to
foods from the other food groups as well.

Milk, Yogurt,
& Cheese
Group
2-3 SERVINGS

Meat, Poultry, Fish,
Dry Beans, Eggs,
& Nuts Group
2-3 SERVINGS

Vegetable
Group
3-5 SERVINGS

Fruit
Group
2-4 SERVINGS

Bread, Cereal,
Rice, & Pasta
Group
**6-11
SERVINGS**

SOURCE: U.S. Department of Agriculture/U.S. Department of Health and Human Services

FIGURE 2   *The Food Guide Pyramid.*
Source: U.S. Department of Agriculture.

The Food Guide Pyramid

The U.S. Departments of Agriculture and Health and Human Services have
developed a set of dietary guidelines. The "Food Guide Pyramid" (see Figure 2), which is based on these guidelines, describes the number of daily
servings you should consume from each of the five food groups to "enjoy
better health and reduce your chances of getting certain diseases." The five
food groups (and the recommended number of daily servings of each) are
the bread, cereal, rice, and pasta group (6 to 11 servings); the vegetable
group (3 to 5 servings); the fruit group (2 to 4 servings); the milk, yogurt,
and cheese group (2 to 3 servings); and the meat, poultry, fish, dry beans,

eggs, and nuts group (2 to 3 servings). In addition, fats, oils, and sweets should be used sparingly.

Sample serving sizes include one slice of bread, 1 ounce (28 g) of ready-to-eat cereal, or ½ cup of cooked cereal, rice, or pasta; 1 cup of raw leafy vegetables, ½ cup of other vegetables, cooked or chopped raw, or ¾ cup (180 ml) of vegetable juice; one medium apple, banana, or orange, ½ cup of chopped, cooked, or canned fruit, or ¾ cup (180 ml) of fruit juice; 1 cup (240 ml) of milk or yogurt, 1½ ounces (43 g) of natural cheese, or 2 ounces (57 g) of processed cheese; and 2 to 3 ounces (57 to 85 g) of cooked lean meat, poultry, or fish (½ cup of cooked dry beans, 1 egg, or 2 tablespoons of peanut butter count as 1 ounce [28 g] of lean meat). We will use these guidelines and serving sizes in the following discussion about nutrition.

Food and Nutrients

Whether you are in motion or at rest, your body needs nutrients to function properly. The nutrients you need include carbohydrates, proteins, fats, vitamins, and minerals. Your body gets these nutrients from the foods you eat. When you combine the right foods, you give your body enough nutrients to function properly. (Water, although strictly speaking not a nutrient, is also necessary for your body to function properly.)

Carbohydrates

Carbohydrates are the main source of fuel in a balanced diet. They energize the brain, the central nervous system, and the muscles. The body converts carbohydrates to glucose, a type of sugar. Some of this glucose is used immediately, while any excess glucose is transformed into another type of sugar called glycogen. Glycogen is stored in the liver and muscles for future use, and can be quickly converted back into glucose as needed. Once the glycogen reservoirs are filled, the remaining glucose is stored as body fat.

Sugars and starches are carbohydrates. Each gram of carbohydrate provides 4 calories. (A calorie is a measure of chemical energy; protein also has 4 calories per gram, but a gram of fat contains 9 calories.) The most common simple sugar is glucose, and when glucose molecules are linked together, they can create a variety of different large molecules, called complex carbohydrates. Starch is the major complex carbohydrate and the major source of glucose in our diet. Fiber, that media and marketing darling of recent years, is a type of complex carbohydrate that may help protect against heart disease and some cancers.

Sugars

Sugars, which are called simple carbohydrates, provide the body with a quick source of energy. The sugars we consume are digested more quickly and easily than complex carbohydrates, because sugars have fewer chemical bonds to be broken down in the digestive process. They can be used immediately by the body as fuel. Refined sugar, brown sugar, corn sweeteners, syrups, honey, and molasses are examples of foods largely composed of sugars. Added sugars are also found in foods like candy, soft drinks, jams, and jellies. Unfortunately, sugars add more calories than nutrients to a diet. However, if you get your daily supply of sugars from fresh fruits and natural fruit purees, you will add more vitamins and minerals to your diet. Try to limit your intake of added sugars to no more than 10 percent of your total daily calories. Another rule of thumb would be to limit your added sugars to 6 teaspoons a day if you eat about 1,600 calories, 12 teaspoons at 2,200 calories, or 18 teaspoons at 2,800 calories.

Starches

Starches are called complex carbohydrates because the digestive process must break them down to release their sugars. Breads, cereals, corn, peas, potatoes, pasta, and rice are examples of complex carbohydrates. Contrary to conventional opinion, complex carbohydrates are relatively low in calories. It's our preparation of these foods that fattens them up. For instance, adding butter (or margarine), sour cream, bacon, and cheddar cheese turns an innocent baked potato into a high-fat, high-cholesterol side dish.

Several studies have shown that when people get most of their calories from such complex carbohydrates as starchy vegetables and whole-grain cereals, they suffer less coronary artery disease than people with high-fat or high-sugar diets. Try to maintain a diet in which your intake of complex carbohydrates is 50 percent or more of your total daily calories. Six to 11 daily servings from the bread, cereal, rice, and pasta group should suffice.

Fiber

High-fiber foods are a form of complex carbohydrates. They can help protect your body against heart disease, cancer, and stomach and bowel disorders. Fiber cannot be digested by humans, and because it binds water and softens stools, it helps speed the elimination of waste (and perhaps cancer-causing agents) from the intestinal tract. Fiber is actually a complex mixture of various substances, which can include cellulose, pectin, and lignin. Pectin, found in the peel of most citrus fruits, has cholesterol-lowering properties. Bran from oats can also help lower blood cholesterol levels by absorbing cholesterol in the small intestine and eliminating it with the body's waste.

Dietary fiber comes in two forms. *Soluble fiber* dissolves in water and is present in most plant foods. Soluble fibers are especially concentrated in vegetables and fruits with edible peels and seeds, in legumes (dried beans and peas), and in oat, corn, and rice bran. *Insoluble fiber* does not dissolve in water and tends to be found in cereals, wheat bran, whole-grain breads, and other grain products including rice and pasta. Your goal should be to eat 20 to 25 grams of dietary fiber daily, including both soluble and insoluble fiber. Table 4 lists the fiber content of many common fruits and vegetables.

Consuming fiber-rich foods may help you lose weight because they provide complex carbohydrates, proteins, vitamins, and minerals and contain little, if any, fat. Foods high in fiber also take up space in the digestive tract, so you tend to feel fuller longer. But introducing too much fiber into your diet too quickly can cause problems like gas, bloating, loose stools, diarrhea, and flatulence. It is best to add high-fiber foods to your diet gradually.

Proteins

Throughout your life, proteins will deliver building materials for the growth, maintenance, and repair of the body's tissues, including the muscles. Proteins are also needed for the production of our body's hormones, enzymes, and antibodies. Excess protein is converted and stored as body fat. It serves as emergency fuel in the absence of carbohydrates and fats.

Proteins are constantly being broken down into their component amino acids, which are used in the body's unending replacement of cells. There are 20 amino acids, and the body manufactures all but nine of them. These nine, called the "essential amino acids," must come from the proteins you eat since the body cannot create them.

There are two general sources of proteins. Foods rich in *animal protein* include beef, pork, fish, chicken, eggs, and dairy products. However, diets containing animal protein tend to increase blood cholesterol levels. Foods rich in *vegetable protein*, on the other hand, seem to lower blood cholesterol levels, reducing the risk of heart disease. Vegetable proteins are found

TABLE 4   *Total Dietary Fiber of Fruits and Vegetables*
(grams per 3.5-ounce portion unless otherwise indicated)

Fruit	Grams of Fiber	Vegetable	Grams of Fiber
Figs, dry (5)	12	Baked beans	9
Prunes, dry (5)	8	Kidney beans	7
Apricots, dry (8)	8	Navy beans	6
Blackberries	7	Lima beans	5
Raspberries	5	Peas	4
Apricots, fresh (5)	4	Corn	4
Dates (5)	4	Sweet potato	3
Banana (1)	4	Carrot, large (1)	3
Pear (1)	4	Potato with skin, large (1)	3
Mango (1)	3	Broccoli (1 stalk)	3
Apple (1)	3	Tomato, large (1)	3
Nectarine (1)	3	Brussels sprouts	2
Orange, large (1)	3	String beans	2
Raisins (¼ cup)	3	Bean sprouts	2
Peach, large (1)	2	Asparagus	2
Plums (3)	2	Summer squash	2
Strawberries	2	Zucchini	2
Blueberries	2	Cabbage	2
Cherries	1	Kale	2
Grapes	1	Onions	2
Grapefruit (1)	1	Cauliflower	2
Cantaloupe (½ cup)	1	Celery	1
Honeydew melon (½ cup)	1	Mushrooms	1
Watermelon (2 cups)	1	Lettuce	1
		Spinach	1
		Radishes (5)	1
		Peppers	1
		Cucumber, large (1)	1

in such foods as broccoli, lentils, potatoes, bulgur, pasta, oatmeal, rice, walnuts, chickpeas (garbanzo beans), soybeans, and kidney, lima, and navy beans.

The World Health Organization, the Food and Nutrition Board of the National Academy of Sciences, and the National Research Council agree that a balanced diet needs only 0.75 grams of protein per kilogram of body weight per day. In more practical terms, you should eat 2 to 3 servings daily from the meat, poultry, fish, dry beans, eggs, and nuts group. Most Americans eat much more protein than that; we also eat more animal protein than vegetable protein by a ratio of two to one. Remember, excess protein is stored as body fat, and, because meats contain saturated fats as well as animal protein, eating them may increase your blood cholesterol. That's why if you have high LDL ("bad") cholesterol levels, or if you have been diagnosed with heart disease, you may want to limit or even eliminate meat from your diet.

Protein and the Vegetarian Diet

A diet devoid of animal protein needs to be carefully planned and monitored. Fruits, vegetables, and grains are considered incomplete protein sources because no individual fruit, vegetable, or grain provides all nine of the essential amino acids (animal proteins, on the other hand, are complete protein sources). Dried beans and peas (legumes) are low in the amino acid methionine, while grains (rice, wheat, corn, and oats) are low in the amino acid lysine. The combination, however, of a legume and a grain in a meal can provide the appropriate amounts of amino acids or "complete protein." In many places throughout the world where meat is scarce or prohibitively expensive, these grain-and-bean combinations account for most of the protein consumed. Nuts and seeds are fine sources of many of the essential amino acids, but they are high in calories and should be consumed sparingly. To ensure the proper intake of all the essential amino acids, some vegetarian diets do include nonfat dairy products including skim milk, nonfat yogurt, nonfat cheeses, and egg whites.

Fats

Dietary fat is a very important component of your daily nutrition, providing you with more than twice as much energy (measured in calories per gram) as either carbohydrates or proteins. Fat helps move vitamins through the body, manufacture hormones, build cell membranes, and create sources of reserved energy for the body. However, fat also interacts with the liver to manufacture cholesterol, thus the amount of fat you consume directly affects your body's blood cholesterol levels. (See chapter 9 for a discussion of cholesterol.) And you need only a small amount of dietary fat to provide the essential fatty acids required to keep your body chemistry in balance.

Most foods contain a mixture of three fats: saturated, polyunsaturated, and monounsaturated. One of these fats usually predominates in the individual foods we eat.

Saturated Fats

Saturated fats are primarily found in foods of animal origin such as meats and whole-milk dairy products, and in tropical oils such as coconut oil, cocoa butter, and palm oil. Saturated fats usually stay solid at room temperature.

Saturated fats are held most responsible for coronary artery disease because they are used by the liver to manufacture cholesterol. The liver normally makes all the cholesterol the body needs to sustain healthy cells and neurological functions. When we eat foods containing saturated fats, however, our livers are prompted to create more cholesterol than needed, and eliminating the excess cholesterol is difficult. Cholesterol, which is moved through the body via the bloodstream, begins to collect in the blood vessels, creating a waxlike substance called *plaque*. This plaque may eventually block the flow of blood to and from the heart and brain, which could result in a heart attack or stroke. That's why excessive cholesterol can be dangerous and why we should attempt to reduce our cholesterol levels by avoiding foods high in saturated fats and cholesterol. For more information about cholesterol, see chapter 9.

Polyunsaturated Fats

Found in vegetable and fish oils, polyunsaturated fats usually stay liquid at room temperature. Oils such as corn, cottonseed, sesame, safflower, and soybean are good sources of polyunsaturated fats.

Polyunsaturated fats are often hydrogenated to produce a solid form of the product, like margarine. Food manufacturers hydrogenate corn, soy, or some other oil by saturating it with hydrogen to make it harden. Hydrogenated oils are found in margarine, shortening, commercially baked goods, nondairy creamers, commercially processed peanut butter, and some ice creams.

The procedure of hydrogenation creates a compound known as a *trans* fatty acid. In the body, these *trans* fatty acids seem to act as saturated fats by raising the LDL ("bad") cholesterol levels and lowering the HDL ("good") cholesterol levels. (See chapter 9 for a discussion of LDL and HDL cholesterol.) Although this is still a controversial subject among scientists, there is evidence from some recent studies that would discourage our consumption of hydrogenated or partially hydrogenated fats.

Monounsaturated Fats

Prominent in olive, canola, and peanut oils, monounsaturated fats don't seem to cause as much of an increase in blood cholesterol levels as other fats do. Foods rich in monounsaturated fats include avocados, olives, and nuts such as pecans, almonds, peanuts, and cashews.

Some cultures consume high amounts of monounsaturated fats and actually have a low incidence of cardiovascular disease. The populations of Greece, Italy, and Spain have a diet high in monounsaturated fats but very low in saturated and polyunsaturated fats. (They consume most of their fat as olive oil.) This "Mediterranean diet" produces some of the lowest incidences of coronary artery disease and breast cancer in the world, and some experts believe that any group (including Americans) that follows such a diet will have a lower incidence of cardiovascular disease.

Most Americans eat a diet that is about 37 percent fat, 15 to 17 percent of which is saturated fat. The American Heart Association and the National Cholesterol Education Program Expert Panel recommend reducing the amount of fat consumed to no more than 30 percent of your total daily calories. And only one-third of that, or 10 percent of your total daily calories, should come from saturated fats. An easier way to keep track of the fats you eat is by knowing that 30 percent of calories from fat is 53 grams of fat in a 1,600-calorie diet, 73 grams of fat in a 2,200-calorie diet, and 93 grams of fat in a 2,800-calorie diet. Although it isn't necessary to monitor your fat intake every day, counting your daily grams of fat consumed from time to time will help keep you below the 30-percent mark. Use the labels on foods you purchase to give you the grams of fat per serving.

If, however, you already have cardiovascular disease, cutting your daily fat intake to 30 percent of your total daily calories may not be enough to stop or even slow the disease process. You may need to reduce your *total dietary fat intake* to 10 percent of your total daily calories, and avoid *all foods* that contain cholesterol. One note of caution, however: Younger children should not be put on a low-fat diet; they need the fat calories to maximize their growth.

Although polyunsaturated fats are better for you than saturated fats, and monounsaturated fats are better than polyunsaturated fats, *all* fats will raise your blood cholesterol levels. Learning to change your eating habits to reduce the amount of high-fat foods you eat is easy and can be fun. When you're finished with this chapter, turn to Part Six of this handbook for some tips on choosing heart-healthy foods and creating a low-fat diet simply by modifying your favorite recipes.

Vitamins

Vitamins are organic substances that perform specific functions required for reproduction and growth. Vitamins regulate your body's metabolism, which controls the amount of energy you use in daily activities like walking, sleeping, and thinking.

Eating foods rich in vitamins helps ensure your good health. Table 5 lists some common vitamins, what they do, and where they're found. *Note*: Diets devoid of animal products probably need vitamin B-12 supplements. Check with your doctor or dietitian.

TABLE 5   *Vitamins: What They Do and Where to Get Them*

Vitamin	Essential For	Good Sources
Vitamin A (and beta-carotene)	Healthy skin, strong teeth and bones in children, maintaining resistance to infection, normal growth, cell structure, normal vision	Fish liver oils, liver, dairy products (vitamin A); carrots, dark-green leafy vegetables (beta-carotene)
Vitamin B-1 (thiamine)	Metabolizing carbohydrates, digestion and appetite, normal function of nervous system	Whole grains, brown rice, beans, peas, organ meats, lean pork, seeds/nuts
Vitamin B-2 (riboflavin)	Normal growth, formation of certain enzymes, cellular oxidation, prevention of sores and inflammation of mouth and tongue	Dairy products, meats, poultry, fish, green vegetables (broccoli, turnip greens, asparagus, spinach)
Vitamin B-3 (niacin)	Activities of enzymes in the metabolism of carbohydrates and fats, detoxification of pollutants and alcohol, nervous and digestive system functions, production of sex hormones, healthy skin	Lean meats, fish, poultry, whole grains
Vitamin B-6 (pyridoxine)	Metabolism of amino acids, manufacture of hemoglobin	Meats, whole grains, wheat germ, brewer's yeast
Vitamin B-12	Nervous system functions, normal development of red blood cells, production of genetic material in cells, use of carbohydrates as well as folic acid in the body	Fish, dairy products, organ meats, beef, pork, eggs
Biotin	Activities of enzymes needed to break down fatty acids in carbohydrates, excretion of wastes from breakdown of proteins	Nuts, whole grains, vegetables, fruits, milk, organ meats, brewer's yeast

(continued next page)

Antioxidant Vitamins and Heart Disease

For years, researchers have been studying the possibility that vitamins A, C, and E might actually prevent heart disease. These vitamins may deter the formation of plaque in the arteries by preventing oxygen from combining with the LDL ("bad") cholesterol. The process by which oxygen and LDL cholesterol combine is called *oxidation*, and the vitamins that hinder or prevent it are thus called *antioxidants*. Vitamin E, in large doses (about ten times greater than that found in most diets), makes LDL cholesterol resistant to oxidation. Vitamin A, beta-carotene, and vitamin C do not completely prevent oxidation but markedly slow the process.

TABLE 5 *Vitamins: What They Do and Where to Get Them* (continued)

Vitamin	Essential For	Good Sources
Folic acid	Important metabolic processes in the body, growth, reproduction, production of red blood cells	Green leafy vegetables, oranges, beans, peas, rice, eggs, liver
Pantothenic acid	Production of adrenal gland hormones, manufacture of sex hormones, activities of enzymes in the metabolism of fats and carbohydrates, utilization of vitamins, normal growth, nervous system functions	Organ meats, eggs, whole grains, brewer's yeast
Vitamin C (ascorbic acid)	Sound skin, bones, teeth, gums, ligaments, and blood vessels; immunity to disease; wound healing; absorption of iron from the digestive tract	Citrus and other fresh fruits, fresh vegetables
Vitamin D	Strong bones; regulation of the absorption of calcium and phosphorus from the digestive tract	Fatty fish, liver, eggs, fortified milk
Vitamin E	Normal neurologic functions, formation of red blood cells, maintaining some enzymes, normal cellular structure, protection against pollutants	Whole grains, vegetable oils, green leafy vegetables, eggs
Vitamin K	Blood clotting	Green leafy vegetables, dairy products

Vitamin A

Vitamin A plays an important role in hormone development, cell differentiation, resistance to infection, and the eye's ability to see in dim light. Vitamin A can be found in liver, egg yolk, fish liver oils, butter, margarine, milk, and cheese. Although these foods are good sources of vitamin A, they are also high in fat. Beta-carotene, a non-fattening source of vitamin A, is found in yellow and orange vegetables such as carrots, sweet potatoes, and pumpkins. Other green and yellow vegetables and fruits containing beta-carotene include cantaloupe, peaches, broccoli, collards, kale, mustard greens, and spinach.

A note of caution about taking vitamin A supplements: Prolonged intake of high doses of vitamin A (greater than 50,000 international units) can be toxic. At those levels, vitamin A may cause, among other things, headaches, vomiting, bone abnormalities, and liver damage.

Vitamin C

The most widely recommended yet highly controversial vitamin supplement is vitamin C. Vital to the formation of collagen in the body, vitamin C increases the body's ability to absorb iron from food. Found in most citrus fruits and in such vegetables as broccoli, cabbage, potatoes, and peppers, vitamin C also promotes wound healing and several enzyme reactions.

A number of studies suggest that taking vitamin C supplements can reduce the severity of the cold virus and cut a patient's recovery time. Other studies indicate that vitamin C may lower the risk of cancers of the stomach and esophagus.

Some researchers recommend high doses of vitamin C (1,000 milligrams per day) to help lower blood pressure and levels of LDL ("bad") cholesterol. But high doses of vitamin C taken over long periods of time can be dangerous to some people. Like all dietary supplements, vitamin C supplements should be taken under a doctor's supervision.

Vitamin E

The body uses vitamin E to form red blood cells and muscle tissue. In recent years, researchers have been conducting studies to evaluate the possible preventive and therapeutic use of vitamin E against heart disease, cancer, cataracts, and Parkinson's disease. Current evidence indicates that vitamin E may help prevent heart disease by reducing the oxidation of LDL ("bad") cholesterol. Vitamin E is prevalent in vegetable oils, green leafy vegetables, wheat germ, and nuts.

Niacin

Nicotinic acid or niacin, one of the B vitamins, has been touted for years as a natural treatment for high blood cholesterol. It can be very effective, dramatically lowering LDL ("bad") cholesterol levels and triglycerides while raising HDL ("good") cholesterol levels. However, because niacin in high doses may have dangerous side effects, it should not be used unless prescribed by your doctor.

A recent study reported in *JAMA* (the *Journal of the American Medical Association*) confirmed high-dose niacin as a cholesterol-lowering agent. Researchers also found, however, that the required high doses of niacin (2,000 to 3,000 milligrams daily) sometimes caused dangerous side effects, including gastrointestinal problems, peptic ulcers, increased blood sugar levels, flushing, precipitated gout attacks, itching, and liver toxicity.

Again, check with your doctor before taking niacin to lower your cholesterol. If you take high doses of niacin, he or she will want to monitor your liver function through routine blood testing.

Minerals and Trace Elements

Minerals are inorganic chemical elements required by the body for many biological processes. Like vitamins, minerals can be found in the foods we eat. Trace elements, too, are inorganic chemical elements, but the body requires only small amounts of these substances. Tables 6 and 7 list some common minerals and trace elements, what they do, and where they are found.

Magnesium, Calcium, and Potassium

Minerals play an important role in the functions of the heart and blood vessels. Magnesium and calcium help to regulate the heart's rhythm. Abnormal levels of magnesium, calcium, and potassium can cause irregular heartbeats, especially in people with preexisting heart problems.

TABLE 6   *Minerals: What They Do and Where to Get Them*

Mineral	Essential For	Good Sources
Calcium	Healthy bones and teeth, nerve conduction, muscle contraction, blood coagulation, production of energy, immunity	Dairy products, green leafy vegetables
Chlorine	Maintaining body's fluid and electrolyte balances, digestive juices	Table salt
Magnesium	Every major biologic process, metabolism of glucose, synthesis of nucleic acids and protein, production of cellular energy	Meats, fish, green vegetables, dairy products
Phosphorus	Strong bones, all cell functions, cell membranes	Dairy products, fish, meats, poultry, vegetables, eggs
Potassium	Many major biologic processes, muscle contraction, nerve conduction, synthesis of nucleic acids and protein, energy production	Fresh vegetables, fresh fruits
Sodium	Osmotic equilibrium in tissues	Table salt, added to foods by manufacturer
Sulfur	Sulfur-containing amino acids	Onions, garlic, eggs, meat, dairy products

TABLE 7   *Trace Elements: What They Do and Where to Get Them*

Trace Element	Essential For	Good Sources
Chromium	Sugar metabolism	Whole grains, spices, meats, brewer's yeast
Copper	Hemoglobin synthesis and function; production of collagen, elastin, neurotransmitters; melanin formation	Organ meats, shellfish, nuts, fruits
Fluorine	Binding calcium in bones and teeth	Fluoridated water
Iodine	Production of energy (as part of thyroid hormones)	Seafood, iodized salt
Iron	Hemoglobin synthesis and function; enzyme actions in energy production; production of collagen, elastin, neurotransmitters	Organ meats, meat, poultry, fish
Manganese	Functions not entirely understood, but necessary for optimal health	Whole grains, nuts
Molybdenum	Functions not entirely understood, but necessary for optimal health; detoxification of hazardous substances	Organ meats, whole grains, green leafy vegetables, milk, beans
Selenium	Functions not entirely understood, but necessary for optimal health	Broccoli, cabbage, celery, onions, garlic, whole grains, brewer's yeast, organ meats
Zinc	Immunity and healing, good vision, hundreds of enzyme activities	Whole grains, brewer's yeast, fish, meats

Magnesium helps the body regulate the conversion of carbohydrates to energy. It also is necessary for the formation of hormones and enzymes that regulate various body processes. Adequate consumption of magnesium may help prevent certain kinds of kidney stones, reduce pain from menstrual cramps, and ward off migraine headaches. A diet deficient in magnesium may increase your chance of developing high blood pressure, a major risk factor for heart attack and stroke. It should not be necessary to supplement the magnesium in your normal diet, however, because magnesium is abundant in whole-grain cereals, legumes, and many fruits and vegetables.

Calcium is needed for healthy bones and teeth. It also plays an important role in muscle and nerve function, blood clotting, insulin secretion, enzyme regulation, and overall bone strength. Some studies have demonstrated that people who consume less than 300 milligrams of calcium per day have two to three times as great a risk of developing hypertension as do those who consume 1,200 milligrams per day. Calcium is found in green leafy vegetables, nuts, milk products, and legumes. Although calcium is also found in canned sardines and salmon, your body may not be able to extract the calcium from these foods.

Potassium is required by the body for many functions. Most adults need about 2,000 milligrams of potassium daily. Potassium can be found in bananas, broccoli, carrots, dates, raisins, dried figs, juices (orange, prune, and tomato), potatoes, spinach, legumes (dried beans and peas), seafood, and meats. Because potassium is found in so many different foods, a varied diet will supply most healthy people with a sufficient amount of this mineral. Consuming too much potassium can cause diarrhea, irritability, muscle cramps, and an irregular heartbeat, so you should not take a potassium supplement unless your doctor prescribes it for a specific purpose. For example, large losses of potassium can occur in people who are taking diuretics; if you are taking diuretics regularly, your doctor may also prescribe a potassium supplement.

Sodium

Although there is no evidence that minerals are *directly* involved in promoting or preventing coronary artery disease, eating too much sodium (salt) can contribute significantly to high blood pressure in some people, and no one *benefits* from eating too many salty foods. Nearly half of our sodium intake comes from salt or sodium compounds added to foods during processing. Luncheon meats, ham, bacon, sausage, snack foods, and many fast foods are major sources of salt for many people. In addition, many recipes for home-cooked meals often call for more salt than is really needed for flavor.

The average American diet provides about 5,000 milligrams of sodium each day. That's twice as much as we need. You should try to limit your total sodium intake to 2,400 milligrams a day, which is roughly the amount contained in a teaspoon of salt—though remember, processed and packaged foods already contain plenty of sodium.

Iron

Iron's main function is to carry oxygen from the lungs to the tissues and cells of the body. Most of the iron in the body combines with protein in red blood cells to form hemoglobin. The remainder is used by enzymes, muscles, and other tissues. Iron is found in a wide variety of plant- and animal-based foods.

Some studies have indicated a relationship between excess iron stores in the body and an increased risk of coronary artery disease or heart attack, but the evidence for such a relationship in the average person is by no means conclusive. Moreover, increased iron intake may lead to hemochromatosis, a disease of iron metabolism that also can be hereditary. In hemochromatosis, progressive iron overload leads to a massive accumulation of iron in the body. If left untreated, hemochromatosis can lead to cardiac disease, cirrhosis, diabetes, arthritis, cancer of the liver, or a combination of these. Early diagnosis and treatment can prevent the progression of the disease.

Consumption of large amounts of iron supplements over time may damage the liver and other organs; it is important, therefore, not to add iron supplements to your daily diet unless you have checked with your doctor. He or she can measure your iron stores to determine whether supplements are necessary.

Vitamin and Mineral Supplements

Please talk with your doctor before taking any supplements. You may need vitamin and mineral supplements if you:

- Consume fewer than 1,500 calories a day.
- Must eliminate, for health reasons, a specific food group from your diet. (Food groups contain similar kinds of foods from which you can choose to maintain a balanced diet. The five food groups are vegetables; fruits; breads, cereal, rice, and pasta; milk, yogurt, and cheese; and meats, poultry, fish, dry beans, eggs, and nuts.)
- Take medications that interfere with your body's ability to absorb or use certain vitamins, such as antibiotics, antacids, diuretics, oral diabetes drugs, anti-inflammatory drugs, and some cancer drugs.
- Become pregnant or are breast-feeding.

WHAT YOU CAN DO

Taking control of your diet is one of the most effective ways you can reduce your risk of developing cardiovascular disease. Learning to select and prepare heart-healthy foods will benefit you throughout your life.

Eat a Heart-Healthy Diet

The first step to healthy eating is to become more aware of your diet. Start thinking heart-healthy, and before you know it, your eating habits will begin to change. The recipes included in Part Six of this handbook will help you get started.

Learn to Read Food Labels

To provide consumers with accurate information about the nutritional content of the foods they buy, the U.S Food and Drug Administration (FDA) recently standardized the language and style of food labeling. The FDA requires that nutrients be arranged in order of greatest importance to health so that consumers may choose an overall healthy diet. See Figure 3 (on the next page) for a sample food label with annotations that explain how to read it.

Because of the abundant food supply in the United States, vitamin deficiencies are no longer a problem, and labels no longer include the familiar Recommended Daily Allowances (RDA) for vitamins and minerals. Instead, the term "Daily Value" has replaced the RDA. The Daily Values for specific nutrients such as fat and sodium, whose overconsumption is related to increased risk of disease, are defined by regulation and based on a diet of 2,000 calories. On the label, "% Daily Value" or "% DV" indicates the percentage of the Daily Value in a single serving of the labeled food. The FDA, which regulates food labeling, redesigned the format and content of the new labels to aid consumers in determining and comparing the nutritional content of food products.

In addition, the FDA has defined numerous basic packaging terms to ensure consistency and accuracy in food labeling and advertising. You can no longer be misled by manufacturers' claims that a food product is "light," "lean," or "fat-free." The FDA requires that food manufacturers adhere to the FDA definitions, which are described in Table 8 (see page 43).

Finally, manufacturers can promote a food product's health benefits only if they can demonstrate a valid relationship scientifically. These are the health claims for food products currently allowed by the FDA:

- That calcium helps prevent osteoporosis (loss of bone substance).
- That reduced consumption of sodium decreases the risk of high blood pressure.
- That reduced consumption of fat helps prevent cardiovascular disease and some cancers.
- That increased consumption of dietary fiber helps prevent colon cancer and heart disease.
- That increased consumption of antioxidants (such as vitamins A, C, and E) helps prevent some cancers.

The new food label will carry an up-to-date, easier-to-use nutrition information guide, to be required on almost all packaged foods (compared to about 60 percent of products up till now). The guide will serve as a key to help in planning a healthy diet.*

Serving sizes are now more consistent across product lines, are stated in both household and metric measures, and reflect the amounts people actually eat.

New title signals that the label contains the newly required information.

Calories from fat are now shown on the label to help consumers meet dietary guidelines that recommend people get no more than 30 percent of the calories in their overall diet from fat.

The **list of nutrients** covers those most important to the health of today's consumers, most of whom need to worry about getting too much of certain nutrients (fat, for example), rather than too few vitamins or minerals, as in the past.

% Daily Value shows how a food fits into the overall daily diet.

Nutrition Facts
Serving Size 1 cup (228g)
Servings Per Container 2

Amount Per Serving

Calories 260 Calories from Fat 120

	% Daily Value*
Total Fat 13g	**20%**
Saturated Fat 5g	**25%**
Cholesterol 30mg	**10%**
Sodium 660mg	**28%**
Total Carbohydrate 31g	**10%**
Dietary Fiber 0g	**0%**
Sugars 5g	
Protein 5g	

Vitamin A 4%	•	Vitamin C 2%	
Calcium 15%	•	Iron 4%	

* Percent Daily Values are based on a 2,000 calorie diet. Your daily values may be higher or lower depending on your calorie needs:

		Calories:	2,000	2,500
Total Fat	Less than		65g	80g
Sat Fat	Less than		20g	25g
Cholesterol	Less than		300mg	300mg
Sodium	Less than		2,400mg	2,400mg
Total Carbohydrate			300g	375g
Dietary Fiber			25g	30g

Calories per gram:
Fat 9 • Carbohydrate 4 • Protein 4

The label of larger packages may now tell the number of calories per gram of fat, carbohydrate, and protein.

Daily Values are also something new. Some are maximums, as with fat (65 grams or less); others are minimums, as with carbohydrate (300 grams or more). The daily values for a 2,000- and 2,500-calorie diet must be listed on the label of larger packages.

* This label is only a sample.

FIGURE 3   *The new food label.*
Source: U.S. Food and Drug Administration.

TABLE 8   *Food Labels: What Do They Mean?*

The FDA requires food labels, when they carry these descriptive phrases, to adhere to certain required definitions.

Free
(Per serving)
For calorie-free: less than 5 calories

For sugar-free: less than 0.5 g of sugar

For sodium-free: less than 5 mg of sodium

For fat-free: less than 0.5 g of fat

For cholesterol-free: less than 2 mg of cholesterol

For free of saturated fat: less than 2 g of saturated fat

Fresh
Raw; never frozen, processed, or preserved

High
Provides more than 20% of the amount recommended for each day, as in "high fiber"

Lean
Cooked meat or poultry with less than 10.5 g of fat (of which less than 3.5 g would be saturated fat) and less than 94.5 mg of cholesterol per 100 g

Extra Lean
Cooked meat or poultry with less than 4.9 g of fat (of which less than 1.8 g would be saturated fat) and less than 94.5 mg of cholesterol per 100 g

Less
Twenty-five percent or less of the sodium, calories, fat, saturated fat, or cholesterol found in the regular product

Light
One-third fewer calories than the regular product; any other use of the term must specify that it is a reference to appearance, taste, or smell, as in "light in color"

Low
(Per 100 g or 3.5 ounces)
For low-sodium: less than 140 mg of sodium

For low-calorie: less than 40 calories

For low-fat: 3 g or less of fat

For low in saturated fat: 1 g or less of saturated fat and not more than 15% of calories from saturated fat

For low cholesterol: 20 mg or less of cholesterol and 2 g or less of saturated fat

More
At least 10% more of the nutrient than in the regular product, as in "more fiber"

Source Of
Provides 10% to 20% of the recommended daily consumption of the nutrient

Source: U.S. Food and Drug Administration.

Follow These Healthy Eating Guidelines

The U.S. Dietary Guidelines are defined by a committee of scientists for the U.S. Departments of Agriculture and Health and Human Services. The guidelines are currently under revision to incorporate the latest nutrition research findings. While we await the new guidelines, let the following suggestions influence your daily eating habits:

▶ 1.   Eat a wide variety of foods. Your body requires about 50 different nutrients. The only way to get them all is to eat a variety of foods every day.

▶ 2. Determine your healthy weight (see chapter 4), and don't eat more than you need to maintain it.

▶ 3. Limit your consumption of fats to no more than 30 percent of your total daily calories. For example, if you consume a daily diet of 2,000 calories, your fat intake for the day should be no more than 65 grams, and if you consume a daily diet of 2,500 calories, your fat intake for the day should be no more than 80 grams. (There are 9 calories in each gram of fat.) In addition, you should limit your consumption of saturated fats to no more than 10 percent of your total daily calories (20 grams of fat in a 2,000 calorie-a-day diet).

▶ 4. Limit your consumption of cholesterol to about 300 milligrams daily. Consult the food labels for the cholesterol content of most foods. (An egg has 213 milligrams of cholesterol.)

▶ 5. Consume at least half of your total daily calories in the form of complex carbohydrates by eating plenty of vegetables, fruits, and grain products. Consume simple sugars sparingly.

▶ 6. Limit your consumption of proteins to no more than 15 percent (some experts say no more than 8 percent) of your total daily calories. Most adults do not need more than 2 ounces (approximately 56 grams) of protein per day.

▶ 7. Limit your daily consumption of sodium to the amount contained in a teaspoon of salt, approximately 2,400 milligrams—but remember that many processed foods already contain excess sodium. Let the new "Nutrition Facts" food labels, which contain an entry for milligrams of sodium, help you stay below the recommended limit.

CHAPTER 4

Weight Control

WHAT YOU NEED TO KNOW

If your self-test showed that you have an unhealthy weight, you're not alone. According to the *Surgeon General's Report on Nutrition and Health*, about one-fourth of all American adults are overweight and nearly one-tenth are obese. Yet a healthy body weight is an important component of good health in general and good heart health in particular. Being even slightly overweight increases your risk of heart disease, and being obese (exceeding one's proper body weight by more than 30 percent) is clearly linked to cardiovascular problems, high blood pressure, stroke, the most common type of diabetes, some cancers, and other illnesses. The operative words here are *healthy weight range*. This doesn't mean that you should be model-skinny: Being too thin for your body type may not be healthy either.

Finding Your Healthy Weight Range

One's healthy weight varies from person to person and depends not only on height, gender, and frame size, but also on what percentage of the total body weight is fat, where the body fat is located, and a personal/family history of medical problems such as high blood pressure.

The following guidelines will help you calculate your own healthy body weight.

Using the Weight Table

To find your healthy weight range, you must first determine the size of your body frame. To do so, place your left thumb and middle finger around your right wrist and squeeze as tightly as possible. If your thumb and finger overlap, you have a small frame; if they just touch, you have a medium frame; if they do not touch, you have a large frame. Turn back to Table 1 in chapter 1, then find your height (without shoes) in the appropriate column for women or men of your frame size, and find your healthy weight range (which includes 3 pounds [1.4 kg] of clothing for women, 5 pounds [2.3 kg] for men). Does your weight fall within this range? Ranges are given because people of the same height may not have identical muscle and bone mass.

Other Factors to Consider

Weight tables only tell part of the story. You can fall within the recommended weights shown on the table and still not be at your healthy body weight, because of your particular balance of fat and muscle. Experienced technicians can use any of several accepted methods to determine precisely what percentage of your total body weight is due to fat. This testing requires special equipment, however, and is usually done for a fee. Fortunately, knowing your exact percentage of body weight due to fat isn't necessary for good heart health. By combining information from the weight table with a few simple tests that you can do at home, you'll be able to judge if an overweight condition is due to muscle mass (and therefore not a problem) or too much fat.

Here are three quick checks that can reveal a lot about the makeup of your body.

▶ 1. *Pinch an Inch.* To determine if you have excess fat, stand straight with your shoulders back. Using your thumb and forefinger, pinch the skin at the side of your waist and estimate the thickness of the fold. If you manage to pinch over an inch, you are probably carrying too much fat.

▶ 2. *The Jiggle Test.* For this test, dress in only your underwear. Stand in front of a full-length mirror and jump lightly up and down. Anything shaking that shouldn't is excess. (Admittedly, this is not a very scientific test, but it does reveal deposits of excess body fat.)

▶ **3.** *Body Shape—Apples versus Pears.* Most men and some women are apple-shaped, meaning that they store fat around their middles. In contrast, pear-shaped people store excess fat on their hips, buttocks, and thighs. People with the apple (or male) pattern of fat storage may be at higher risk for heart attack.

Body Shape

In order to determine your own body shape, first measure your waist at about the level of your navel. Stand relaxed and don't pull in your stomach. Next, measure your hips at the largest part of your bottom. Divide the waist measurement by the hip measurement to get your waist-to-hip ratio. A ratio above 1 (waist larger than hips) indicates an apple shape. A ratio below 1 (hips larger than waist) indicates a pear shape.

Many experts hold that a woman's waist measurement should not be greater than 80 percent of her hip measurement (a waist-to-hip ratio of 0.8) for optimum heart health.

Men with a waist measurement larger than their hip measurement are showing the normal male apple-type distribution of body fat, which has been linked to an increased risk of heart disease. Men should strive for a waist measurement below 95 percent of their hip measurement (a waist-to-hip ratio of 0.95).

Women and Weight

An 8-year Brigham and Women's Hospital study indicated that the relationship between body weight and heart disease may be stronger among women than men. For a woman, being even slightly overweight appears to dramatically increase risk.

As with men, risk of heart disease appears to be greater for women who have the apple shape with fat distributed around the waist. Reasons for this increased risk are unclear. Some believe fat from around the waist fuels cholesterol levels more than fat from the hips or thighs. Also, the apple shape could indicate a shortage of estrogen, since sex hormones, including estrogen, influence where body fat is deposited. And estrogen may be a protector against heart disease; after its decline at menopause, women's risks increase.

The Right Weight

It's important to remember that most people need not be thin to be healthy. If you fall inside your healthy weight range according to Table 1, cannot pinch more than an inch or so of fat from around your waist, and have a desirable waist-to-hip ratio, you're at the right weight in terms of good health. If not, you need to begin a weight-control program—one that focuses on losing body fat and increasing muscle mass rather than just shedding pounds.

Dieting Is Not *Weight Control*

Dieting is not the same as weight control. For most people, dieting leads to a yo-yo effect in which the dieter's weight goes down with starvation but shoots back up again when the diet stops. Weight gain follows weight loss in an unending up-and-down cycle. The long-term effects of this yo-yo pattern (also known as *weight cycling*) are not fully understood, but if you are not obese (more than 30 percent over your healthy body weight), you should attempt to maintain a stable weight. If you are obese and you want to lose weight, you should be prepared to commit yourself to an effective, lifelong weight control program, including changes in behavior, diet, and physical activity.

WHAT YOU CAN DO

Many of us struggle with our weight, and controlling it can be difficult. But weight control is important to the health of your heart, so act now.

Take a Practical Approach to Weight Control

Controlling your weight involves so much more than counting calories. Certainly as important, if not more so, is maintaining a well-balanced diet that reduces your consumption of fat, cholesterol, and sodium. As we gain more understanding of what constitutes sound eating habits, the link between diet and good heart health becomes even more pronounced. For more information on diet and nutrition, read chapter 3. Then review the menus and recipes in Part Six of this handbook to see how delicious a heart-healthy cuisine can be.

Exercise is another important part of an effective weight-control program. Table 9 lists a variety of aerobic activities and the average calories burned per hour by a 150-pound (68-kg) person in each activity. (The figures are approximate, as they are averaged from several sources.) The number of calories burned also varies by body weight. For example, a 100-pound (45-kg) person burns one-third *fewer* calories than a 150-pound (68-kg) person, so you would multiply the number of calories for a given activity by 0.67. For a 200-pound (90-kg) person, multiply by 1.33, because someone weighing 200 pounds (90 kg) burns one-third *more* calories than an individual who weighs 150 pounds (68 kg). Regardless of your weight,

TABLE 9   *How Many Calories You Burn In 1 Hour*

Activity	Calories Burned per Hour (by a 150-pound [68-kg] person)
Bicycling, 6 mph (10 km/h)	240
Bicycling, 12 mph (19 km/h)	410
Cross-country skiing	700
Jogging, 5½ mph (9 km/h)	740
Jogging, 7 mph (11 km/h)	920
Jumping rope	750
Running in place	650
Running, 10 mph (16 km/h)	1280
Swimming, 25 yds/min (23 m/min)	275
Swimming, 50 yds/min (46 m/min)	500
Tennis (singles)	400
Walking, 2 mph (3 km/h)	240
Walking, 3 mph (5 km/h)	320
Walking, 4½ mph (7 km/h)	440

Source: National Heart, Lung, and Blood Institute and the American Heart
Association, *Exercise and Your Heart: A Guide to Physical Activity,* 1993.

however, the more strenuous the exercise, the more calories you will use. Read chapter 15 to learn more about an easy-to-start exercise program, and remember that all these activities can improve your cardiovascular fitness, too.

Control Your Weight—You Can Do It

Unless you are one of a very small group with certain medical problems, you *can* control your weight if you truly have the desire. You must, however, be ready to make a firm commitment to making some adjustments in how you live. You have to replace ingrained unhealthy eating habits with healthier ones. However, these changes can be made gradually over a period of time, so that you can integrate new habits into your daily routine with a minimum of stress and strain. In this way, your new habits can become a permanent part of your heart-healthy life.

You'll find a workable weight-control plan that delivers a variety of health benefits described in Part Five of this handbook. If you have a problem with excess body fat, this blueprint may be just what you need to achieve a healthier weight. You can find other sources under "Fitness" and "Nutrition" in the "Resources" appendix.

CHAPTER 5

No More Smoking and Tobacco

WHAT YOU NEED TO KNOW

If you smoke or use tobacco in any form, you owe it to your heart to read this chapter.

Tobacco is one of the most widely used and accepted substances in the world. A large portion of the earth's population smokes, and frequent daily use is entrenched in the social routines of most societies.

What are the truths about this common habit? Is smoking really all that bad for you? Yes, it is. Research has consistently shown that the use of tobacco poses a significant threat to your heart and to your good health in general.

You probably know that the Surgeon General's warning about the hazards of smoking is printed on every pack of cigarettes and in every cigarette ad published or displayed in the United States. But chances are you don't really *see* the Surgeon General's warning anymore, in the sense that its truth no longer registers. In fact, given the health risks that cigarettes pose, the government has gone rather easy on them. So even if you're just a light smoker, please read this chapter.

The Truth about Cigarette Smoking

In the United States, one out of every five deaths is attributable in some degree to cigarette smoking. That's over 400,000 people every year. And at least one-third of those deaths are related to heart disease.

Indeed, for some people, smoking even a moderate number of cigarettes a day can triple their chance of developing a cardiovascular disease. Why is this risk so high? Because when cigarette smoking is added to another risk factor—such as high blood pressure, high cholesterol, heredity, or obesity—the *compounded* risk is far greater than either one by itself.

From the standpoint of cardiovascular health, the main active agent in tobacco is nicotine (although tars and other substances are also harmful). Nicotine is an addictive drug that exerts profound effects on heart rate, blood vessel size, and the efficiency of the circulatory system. Nicotine increases blood pressure and heart rate at the same time that it constricts arteries and reduces the amount of oxygen in the blood. Smoking is also the main cause of chronic lung diseases, which put a considerable further strain on the heart.

Even switching to low-tar, low-nicotine cigarettes doesn't decrease the harmful consequences of smoking. Smokers of "light" cigarettes may actually *increase* their risk of heart disease because they are inclined to inhale more deeply, hold the smoke in their lungs longer, and smoke more cigarettes—all in an attempt to get the nicotine their body craves.

Smoking in the United States Today

The number of smokers in the United States has declined since 1964, when a committee formed by the U.S. Surgeon General issued the first report on the dangers of smoking. Figures from the U.S. Centers for Disease Control and Prevention (CDC) indicate that in 1966, about 50 percent of all American adults smoked cigarettes. Today, the CDC's estimate is down to about 26 percent. Approximately 25.5 percent of all White adults are smokers; this compares with about 29 percent of all Black adults. A significant number of middle-aged men of all races appear to have broken the smoking habit. Since middle-age is the period when heart attacks become more common among males, that's a very positive sign. Unfortunately, smoking among women is on the increase. If trends continue, more women than men will be smoking by the twenty-first century.

Smoking among teenagers has declined, but at a slower rate than among adults. In 1976, an estimated 29 percent of all teens smoked cigarettes. Today, the figure is 17 percent. The American Heart Association's tenth annual statistical report indicated that 2.2 million American children, ages 12 to 17, smoke cigarettes. And 3,000 American children in this age range begin smoking cigarettes every day. Increased cigarette use among teen girls seems to have been the major difference—which seems to increase the trend toward equal-opportunity heart disease (see the section on "Smoking and Women," below).

A message to the young: It's much easier never to start smoking than it is to break the habit later. It's also easier to stop now than it will be after years of smoking.

Why Smoking Is Bad for You

Although we know that smoking contributes to the development of heart disease, we don't yet completely understand all facets of the connection. But we do know of many specific adverse effects that smoking has on the human body. And while nicotine is the main active agent in cigarette smoke, there are many other chemicals and compounds, including tars and carbon dioxide, that are also potentially harmful to your heart.

Eight Reasons Not to Smoke

▶ 1. Smoking increases heart rate, constricts major arteries, and can create irregularities in the timing of heartbeats.

▶ 2. Smoking raises blood pressure. And elevated blood pressure, especially in those who have hypertension or continually high blood pressure, increases the risk of stroke and damages the heart's blood vessels and the kidneys.

▶ 3. According to some studies, smoking promotes a roughening effect on arterial walls. This irregularity has been linked to the formation of plaque, the substance that clogs arteries.

▶ 4. Smoking promotes hardening of the arteries by contributing to plaque development. This occurs because smoking lowers the HDL ("good") cholesterol levels in the blood. Low levels of HDL cholesterol have been found in those most susceptible to heart disease.

▶ 5. Smoking increases levels of *fibrinogen*, a blood component that assists in blood clotting. Studies have indicated that increased fibrinogen may result in the formation of blood clots. These clots may then lodge in arteries narrowed by plaque, stopping blood flow to the heart—the result is a heart attack.

▶ 6. Smoking may trigger the release of certain types of fats into the bloodstream, enhancing plaque development.

▶ 7. Smoking causes platelets in the blood to collect into clumps or clusters, which then impede blood flow through narrowed vessels.

▶ 8. Smoking has an adverse effect on a number of other organs and tissues, including the lungs. Research points to a direct link between cigarette smoking and increased risk of developing many cancers.

Smoking and Women

After a period of decline, cigarette smoking among women is again on the rise. Eventually the number of women who smoke cigarettes might possibly equal or surpass the number of male smokers. This trend may already have contributed to lung cancer replacing breast cancer as the largest cause of cancer-related deaths among women.

Women who smoke face the same risks as men do—and more. Women who smoke also lose some of their natural defenses against heart and artery disease: Smoking as few as four cigarettes a day doubles their risk of developing coronary heart disease, while women who smoke a pack a day have five to ten times the risk. Part of the reason for this increased risk is that smoking lowers the level of estrogen in a woman's system. Estrogen helps prevent the buildup of plaque in blood vessels and is thought to be the main reason heart attacks aren't common in women until after menopause. Smoking also lowers the level of HDL ("good") cholesterol in both men and women, promoting artery-clogging plaque buildup. (For more information on cholesterol, see chapter 9.)

Research has also indicated that women smokers who use oral contraceptives, especially those over 35, have higher rates of coronary heart disease than nonsmokers. For reasons not yet fully understood, smoking and the use of oral contraceptives can increase both blood pressure and cholesterol levels, thus intensifying these risk factors.

Smoking and the Heart Patient

Since smoking increases heart rate, constricts arteries, raises blood pressure, and promotes irregularities in the heartbeat, the best advice we can give is that if you have a heart or circulatory problem, *don't smoke.*

If you are a smoker and have had a heart attack, stopping smoking may be the best protection against another attack.

People who continue to smoke after heart bypass surgery are twice as likely to experience a heart attack, stroke, or chest pain within 10 years of their operation than those who stop.

If you are a heart patient and a smoker, talk to your physician about quitting: Discuss the effects of various smoking-cessation aids, such as nicotine patches and chewing gums, as well as other withdrawal methods. Also, read chapter 17 of this handbook, which offers a personalized action plan for quitting smoking.

Benefits of Not Smoking

The good news is that when you quit smoking, your body will in time repair the heart-related damage that smoking caused. Even heavy smokers have a chance to bring their cardiovascular system back to normal by stopping. In fact, several studies have shown that within 5 to 10 years after their last cigarette, ex-smokers face the same risk for heart disease as those who never smoked. Within 20 minutes after the final puff, nicotine-induced narrowing of blood vessels stops. This is great news for heart health; however, science still doesn't know the amount of time required for the lungs to fully recover from the effects of long-term smoking.

Effects of Secondary Smoke

A great deal of concern has arisen in recent years over the problem of cigarette smoke in the air being breathed by nonsmokers. Studies conducted by the Environmental Protection Agency have suggested that this secondary (or secondhand) smoke may be as damaging as smoking itself. Other research has presented a milder view, although the American Heart Association considers secondary smoke a major cardiovascular risk factor. Cigarette smoke is an airborne pollutant, and like any pollutant, should be avoided. There are *no* health benefits to be derived from exposure to smoke, so it would be wise to take reasonable steps to minimize your intake of secondary smoke, including insisting on a smoke-free work area and banning cigarettes from at least a part of your home.

Other Tobacco Products

Since cigarettes are the most prevalent form of tobacco, cigarette smoking has been the focus of most of the studies on the effects of tobacco use.

However, here is what we know about the health hazards of other forms of tobacco.

Pipes and Cigars   While it is true that your risk of developing coronary disease is lower if you are a pipe or cigar smoker than if you are a cigarette smoker, pipe and cigar smokers are still at considerably higher risk than nonsmokers.

The amount of smoke inhaled seems to be responsible for the major differences in toxicity. Pipe and cigar smokers generally inhale less tobacco smoke. However, smokers who switch from cigarettes to a pipe or cigar often do *not* benefit from lowered risk because they continue to inhale larger amounts of smoke.

Inhaling or not, the nicotine in tobacco is still absorbed through the lining of the mouth, harming the heart. In addition, cigar and pipe smokers face a greater chance than nonsmokers of developing mouth or throat cancers, which are caused by a variety of chemicals and compounds in tobacco smoke.

Smokeless Tobacco   Snuff, chewing, and other forms of smokeless tobacco also are not safe ways to maintain a nicotine habit. Although research on the effects of smokeless tobacco use continues, the cardiovascular risk appears to be lower than for cigarettes, but the chance of developing cancer of the mouth or throat is higher than for non-tobacco users. Moreover, there are no positive health benefits to be gained from sniffing or chewing tobacco.

WHAT YOU CAN DO

Do your heart a favor by avoiding smoking and tobacco in all its forms.

Break the Smoking or Tobacco Habit

You *can* break your dependence on tobacco—and on nicotine, the most addictive agent in tobacco. For many people, this is a difficult task. Even so, if you truly want to quit smoking, you can. The stop-smoking program we've outlined in Part Five of this handbook can help. Our program also addresses the problem of weight gain experienced by some who break the cigarette habit. Remember, though, that the health benefits gained from quitting smoking far outweigh the minor risk of gaining (often only temporarily) a few unwanted pounds.

Also, keep in mind that you have a strong ally in your physician. Your doctor can give you advice and support, talk about options—such as nicotine patches or chewing gum—that may help, direct you to a number of successful smoking-cessation programs, and explain in detail the benefits of not smoking. Other sources for information are listed under "Smoking" in the "Resources" appendix.

If you smoke, our best advice is—*quit*. Remember that every time you light up, you increase the risk of shortening your life—and perhaps the lives of those around you who are exposed to your smoke.

Avoid Secondary Smoke

Even though the risks faced by nonsmokers who inhale smoke from others' cigarettes are probably less than for the smokers themselves, you may wish to avoid breathing this secondary smoke. Here are some suggestions.

- Ask to be seated in nonsmoking sections in restaurants and book smoke-free rooms in hotels.
- If you are troubled by others smoking in your workplace, discuss your concerns with your supervisor. If that doesn't help, use a small electric or battery-powered fan to blow air out of or away from your workstation.
- If you are joining a carpool, ask about smoking rules before making a commitment.
- If you live with a family member or friend who smokes, establish smoking and nonsmoking areas in your home.

As you try to avoid others' smoke, remember that a little courtesy can achieve more than a lot of scorn.

CHAPTER 6

Moderate or No Drinking and No Illegal Drugs

WHAT YOU NEED TO KNOW

Medical researchers have spent several decades investigating the effects of alcohol and common illegal drugs on the health of the heart. They have no doubt that illegal drugs are bad for your health. However, the evidence on alcohol is not so clear-cut.

Alcohol and Your Heart—The Pros and Cons

Studies have consistently shown that *modest* alcohol consumption actually *protects* against heart disease and heart attack. *Moderate* drinkers have a much lower risk of developing coronary artery disease. The best guess as to why alcohol is helpful is that it tends to raise a person's HDL ("good") cholesterol levels. An increase in HDL levels allows more LDL ("bad") cholesterol to be moved through the liver for excretion. (See chapter 9 if you need more information on cholesterol.)

The American Heart Association suggests that moderate consumption is 1 ounce (30 ml) of alcohol per day—roughly the amount found in one cocktail (made with 2 ounces [60 ml] of a 100-proof spirit), one 8-ounce (240-ml) glass of wine, or two 12-ounce (355-ml) glasses of beer. Drinking more than 1 ounce of alcohol a day does *not* enhance the health benefit. In fact, an elevated level of alcohol consumption *increases* the risk of high blood pressure and can lead to strokes. Moreover, heavy drinking among pregnant women has been shown to damage the fetus in the womb (see the section on "Alcohol and Pregnancy," below). Therefore, please do not consider this medical advice to begin consuming alcohol *if you don't already do so*. There are other factors to be considered, not the least of which is that alcohol is easily and frequently overused and abused.

Excessive Drinking and Your Heart

The degree of alcohol consumption that can be classified as overindulgence varies from person to person. Factors such as sex (because some studies indicate alcohol affects women more quickly than men), body weight, and diet all play roles in how alcohol affects your system. However, overindulging on a frequent, regular basis can cause serious cardiovascular problems. In addition to the increased incidence of high blood pressure and stroke mentioned earlier, about one-third of all cases of cardiomyopathy are caused by excessive drinking. Cardiomyopathy is a serious disease in which the heart muscle becomes enlarged and flabby. The result is poor circulation and, possibly, heart failure. Fortunately, early detection of this disease and abstention from further alcohol abuse can reverse the process, allowing a damaged heart to return to normal.

Furthermore, drinking large amounts of alcohol in a short period of time, an activity known as binge drinking, can trigger arrhythmias, or irregularities in the natural rhythm of heartbeats. (See chapters 26 and 27 for more information on cardiomyopathy and arrhythmias, respectively.)

Many medical professionals now feel that excessive drinking is a disease in and of itself. Certainly, alcoholism causes great losses to our communities. A report from the Robert Wood Johnson Foundation indicated that alcohol abuse cost the United States $99 billion in 1990 alone! Quite aside from the cardiovascular health concerns, alcoholics do themselves great bodily harm. Malnutrition, for instance, is common among alcoholics, partially because excessive alcohol use tends to quell the appetite.

All factors considered, the best advice for those who drink is to limit your consumption of alcohol to a maximum of one or two drinks a day, depending on what you're drinking. And if you find that you cannot control your alcohol intake, *seek help immediately*. Your doctor or other health-care provider is a good place to start.

Alcohol and Medications

Alcohol interacts with a variety of over-the-counter and prescription medications, often intensifying their effects. If you're taking any prescription medications, be sure to ask your doctor or pharmacist if it is safe to drink alcohol (even in moderation). If you are taking an over-the-counter medication, be sure to read the warning label before drinking alcohol. In fact, you probably should review your entire medication list with your doctor, just to be safe.

Alcohol and Disease

If you have any form of diabetes, avoid alcohol because it is metabolized as sugar. Likewise, if you have high blood pressure, alcohol will only worsen your condition. And since the amount of alcohol in the blood is controlled by the liver, if you have liver damage or cirrhosis, *definitely don't drink*.

Alcohol and Weight Control

At 7 calories per gram, alcohol is also highly caloric. A 12-ounce (355-ml) beer, for example, has about 145 calories. If you have begun a weight-control program, you should be careful about your alcohol consumption.

Alcohol and Pregnancy

You have probably noticed the Surgeon General's warning to pregnant women on the labels of alcoholic beverages. If you have not, please take note: If you are pregnant, you should sharply restrict your consumption of alcohol, which can cause serious damage to the human embryo and fetus. Recent evidence indicates that pregnant women who drink *to excess* may give birth to infants with fetal alcohol syndrome, a serious condition characterized by face and body abnormalities and, in some cases, impaired intellectual capabilities. Also, if you are breast-feeding your baby and drink, the alcohol will be present in your milk, although the alcohol clears from your milk at the same rate that it clears from your blood.

Again, what constitutes drinking to excess varies from individual to individual. And although drinking moderately during pregnancy may not harm *your* heart, it can, nonetheless, harm your unborn baby. If you drink and are pregnant, please discuss what's best for both you and your unborn baby with your doctor.

Illegal Drugs and Your Heart

Marijuana and cocaine (in any of its derivative forms) are two of the most commonly used illegal drugs. At least part of the reason for their popularity stems from the manner in which they are taken into the body: Neither requires injection into the bloodstream. A third class of narcotics does require intravenous injection, an act that can offer a unique threat to heart health in and of itself.

Marijuana

THC (*tetrahydrocannabinol*), marijuana's active ingredient, affects the cardiovascular and central nervous systems by increasing heart rate, blood pressure, and body temperature. Also, even though marijuana contains no nicotine (the most active agent in tobacco), other components of marijuana smoke (such as carbon monoxide) produce effects similar to those experienced by tobacco smokers. Therefore, although research is somewhat limited, we do know that smoking marijuana increases the risk of heart attack, stroke, and some forms of cancer.

As with most street drugs, however, marijuana has been found to have some medically acceptable applications. It is used, for instance, to reduce pressure in the eye as treatment for glaucoma and to counter the nausea often associated with cancer chemotherapy. Even in these instances, though, the specific ingredient that produces the benefits is extracted from the plant and prescribed as a medication to be ingested. Smoking the drug is still discouraged by most physicians.

Cocaine

Although many users believe it is safe and nonaddicting, cocaine—particularly in the form of "crack"—is, in fact, a powerful, addictive drug that has a direct effect on the heart. Cocaine increases blood pressure and constricts blood vessels. It also stimulates the formation of blood clots in the vessels, disrupts normal heart rhythm, and can bind directly to heart muscle cells, thereby weakening the heart's ability to pump blood. A variety of cardiovascular conditions and diseases have been associated with cocaine use, including hypertension, arrhythmias, cardiomyopathy, strokes, aneurysms, myocarditis, and heart attacks.

Even first-time cocaine users may experience seizures or heart attacks that can be fatal. Furthermore, pregnant women who use cocaine increase the possibility of miscarriage or premature delivery, as well as the chance that their babies will be born with a congenital heart defect.

Cocaine abusers who take the drug intravenously are also at risk for illnesses such as hepatitis and AIDS; and pregnant women who become infected with AIDS can pass the virus on to their unborn babies.

Recovery from cocaine addiction takes professional intervention and requires an enduring commitment on the part of the addict. The drug is in no way part of a heart-healthy life.

Injecting Drugs   Besides suffering the ill effects of the illegal drugs themselves, those who use nonsterile syringes to inject the drugs also impair their health by injecting bacteria, other microbes, and sometimes fungi into their bloodstream. These may form growth colonies in the heart, producing a disease called endocarditis, an infection of the cells lining the valves and cavities of the heart that can result in dramatically impaired heart function or death.

There is also some evidence that injecting drugs into a vein or artery is in itself damaging to the heart because of solid foreign matter and particles in the drug that may scratch or roughen the inside of the heart and vessels.

WHAT YOU CAN DO

You can do a world of good for your heart by acting now to control any alcohol or drug problem you may have.

Use Alcohol in Moderation and Abstain from All Illegal Drugs

The best course to heart health calls for moderation if you drink alcohol and complete abstention from illegal drugs. In addition to the specific harmful physical effects already discussed, because alcohol and illegal drugs impair your judgment, they can be dangerous to both your heart health and your overall well-being in general.

Although limited alcohol consumption may generate some heart-health benefits, if you don't drink, there is no prevailing health reason to start. And if you do drink alcohol, there are clear health reasons always to do so in moderation.

Conversely, the most commonly available illegal drugs, including marijuana, cocaine, and others, offer *no* heart-health advantages whatsoever and can do serious harm to your cardiovascular system. Avoid them at all times.

Be Honest with Your Physician

If you use alcohol or any illegal drug, even on a casual basis, tell your physician. It's important information, because combining alcohol or illegal drugs with certain prescription and even over-the-counter medications can have disastrous effects. Conversations with your doctor are strictly confidential; his or her goal is to help you—not to get you in legal trouble.

The following discussion offers some helpful guidelines toward ending your alcohol or drug dependence. If you want to end your dependence on these substances, read this information and see your doctor for assistance. It's possible to make the transition alone, but it's easier, and often quicker, to enlist the aid of a medical professional.

Be Realistic about Abstention Programs

Most heavy users of alcohol and illegal drugs suffer from some degree of dependence on those substances. Their addiction has both mental and physical aspects. And despite the best intentions of the user, addictions are extremely difficult to overcome. Breaking away from substance abuse is a medical problem and usually requires changes in attitude as well as lifestyle.

Not only is there no totally effective self-help program for substance abusers, there is also no totally effective group activity or therapy available, although many have been helped by such group programs as Alcoholics Anonymous. For many, the difficulty of recovery is increased by negative social attitudes toward abusers and addiction. Nevertheless, literally millions of alcoholics and drug abusers have recovered from their addiction, reclaimed their health, and rejoined the ranks of productive society. You can, too.

Know the Three Prerequisites for Ending Addiction

In analyzing the attitudes and experiences of those who have managed to recover from their addictions, we can identify three common elements.

▶ 1. *Admitting Addiction.* Those successful in recovering from substance abuse were able to admit to themselves that they had a problem and that it was too large for them to solve without assistance. This admission of helplessness has become a key element in many of the more successful treatment programs.

▶ **2.** *Desiring to End the Addiction.* Those successful in recovering from substance abuse strongly desired to end their addiction. The basis for this desire varies greatly, ranging from a need to reestablish themselves among loved ones to anger over the way their affairs were handled while they were incapacitated. The reasons, however, are consistent in one sense: They were of vital importance to the recovering substance abuser.

▶ **3.** *Accepting Help.* Those successful in recovering from substance abuse sought and received some form of assistance in making the recovery. Although sometimes able to refrain temporarily from their addiction through their own efforts, most substance abusers found that they needed some form of assistance to achieve complete, long-term recovery. Those who succeeded in their efforts also had adequate medical care and the services of a physician.

Get Help

In addition to the many private organizations, medical practices, and hospitals to which they can turn for help, substance abusers may find free aid through city, county, state, and federal sources. Many of these resources provide psychological counseling and other programs tailored to individual requirements. The names and phone numbers of some group assistance organizations can be found under "Drugs" and "Alcohol" in the "Resources" appendix.

If you've reached the point where you believe you may have a substance abuse problem—or even if you're not sure—you need to seek and obtain professional assistance. You can start by talking with your doctor. Be assured that you *can* recover and that help *is* available. Act now. The longer you delay, the more harm you're doing to your heart and body.

PART THREE

Controllable Health Factors

Stress

Hypertension

Cholesterol and Triglycerides

Diabetes

CHAPTER 7

Stress

WHAT YOU NEED TO KNOW

You wake up in the middle of the night, your mind churning, and have trouble getting back to sleep. In the morning, your muscles are stiff, and you have a headache you'll keep all day. You're tense and agitated, and irritable with friends and coworkers. You know the symptoms: You have the disease for modern times—stress.

Is "stress" simply a much-used, and sometimes misused, diagnosis, a convenient catchall when we don't have another explanation for what ails us? In common usage, we know what stress means: the world is more than we can handle. But in medical terms, what exactly is stress, and what does it have to do with the health of the heart?

Stress itself is not a thing; it is our *reaction* to things. *Stress* can be defined as our mental, emotional, and physical responses to the irritants, challenges, and threats—individual and accumulated—in our lives. Stress is, above all, *personal*. While any of us might have our equilibrium disturbed by a major life event such as a divorce or job change, *how much and in what way* such things affect us can vary considerably. In addition, some of us will be distressed by such minor annoyances as losing our car keys, waiting a long time for an appointment, or being stuck in traffic; while others will hardly be bothered. And the same person could respond differently at different times, depending on whether that person was having a good or bad day.

Given that we all experience stress at times, and feel differently about it (and differently at different times), the most important personal aspect of stress is how we choose to respond. We use the word *choose* deliberately and with some caution. All of us can, to some extent, control our responses to the things that cause us to feel stress. First of all, we should recognize that stress itself need not be a bad thing. Certain pressures can be challenges that trigger excitement, exhilaration, and mental alertness. The intensity of our response—whether to a ball game we care about, a deadline on a tough assignment at work, or whatever brings us to full attention—can lead to joy and satisfaction, as well as peak accomplishment.

However, our main concern here is dealing with the physical aspects of the stress response (as much as they can be separated from the mental and emotional aspects) and how they affect the health of your heart.

The Effects of Stress on Your Body

You may have heard of the *fight-or-flight response*. That's the psychologist's term for our primitive or animalistic reaction to a dangerous (or stressful) situation, in which we prepare ourselves to take quick action to either meet or run from a perceived threat. That threat, we should note, could be mental (an impending deadline) or emotional (an impending divorce or death of a loved one) as well as physical (an impending car accident). There are many dangers in the modern jungle with which we must contend.

In less than a second, when confronted with such a stressor, your nervous system and hormones from your adrenal gland (chiefly epinephrine, also called adrenaline) automatically trigger a number of physical changes, to facilitate your capacity to fight or take flight. Typically, your heart rate increases, your blood pressure rises, the clotting ability of your blood is enhanced, the blood vessels in your skin constrict, your muscles tense, additional blood flows to your muscles and brain, and your body releases stored fat and changes it to fatty acids for quick conversion to energy.

These physical adaptations in response to stress are observable, quantifiable, and established. What is less clear is the *causal* relationship, if any, between the physiological responses to stress and heart disease. Stress itself is very hard to measure and, as we have noted, people's responses to stress are personal and highly variable. Given those caveats, here is what we know.

Stress and Heart Disease

People with heart disease commonly report that they suffer heart pain during emotionally charged situations. Heart attacks are also common during these periods. We can identify several links.

▶ 1. The rapid increase of heart rate and blood pressure associated with the stress response generates a greater demand by the heart for oxygen and can bring on an attack of angina pectoris, or chest pain, in people who already have heart disease.

▶ 2. The combination of excess hormones and intensified blood circulation during the stress response can actually injure the lining of the arteries. As these injuries heal, the arterial walls harden or thicken, thus becoming more susceptible to the buildup of plaque. In time, deposits of plaque can increase to the point where the artery is narrow and blood flow impaired.

▶ 3. The increased likelihood of the blood to clot during the stress reaction may, in fact, lead to formation of a clot, blocking a partially constricted artery and resulting in a heart attack.

While these links allow us to conclude that stress can *contribute* to the risk of heart attack by producing the physical effects discussed, we are unable to state conclusively that stress *causes* heart disease. We can say, however, that certain heart conditions can be *exacerbated* by stress.

Myocardial Ischemia

"Ischemia" is a condition in which insufficient blood and oxygen reach tissues. When those tissues are heart muscle (myocardium), the result is *myocardial ischemia*. Myocardial ischemia is a product of coronary artery disease—specifically, blockage of the coronary arteries. As we have noted, the stress reaction makes the heart work harder, which produces a greater need for oxygen in the coronary arteries. If that need is not met—as it would not be if the arteries were blocked—the result is myocardial ischemia, and the stressed individual suffers chest pain (*angina*).

It may be that you have enough blood flow to handle normal heart activities but not enough to support the heart muscle during periods when greater than typical cardiac output is required. Your myocardial ischemia could be sufficiently intensified during the stress reaction for you to recognize it through the symptom of chest pain. Therefore, if you are in a stressful situation and suddenly experience chest pain, especially if accompanied by pain radiating down your left arm, consider yourself alerted. Try to stay calm and seek medical assistance immediately.

You cannot, however, rely on pain as a warning sign. In all too many cases, and especially during a stressful situation, you don't feel chest pain even if you have myocardial ischemia. Why not? Perhaps the blockage was brief and less severe. Perhaps you have a particularly high pain threshold. Or perhaps the excitement of the moment, along with the adrenaline rush, blanketed the pain sensation. In any case, the blockage of coronary arteries and the resulting inadequate blood and oxygen flow (*ischemia*) are still there. When the ischemia occurs without pain, it is called *silent ischemia*—which several researchers contend is a factor in many heart attacks that strike with no apparent warning.

How can you tell if you are at risk for myocardial ischemia? See your doctor and ask whether a stress test might be in order. (Essentially, *stress tests* are monitored exercise sessions, in which you are hooked up to machines that measure heart function and oxygen consumption while you walk on a treadmill or pedal a stationary bike.) In the meantime, use the information presented here and in chapter 18 to avoid and/or reduce the levels of stress in your life. You might also consider the impact of your personality type.

Is "B" Better Than "A"?

What medicine knows about the effects of stress on the heart is in the arena of sudden, intense, one-time events triggering a severe physical reaction. We are less sure of the relationship between ongoing, accumulated stress and the underlying coronary artery disease associated with heart attacks. Medical and psychological studies into personality types and their reaction to the environment are an effort to discover the long-term effects of stress on health.

The first major advance in this field occurred in the mid-1960s when Meyer Friedman and Ray Rosenman posited the concept of the "type-A" personality. They described type-A people as highly competitive, intense, and success/achievement-driven. These can be useful qualities, of course, because they can lead to personal and societal productivity and accomplishment. However, type-A people are also impatient, easily provoked to hostility, and work-obsessed. Besides being irritating, these traits can also be dangerous to one's health—or so some research has indicated.

To see how, we have to describe another personality type: "B." These folks, in contrast, are more relaxed, unhurried, and likely to be satisfied with their degree of success. They can still be achievement-oriented—they're not societal dropouts—but they're not as driven as type A's. And they may find their rewards in this lifetime. According to research based on one large study, type-B people have half the risk for developing coronary heart disease as type-A people.

However, the original personality-type study, though clearly groundbreaking, was flawed in that its study group was restricted to men of certain occupations. And subsequent studies have failed to corroborate that type A's die earlier than type B's, perhaps because their study groups were greatly expanded to include more occupations and women, perhaps because it is difficult to quantify individual levels of stress. Current research is unbundling the large package of type-A personality traits and concentrating on the ramifications of specific behaviors: Researchers are focusing on people who respond to stressful situations with anger, explosive actions, and frustration. And the early results have pointed to a connection between such behaviors and heart disease.

Does this mean that you should never get angry or frustrated? Of course not. However, should you worry if you are angry and frustrated much of the time? Perhaps. Again, the amount and intensity of one's anger and frustration is hard to measure. The research into the relationships among personality, stress, and heart disease does seem to indicate, however, that how you habitually respond to stressful situations could affect your health. A physical examination by your doctor can help you decide how concerned you should be. In any case, learning how to identify, control, and even reduce your stress is obviously of value—both to the quality of your life and to the health of your heart.

Occupational Stress

Since stress may be a risk factor for heart disease, we are tempted to conclude that jobs with the highest stress have the highest mortality rates. However, people's responses to stressful situations are highly individualized; what stresses your neighbor may not stress you. If that weren't true, probably no one could endure life as a police officer, air traffic controller, emergency-room nurse, or inner-city schoolteacher. Furthermore, measuring stress has proven elusive, so establishing a scientific correlation to heart disease is very difficult.

Nevertheless, medical researchers and social scientists keep trying. For instance, a noted study of the Chicago Western Electric facility found that job stress was highest for employees whose jobs offered little latitude in decision making but placed considerable psychological demands on them. In other words, they had plenty of responsibility but not enough authority. However, the research was able to find only limited hard evidence linking those job characteristics and coronary heart disease.

Researchers in Europe have had more success establishing connections between heart disease and life at work. For instance, at greater risk were men who were incapable of relaxing after the job, people whose careers were disrupted by conflicts, and workers who were given increased responsibility at a young age. In contrast, people who had jobs that offered or placed on them status, moderate responsibility, reasonable expectations, and opportunity for social interaction during working hours had a better chance at good health.

Does all this boil down to: If you like your job and can handle the work, your heart is not at risk from your occupation? That's probably too simple, but the truth seems to be that your particular fit with your job/occupation is more important than the job/occupation itself. However, as we've all experienced, job conditions are likely to change from time to time, often without much warning. Our work life is critical to our well-being, and how we adapt to changes in that environment is also important to the health of our hearts.

WHAT YOU CAN DO

As we have noted, all stress is not bad; meeting mental, emotional, and physical challenges can build character, lead to achievement, and even be enjoyed. Such happy outcomes, however, require that you be able to respond in a positive manner and that you not be overwhelmed by too many stressful situations.

Check Your Stress Level

How can you tell how much stress is too much? In the midst of a busy life, it's not always easy to recognize when the world is becoming more than you can handle. One way is to see if you are exhibiting any of the com-

TABLE 10　　　　*Symptoms of Stress*

Sudden heart pounding	Headaches	Overreaction to what happens around you
Cold, clammy hands	Upset stomach or heartburn	
Drumming fingers or tapping foot	Sudden anger	Irritability
Nervous coughing	A constant feeling that there isn't enough time	Impatience
A general feeling of fatigue	Sudden tears for no apparent reason	Grinding teeth
Dry mouth		Binge drinking
Difficulty breathing	Sudden sense of impending bad news or doom	Binge eating
Muscle aches		Chain-smoking
Clenched jaws or other tight facial muscles	Frustration	Nail biting
	Depression	Constant picking at fingernails or face
Stiff neck	Anxiety or anxiousness	Trying to do two or three things at once
Tics at the mouth or eyebrows	Talking too much	
Sudden sweating	A sudden inability to express yourself	Fiddling with, twisting, or pulling out hair
Turning red-faced		

mon symptoms of stress listed in Table 10. A good guideline is that if you identify at least three of these symptoms over a period of a week or so, you may be experiencing too much stress.

Reduce Stress When You Can

If you've decided you've got too much stress in your life, you can adopt any or all of several lifestyle changes to lighten the strain. For instance, you might:

- Travel more slowly, both walking and driving.
- Give yourself more time to complete tasks.
- Remind yourself to relax in frustrating situations.
- Be prepared with things to do or read during long waits for meetings or appointments.
- Maintain good social relationships; make time for fun with friends and family.
- Don't set unrealistic expectations for yourself—or others.
- Improve communication by becoming an active listener.

- Be assertive, rather than passive or aggressive, to get what you want.
- Think positively.
- Don't make everything a crisis.
- Keep organized to minimize crisis situations.
- Avoid dependence on caffeine, nicotine, or alcohol.
- Get enough rest.
- Spend time on your hobbies (if you don't have any, find some).
- Start and stick to an exercise program.
- Practice relaxation techniques.

Exercise and stress-management programs, including numerous relaxation techniques, are described in detail in Part Five of this handbook.

Avoid Stress Where Possible

Certain stressful situations are beyond your control; others are not. By managing those stress-producing elements that *are* within your control, you will reduce the overall effects of stress on your life. Fortunately, this task will likely be a lot easier than you think. You must first ask yourself why you are feeling stressed. When you can identify the sources of your stress, you can develop ways to avoid them.

For example, say you are agitated right from the start of the day because you always seem to be running late. Once you understand that lateness is the source of your stressful feelings, you can eliminate the problem with a simple schedule change. Instead of rushing through breakfast and hurrying for the bus, try getting out of bed a little earlier. (Maybe that means going to bed a little earlier, too. Your rest is important.) Give yourself time—5 to 10 minutes might be enough—for a more leisurely prework morning. Thus, by modifying your behavior, you can avoid some stress.

Avoiding stress in this manner is part of a total stress-management program. See chapter 18 for a description of the complete program. If you're troubled by stress or feel you live in a world of unrelenting pressure and tension, it's time to act. As a heart owner, you have an obligation, to your heart and yourself, to improve your chances for good health and a happier life.

CHAPTER 8

Hypertension

WHAT YOU NEED TO KNOW

If you answered yes to having high blood pressure on your self-test, or even if you haven't had it measured recently, you owe it to yourself to read on. Why? Because hypertension, the medical name for high blood pressure, is a silent killer. According to the American Heart Association, as many as 50 million Americans aged 6 and older have high blood pressure, including one of every four adults. And since you can have high blood pressure without any noticeable symptoms, many people don't even realize they have it.

It's important for you to know that, in general, hypertension can be completely controlled. Furthermore, in most cases, managing the disease does *not* require medication. It *does* require you to eat a low-fat, low-sodium diet and to drink alcohol in moderation if at all. Following a fitness program also helps, as does reducing stress related to high blood pressure. Finally, if you smoke, you need to quit.

What Is Hypertension?

The name *hypertension* wasn't given to this condition because the people who have high blood pressure are hyper or always very tense. Many relaxed, easygoing people have the disease. The term *hypertension* indicates a problem in the mechanism that regulates blood pressure in the circulatory system ("hyper" means too much or excessive; "tension" refers to pressure).

Your heart pumps blood through a vast network of arteries, capillaries, and veins. The force exerted by the moving blood against an arterial wall is measured as blood pressure. Your blood pressure is controlled by very tiny arteries called *arterioles*. Should these arteries constrict, or become smaller, the heart has to work harder to pump blood through the reduced space, thus increasing blood pressure. In nearly all cases, we don't know *why* the arterioles constrict (see the section "Two Kinds of Hypertension," below). But we do know that high blood pressure poses a number of serious health risks.

Just How Serious Is Hypertension?

Hypertension is among the most common and most dangerous of the risk factors for cardiovascular diseases. It is the leading cause of strokes and is a major risk factor for heart attack and kidney failure.

Fortunately, dramatic strides have been made in the treatment of hypertension since the late 1950s, and today hypertension can be controlled in most people. So it's important to check your blood pressure periodically and seek treatment if it's too high.

Here are four of the main ways hypertension can harm your health.

▶ 1. *Hardening of the Arteries.* A healthy person's arteries are muscular and elastic. They stretch or contract as the heart pumps blood through them. If you have high blood pressure, the additional pressure inside your arteries can cause the muscles that line the walls of the arteries to thicken. Thickening causes the arteries to narrow, increasing the risk that a blood clot might partially or completely block the flow of blood to the heart or brain (thus causing a heart attack or stroke). In addition, high blood pressure can affect the elasticity of your arteries, which may compound the problem of narrowing.

▶ **2.** *Enlarged Heart.* High blood pressure increases the workload of the heart. So, like any heavily exercised muscle, the heart grows bigger. Eventually, however, the extra exertion takes its toll, and your heart is unable to maintain the necessary flow of blood. As a result, you experience weakness and fatigue and are unable to exercise or perform physical activities. In time, this can cause your heart to fail.

▶ **3.** *Kidney Damage.* Prolonged high blood pressure can also bring about kidney damage. About a quarter of the people who receive kidney dialysis require it because of hypertension.

▶ **4.** *Eye Damage.* In people who have diabetes, hypertension can also harm the retina of the eye by damaging the capillaries and causing bleeding. This condition, called *retinopathy,* can lead to blindness.

Two Kinds of Hypertension

There are two basic kinds of hypertension: primary and secondary.

Primary Hypertension

About 90 to 95 percent of all high blood pressure cases are considered *primary,* or essential, *hypertension.* Although we don't know the actual cause of primary hypertension, we can identify a number of factors that correlate (or are associated) with the condition. You are at increased risk to develop high blood pressure if you:

- Have a family history of hypertension.
- Are Black.
- Are male.
- Are over 60.
- Face high levels of stress.
- Are obese.
- Use tobacco products.
- Use oral contraceptives.
- Eat a diet high in saturated fats.
- Eat a diet high in sodium (salt).
- Drink more than a moderate amount of alcohol.

■ Are physically inactive.

■ Have diabetes.

Researchers have also recently identified a gene that appears to be linked to a predisposition for hypertension. Such a genetic relationship, however, doesn't mean that you or your children are *certain* to become hypertensive if you have the gene. It does mean that you are *more likely* to develop high blood pressure and so should more conscientiously monitor your blood pressure.

A condition known as *isolated systolic hypertension*, mostly found in older people, can produce high systolic readings and low or normal diastolic readings, such as 160/90. If your systolic blood pressure is consistently at or over 160 and your diastolic blood pressure is less than 90, you should see your physician. (See "Understanding Your Blood Pressure Reading," below, for an explanation of these terms.)

Secondary Hypertension

The remaining 5 to 10 percent of all high blood pressure cases are considered *secondary hypertension,* which means that the elevated blood pressure is the result of another condition or illness.

Many cases of secondary hypertension are directly related to kidney (renal) disorders because the kidneys regulate body fluid levels and the body's balance of sodium and water. Kidney infections, a narrowing of the arteries that carry blood to the kidneys, and other kidney malfunctions can disrupt the body's fluid balance, potentially leading to hypertension.

Other conditions that can cause secondary hypertension include parathyroid gland abnormalities, acromegaly, tumors in the adrenal or pituitary glands, reactions to drugs prescribed for other medical problems, and pregnancy.

If you have kidney trouble or any of these other conditions, be sure to have your blood pressure monitored frequently. For the same reason, if you develop high blood pressure, your doctor will want to check for contributing illnesses and conditions.

Understanding Your Blood Pressure Reading

Blood pressure has two phases. The first phase occurs when the heart contracts, squeezing blood into the aorta, the large artery that then carries the blood into the arterial system. The second phase follows, when the heart relaxes, readying itself to contract again. During this short intermission, some blood continues to flow because of pressure remaining in the vessels.

The highest pressure, called *systolic pressure,* occurs when the heart contracts, forcing blood into the arteries. The lowest pressure, called *diastolic pressure,* occurs when the heart relaxes.

Blood pressure is expressed as a pair of numbers with a slash (/) between them. The first number, or the number on top, is the systolic reading; the second number, or the bottom one, is the diastolic reading. The numbers reflect pressure in terms of millimeters of mercury (mm Hg)—that is, how high the pressure inside your arteries would be able to raise a column of mercury. A reading of 120/80 (said as "one-twenty over eighty") means that your blood exerts a pressure of 120 mm Hg against your arterial walls when your heart contracts, and a pressure of 80 mm Hg when it relaxes.

What Is Normal Blood Pressure?

A systolic reading of 120 to 130 and a diastolic reading of 80 to 90 is considered normal for a healthy adult at rest. Blood pressure varies, however, with any activity and with age.

The level of blood pressure needed to maintain proper circulation is constantly changing as we move. Less blood pressure is required when you're lying down, for example, than when you're standing. Even the act of sitting up from a prone position produces an instant need for more blood pressure to push your blood upward against gravity and to maintain an adequate supply to your brain.

Moreover, both systolic and diastolic pressures vary with age, so the blood pressure readings that are considered normal also vary with age. In general, the younger you are, the lower your blood pressure should be. Table 11 shows the National Institutes of Health guidelines for blood pressure levels for adults 18 and older; Table 12 shows blood pressure levels that indicate hypertension in children by age group. (Both tables can be found on the next page.)

If your (or your child's) blood pressure reading is above the high-normal ranges shown in the tables, you should talk to your doctor.

How Is High Blood Pressure Detected?

Since no one can feel high blood pressure and most people who have it don't show any symptoms of heart disease, a checkup or physical examination is the only way to detect the condition. The process can be as simple as having your blood pressure measured by a trained specialist. However, a complete physical evaluation will give a more accurate picture of your health. In any case, if you are over 18 and have a one-time reading higher than 139/89, you should have the reading confirmed within 2 months and, if it remains high, see your physician.

TABLE 11   *What Does Your Blood Pressure Reading Mean?*[1]

Systolic Pressure	
Under 130	Normal
130–139	High normal
140–159	Mild hypertension
160–179	Moderate hypertension
180–209	Severe hypertension
210 or over	Very severe hypertension

Diastolic Pressure	
Below 85	Normal
85–89	High normal
90–99	Mild hypertension
100–109	Moderate hypertension
110–119	Severe hypertension
120 or over	Very severe hypertension

[1]These guidelines are for adults 18 and older.

Adapted from "The Fifth Report of the Joint National Committee on Detection, Evaluation, and Treatment of High Blood Pressure," *Archives of Internal Medicine,* 1993; 153:154–83.

TABLE 12   *What Does Your Child's Blood Pressure Reading Mean?*[1]

Child's Age	Normal (below 90th %tile)	High Normal (90th–94th %tile)	High (95th–99th %tile)	Very High (above 99th %tile)
Infants under 2	below 104/70	104–111/70–73	112–117/74–81	118+/82+
3–5 years old	below 108/70	108–115/70–75	116–123/76–83	124+/84+
6–9 years old	below 114/74	114–121/74–77	122–129/78–85	130+/86+
10–12 years old	below 122/78	122–125/78–81	126–133/82–89	134+/90+
13–15 years old	below 130/80	130–135/80–85	136–143/86–91	144+/92+
16–18 years old	below 136/84	136–141/84–91	142–149/92–97	150+/98+

[1]If your child's blood pressure falls in any of the high ranges above, discuss options for controlling the high blood pressure with your family doctor.

Note: Numbers to the left of the slash mark indicate systolic pressure, numbers to the right of the slash mark indicate diastolic pressure. Note that adult classifications differ.

Adapted from "The Fifth Report of the Joint National Committee on Detection, Evaluation, and Treatment of High Blood Pressure," *Archives of Internal Medicine,* 1993; 153:154–83.

A Complete Blood Pressure Checkup

When you visit your physician, you'll find that a typical checkup has three stages:

▶ **1.** *A Brief Review of Your Family Medical History.* This is important because of the suspected genetic link in the incidence of high blood pressure. Your own past medical history and any symptoms are also vital. Give your physician as many details as you can about the status of your health.

▶ **2.** *Several Painless Blood Pressure Readings.* Your blood pressure will probably be measured more than once during the checkup. It's often important to take different readings—while you are seated then standing, or from one arm then the other—because even these small changes can affect the reading.

▶ **3.** *A Few Routine Tests.* These tests provide your physician with the information needed to evaluate your condition thoroughly.

- Your physician may use a flashlightlike device, called an ophthalmoscope, to look at the blood vessels in your eyes, the only place where blood vessels are visible. This inspection allows the doctor to check for thickening, narrowing, or hemorrhages.

- Your physician will also place a stethoscope at various places on your body to listen to blood flow. This is a process called auscultation, in which the doctor listens to sounds made by the heart and blood flowing through the arteries. Trained ears can detect valuable information.

- Your pulse can be checked at different points, including your wrist, neck, groin, and ankle.

- Your reflexes will be tested.

- Your height and weight will be recorded.

- Your physician will palpate, or feel for the size and condition of, internal organs.

- An X ray of the chest area may be needed to evaluate heart size, disease in the lungs, and other conditions.

- An *electrocardiogram,* which measures the electric activity of the heart and gives an indication of the thickness of the heart muscle, may also be needed.

- Your physician may learn further details about your health from an analysis of your urine and blood samples, which can indicate kidney damage, kidney performance, diabetes, and the presence of bladder infections.

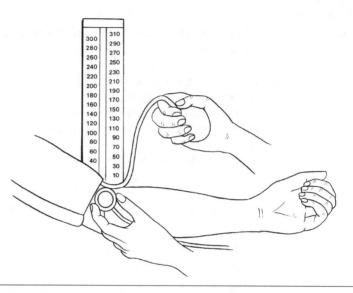

FIGURE 4   *Getting your blood pressure checked.*

*How Blood
Pressure Is
Measured*

Blood pressure is measured by an instrument called a *sphygmomanometer* (pronounced: sfig-moe-ma-*nom*-a-ter). Fortunately, the device is simpler to operate than the name is to say. You've probably had the procedure many times, even if you didn't know the name of the device. These are the steps and what they mean (also see Figure 4):

▶ 1.   A rubber cuff is wrapped around your arm just above the elbow. The cuff is attached by a hose to a column of mercury in a glass tube. The tube is marked in millimeters.

▶ 2.   Air is pumped into this cuff, squeezing your arm until blood flow through the main artery in the arm is cut off by the pressure. The gauge reading will be above your anticipated systolic pressure.

▶ 3.   A stethoscope is placed on your skin over the artery so that the person measuring the blood pressure will be able to hear the sounds of your blood moving.

▶ 4.   Air pressure in the cuff is gradually released and the column of mercury drops.

▶ 5.   At the exact instant the person making the measurement hears the "thump" of blood beginning to flow in the artery, the measurer notes the height of the column of mercury, which is the pressure level at which the heart can force blood past the squeezing cuff. This is the systolic reading.

▶ 6. The measurer observes the descending column of mercury until the last sound of blood flow in your artery can be detected. Again, the height of the column of mercury indicates the pressure in the cuff at that point, which is the diastolic reading.

How Often Should Blood Pressure Be Checked?

Since uncontrolled hypertension can be so destructive, yet most people don't know whether they have it, periodic blood pressure checks are vital to heart health. Table 13 offers guidelines for how often you should have your blood pressure checked. If your doctor discovers signs of hypertension, he or she will counsel you on how frequently you should have your blood pressure rechecked in the future.

While it's possible to monitor blood pressure constantly over a 24-hour period, doing so may not be of much value to most people. In fact, most hypertensive people don't even need to measure their blood pressure at home. Many do, though, because they find that self-monitoring keeps them aware of the problem and helps them follow their control program. Consult your doctor on whether you should invest in a home-monitoring device.

TABLE 13   *How Often Should You Have Your Blood Pressure Checked?*

Up to Age 18:	
Check blood pressure every 2 years unless an unusual reading occurs.	

Over Age 18: If the Reading Is	Recheck
129 or below/84 or below	in 2 years
130–139/85–89	within 1 year
140–159/90–99	within 2 months
160–179/100–109	within 1 month
180–209/110–119	within 1 week
210 or above/120 or above	immediately

Adapted from "The Fifth Report of the Joint National Committee on Detection, Evaluation, and Treatment of High Blood Pressure," *Archives of Internal Medicine,* 1993; 153:154–83.

If you do monitor your own blood pressure at home, it's a good idea to take your home-monitoring device to your physician's office to verify its accuracy by comparing readings.

Where Should Blood Pressure Be Checked?

Having your blood pressure checked at company screenings or health fairs can serve a useful purpose if it identifies a potential problem. However, the atmosphere may be too busy and you may be too involved with the action for a reading to be reliable. Remember, activity and stress can elevate readings.

The same warning holds true for coin-operated blood pressure machines in highly trafficked public areas. Such machines also may not be accurate because of improper or infrequent maintenance. With all that in mind, for your regular readings, have your blood pressure checked in a calm setting by a trained professional. Nonetheless, you may still have to consider the impact of your surroundings.

White-Coat Hypertension

Most of us are a little nervous in the doctor's office. Some people get a bit more agitated when a doctor, nurse, or physician assistant (someone in a white coat or uniform) attaches them to a machine. Because stress elevates blood pressure, these people may find their blood pressure readings in the doctor's office higher than they get in a more relaxed atmosphere at home or work.

This discrepancy is called *white-coat hypertension,* and medical opinions differ as to what it means for the patient. Some physicians think that if the pressure is normal or nearly so most of the time, sharp elevations shown during measurement are no reason for alarm. Others believe that since we live in a stress-laden world, the elevated pressures may occur frequently enough outside the doctor's office to ravage the body, and should be treated. Our position is that if you're getting consistently high readings, regardless of the cause, you should consider them a significant signal to consult your doctor. Using a device that monitors your blood pressure while you go about your daily activities can be helpful in determining the seriousness of this problem.

Hypertension during Pregnancy

During their final trimester of pregnancy, many women develop high blood pressure. This condition represents a significant change, because blood pressure during the first six months of pregnancy tends to fall into the low-normal range. (Typical readings for the first two trimesters are 90–100/70–75.) You and your physician should therefore keep close watch over your blood pressure throughout your pregnancy. Readings in the range of 135–140/85–90 during the final trimester may require treatment.

The good news is that after childbirth, your blood pressure usually returns to prepregnancy levels. Nonetheless, your blood pressure should be monitored for an additional 2 to 3 months.

WHAT YOU CAN DO

Hypertension is serious. But it *is* treatable. You owe it to your heart to find out if you have it—and to act to control it.

Seek Treatment for Hypertension

Unless you have a severe case of hypertension, a diagnosis of high blood pressure doesn't mean that you'll have to start taking medication. Instead, there are a number of changes you can make in the way you live that will help control your blood pressure. Then, if your body still needs more help, medications are available.

Drug-Free Ways to Control Hypertension

Ordinarily, a physician will ask you to modify activities and habits that you can control. The following changes may bring your blood pressure back to normal:

- Reducing your intake of sodium (salt) and fat.
- Beginning a regular exercise program.
- Managing stress in your life.
- Quitting smoking.
- Drinking alcoholic beverages in moderation, if at all. (Remember the guidelines for moderate alcohol consumption: Your daily alcohol intake should be no more than 2 ounces [60 ml] of 100-proof whiskey, one 8-ounce [240-ml] glass of wine, or two 12-ounce [355-ml] glasses of beer.)

For help incorporating these heart-smart changes into your life, see the programs described in Part Five and the recipes described in Part Six of this handbook.

If you begin to alter your activities with the aim of reducing your blood pressure, you should have your blood pressure monitored regularly (look back at Table 13 to find guidelines on how often, or follow your doctor's directions) for 3 to 6 months. If your doctor sees enough improvement and your blood pressure stabilizes below the 130/90 threshold, you will probably *not* have to take medication. If, however, your blood pressure remains above 130/90, your doctor may recommend drugs.

If drugs are prescribed, they are usually in addition to, not in place of, changes in diet, exercise, stress management, and smoking and drinking habits. If you maintain heart-healthy habits in all these areas, your physician may be able to prescribe smaller doses of drugs.

Medications for Hypertension

One key to the dramatic reduction in deaths from stroke in the United States is the constant improvement in drugs used to treat hypertension. Drugs prepared from the plant genus *Rauwolfia* were the first to be used to treat high blood pressure. Unfortunately, many patients were plagued by such undesirable side effects as depression and impotence. In response, scientists developed dozens of different kinds of drugs that may be used alone or in combination to reduce or eliminate some of these problems.

Today, although some hypertension medications have side effects, in most of those cases, a physician is able to formulate an effective alternative drug therapy.

There are eight main types of drugs commonly used to treat hypertension. Each works by a different mechanism, as explained below.

▶ 1. *Diuretics.* Diuretics, which are sometimes referred to as "water pills," act to reduce excessive amounts of water and sodium chloride in the body and tissues. This reduction, in turn, relieves edema (swelling) from water-swollen tissues, reduces overall fluid volume (including blood volume), and relaxes the walls of small arteries in the body. As a result, blood pressure decreases and heart function improves because the heart doesn't have to work as hard to pump.

Of the different types of diuretics, the most common are thiazides, loop diuretics, and potassium-sparing diuretics. Although each type works in a different manner, all diuretics act on the kidneys to reduce the amount of sodium and water in the body (and bloodstream) by increasing urine output.

Thiazide diuretics are prescribed most often, but because they may cause a deficiency of potassium, they are often given with potassium-sparing diuretics, which help prevent excessive potassium loss. Loop diuretics, which act quickly and are more powerful, are usually reserved for people whose hypertension cannot be controlled by thiazide, especially those with associated kidney dysfunction. Loop diuretics are also most often prescribed in combination with a potassium supplement, because they also can cause potassium loss.

▶ **2.** *Beta-Blockers.* First used to treat angina, beta-blockers also help reduce blood pressure because they slow the heart rate and decrease the force of its contraction. In this way they reduce the amount of blood being pumped in a given period of time. Beta-blockers are not as effective for Blacks and are seldom recommended for patients with heart failure, asthma, diabetes, or circulation problems in the hands or feet. Most patients have few side effects when these drugs are prescribed in low doses or when they are combined with one of the other types. However, beta-blockers have been known to cause impotence, depression, and lethargy.

▶ **3.** *Calcium Channel Blockers.* Calcium channel blockers slow the rate at which calcium passes into muscle cells, primarily in the arterial wall. By hindering the muscles that constrict arteries, thus keeping those arteries more open, calcium channel blockers allow blood to flow more freely. Calcium channel blockers are tolerated well by most patients.

▶ **4.** *Angiotensin-Converting Enzyme (ACE) Inhibitors.* ACE inhibitors lower blood pressure by blocking the formation of angiotensin II and therefore *renin,* a natural substance that constricts or closes blood vessels. They also decrease the retention of sodium and water. ACE inhibitors are frequently prescribed for patients with kidney disease, heart failure, or diabetes, and are occasionally supplemented with diuretics. They do not seem as effective when administered to Blacks.

▶ **5.** *Alpha-Blockers.* Alpha-blockers interfere with the receptors that function to constrict the smaller arteries in the body. They counteract the hormone responsible for increased blood pressure during the fight-or-flight reaction to a perceived or actual threat (for more information on the fight-or-flight response, see chapter 7). A notable side effect, however, especially in older people, results in a drop in blood pressure when the person on the drug moves suddenly or stands abruptly. This plunge in blood pressure can result in fainting and falling.

Drugs that combine alpha- and beta-blockers are also now available.

▶ **6.** *Other Vasodilators.* Vasodilators open arteries and can produce a sharp, rapid drop in blood pressure. They may be administered by injection to meet hypertension emergencies.

▶ **7.** *Peripheral Adrenergic Antagonists. Peripheral adrenergic antagonists* are the lowest-priced antihypertension medications. These drugs, however, are associated with slowed mental activity and languor. But these symptoms are less likely to occur with small doses. This class of drug is usually given along with a diuretic.

▶ **8.** *Centrally Acting Drugs*. Centrally acting drugs block impulses from the brain to the sympathetic nervous system, resulting in an opening of arteries and often a slowed heart rate. These drugs are usually prescribed along with another antihypertension medication and can produce such side effects as tiredness, weakness, constipation, sleepiness, depression, and dry mouth.

As researchers gain more knowledge about the biochemical processes that govern blood pressure, even more effective drugs will be developed. These medications will provide new alternatives to people on a lifetime treatment program.

What to Ask
Your Physician

If you have high blood pressure, talk to your doctor about this condition. Don't be afraid to take notes.

If you are being treated without medication, be certain you understand exactly what you should do in terms of diet, exercise, and stress management. And be sure your physician knows of any drugs you're taking for another condition or illness, including over-the-counter medications you might use for allergies or colds.

If your doctor recommends medication to control your hypertension, be sure you understand the answers to the following questions before leaving your doctor's office:

- When should I return for another consultation or blood pressure reading?
- What should I do if I forget or miss taking my medication?
- Are there any specific foods or drinks I should avoid while on the medication?
- Should my medication be taken on a full or empty stomach?
- Will my antihypertensive drugs be safe to take with my other medications?
- Are there any over-the-counter medications I should avoid? (These might include some brands of cold remedies.)
- What are the side effects of my prescribed medication?
- Will the side effects pass with time?
- Are there any activities (such as strenuous physical exercise, driving, and so on) I should avoid while taking the medication?

If the cost of a recommended medication creates a financial problem for you, say so! Often the doctor can prescribe an equally effective, less-expensive alternative or a generic equivalent.

If you experience any side effects from the medication, tell your physician immediately. There may be an alternative medication that won't give you problems, or additional drugs you can take to manage them. People often suffer needlessly because their doctors don't know about their difficulties.

Recognize that It's Not Too Late

It's rarely too late to benefit from controlling high blood pressure. Much heart damage, for example, is reversible if blood pressure is returned to a normal range. The same is true for kidney damage.

It's important to remember, though, that high blood pressure can be controlled but not cured. If you have high blood pressure and are under treatment, your blood pressure will rise if you abandon that treatment. If your blood pressure is regulated by antihypertensive medications, it's important that you take the prescribed dosages at the stated intervals. If you skip or decide to reduce your drug intake, or follow your physician's advice only on a now-and-again basis, the treatment *won't* work: Your blood pressure will remain high, and your good health will be endangered. If you *do* follow your treatment, however, you can keep your blood pressure at levels compatible with a healthy heart.

If you haven't had your blood pressure checked by a professional, do so without delay. Only if you know about a hypertension problem can you attempt to control it.

CHAPTER 9

Cholesterol and Triglycerides

WHAT YOU NEED TO KNOW

If your self-test showed that your total blood cholesterol is high, or you don't know what your cholesterol level is, the information here may inspire you to act.

In 1784, a French chemist distilled a white, waxy powder from a gallstone. This material went unnamed until 1816, when another French scientist described the substance by combining the Greek words *chole* (bile) and *steros* (solid). In the early 1900s, researchers began studying cholesterol in earnest and to date, 13 different Nobel Prizes have been awarded for work relating to this substance.

Why all this attention to cholesterol? Because elevated levels of cholesterol and other lipids (fatty substances) in the blood have been linked to an increased risk for cardiovascular disease.

What Is Cholesterol?

Cholesterol is one of a group of fatty or oily compounds called *lipids*. As unpleasant as that may sound, however, cholesterol is essential to the proper functioning of the human body. It is used by our glands to make hormones. It also assists the liver in making bile (a greenish fluid that then gets stored in the gallbladder), which is needed to digest fats. The biggest role of cholesterol, however, is in the formation of cell walls or membranes: Every cell membrane is composed partly of cholesterol.

Like all animals, we humans are able to manufacture internally all the cholesterol we need. It is made in the liver and released into the bloodstream. What happens after it reaches the bloodstream explains why people speak of "good" and "bad" cholesterol.

Good and Bad Cholesterol

Because blood is water-based and cholesterol is oil-based, the two cannot mix directly. For cholesterol to be carried in the bloodstream, it must be covered by a molecular "wet suit" made of protein. This protein coating keeps the oily cholesterol and other lipids from coming into contact with the watery portion of blood and allows the cholesterol to flow freely in the bloodstream. These protein-coated lipids are called *lipoproteins*.

Most cholesterol is transported to the body's cells in particles called *low-density lipoprotein* (LDL). The cholesterol contained in these particles is called *LDL cholesterol*. Because high levels of LDL are closely linked to increased risk for heart disease, LDL cholesterol is known as "bad" cholesterol.

Cholesterol in *high-density lipoprotein* (HDL) is called *HDL cholesterol*. Because high levels of HDL are linked to decreased risk for heart disease— that is, HDL appears to protect against heart disease—HDL cholesterol is known as "good" cholesterol.

When LDL levels are high, the excess cholesterol in those particles can be deposited on the artery walls. Once there it helps form *atherosclerotic lesions*. HDL particles, however, "pick up" cholesterol from lesions in the artery walls and return it to the liver.

Population studies clearly show that as the level of LDL ("bad") cholesterol rises, the incidence of heart disease increases; and as the level of HDL ("good") cholesterol rises, the incidence of heart disease decreases.

Cholesterol and Plaque

Too much LDL ("bad") cholesterol in the blood leads to deposits of fatty streaks in the arteries, where such deposits contribute to a buildup called *plaque*. Well over a hundred years ago, scientists in Russia discovered that plaque, a solid, fatty substance, was over 60 percent cholesterol. Deposits of plaque can narrow arteries and reduce blood flow, a condition called *atherosclerosis*. If the plaque buildup blocks a coronary artery completely or causes a blood clot, then the flow of blood to the heart muscle stops suddenly, resulting in a heart attack. If an artery to the brain is clogged by plaque, blood flow to the brain could be interrupted, resulting in a stroke.

If arteries in the legs are blocked, lack of circulation can cause a painfully serious condition called *claudication.*

Checking Your Cholesterol Levels

Because the amount of cholesterol in your bloodstream has such a profound effect on the health of your heart, you should have your cholesterol levels checked regularly. The current recommendation for a person over 20 who has no symptoms of heart disease is to check cholesterol levels at least once every 5 years. More frequent checks, perhaps once every 2 or 3 years, should be considered for men over 45 and women over 55. At any age, if your levels are high or if you have heart disease, have all three cholesterol readings (total, HDL, and LDL) checked annually or as instructed by your physician.

The test for total cholesterol and for HDL cholesterol is simple and requires no fasting ahead of time. One small blood sample can be used to measure both HDL and total cholesterol levels. LDL cholesterol levels *can* be from the same blood sample, but only if you have fasted for about 12 hours before the test.

To ensure accurate readings, the laboratory must use a standard procedure approved by the Centers for Disease Control and Prevention. Quick tests at health fairs or in shopping centers and the new home-testing kits, which measure total cholesterol from a drop of blood squeezed from a pricked finger, may not always provide laboratory-grade results. If you have an unusual reading from any source, you should have the results reviewed by a physician.

How Much Is Too Much Cholesterol?

For adult men and women, it is generally accepted that your total blood cholesterol level should not exceed 200 milligrams (mg) for each tenth of a liter (deciliter or dL) of blood (or 5.2 mmol/L).

This number was arrived at after extensive research on populations of both women and men. The Framingham Heart Study showed that men and women whose total cholesterol is 300 mg/dL (7.8 mmol/L) have a 3 to 5 times greater risk for cardiovascular disease than men and women whose total cholesterol is 200 mg/dL (5.2 mmol/L).

The data from Framingham and other studies don't prove that keeping blood cholesterol at a specific minimum level *prevents* coronary heart disease. But they do clearly indicate that total cholesterol levels above 240 mg/dL (6.2 mmol/L) increase the risk that a person will develop heart disease.

TABLE 14 *Protective Cholesterol Levels*
(for adults with no previous signs of heart disease)

	Total Cholesterol		LDL Cholesterol		HDL Cholesterol	
	(mg/dL)	*(mmol/L)*	*(mg/dL)*	*(mmol/L)*	*(mg/dL)*	*(mmol/L)*
Men	200 or less	5.2 or less	130 or less	3.4 or less	60 or more	1.2 or more
Women	200 or less	5.2 or less	130 or less	3.4 or less	60 or more	1.4 or more

While the 200 mg/dL (5.2 mmol/L) maximum serves as a simple goal, individual differences can complicate the meaning of any individual reading. A person with a total cholesterol level above 200 mg/dL (5.2 mmol/L) may have an exceptionally high HDL ("good") cholesterol level, making the total number less dangerous. Conversely, a reading under 200 mg/dL (5.2 mmol/L) may be due to low HDL ("good") and high LDL ("bad") cholesterol levels, making the total level more risky than usual. The higher the proportion of HDL ("good") cholesterol, the better for your cardiovascular health.

Women, especially those under 50 who have not yet begun menopause, tend to have higher concentrations of HDL ("good") cholesterol than men. According to study findings, women aged 20 and older average about 56 mg/dL (1.5 mmol/L) of HDL. Men of comparable ages average only 47 mg/dL (1.2 mmol/L). These higher HDL levels may explain why women typically develop heart disease about 6 to 10 years later than men.

Table 14 shows protective cholesterol levels for adult men and women.

You may have had a simple blood test that yielded only a total cholesterol count. That may be all you need to know if your total cholesterol is below 240 mg/dL (6.2 mmol/L) and you have no symptoms of heart disease. However, several studies have indicated that the ratio of total cholesterol to HDL cholesterol (one of several calculations known as *lipid ratios*) is the most efficient predictor of the risk for coronary heart disease. Therefore, you should get a full measurement of HDL and LDL cholesterol levels (*and* triglycerides; see below) if:

■ Your total cholesterol is greater than 240 mg/dL (6.2 mmol/L).

■ You have other risk factors for heart disease (such as high blood pressure, diabetes, or smoking) and your total cholesterol is greater than 200 mg/dL (5.2 mmol/L).

■ You have had symptoms of heart disease or other atherosclerotic disease such as stroke.

Heredity and Cholesterol Levels

A tendency toward high cholesterol levels can be inherited. *Familial* (inherited) *hypercholesterolemia* (elevated blood cholesterol) affects one in every 500 Americans. It is a good idea for parents who have cholesterol levels above 240 mg/dL (6.2 mmol/L) to have their children's cholesterol levels tested as well. The children may have inherited a gene that affects the way cholesterol is removed from their bloodstream.

What Are Triglycerides?

Triglycerides are fats. Most of the fat you eat is in the form of triglycerides. Different from cholesterol, which is a building block of cells, triglycerides are used by your muscles and provide your body with energy. Excess triglycerides are stored as body fat for future use or are recycled by your liver.

Triglycerides and Your Heart

There are different opinions about how triglyceride levels affect coronary heart disease. It is common for patients with some forms of heart disease to have high triglyceride levels. It is also common for those with high triglyceride levels to have high blood pressure, lower levels of HDL cholesterol, and diabetes, and to be obese. Since these conditions are all known risk factors for coronary heart disease, high levels of triglycerides are obviously *associated* with heart disease. However, it has been difficult to establish that they cause heart disease. Therefore, elevated triglyceride levels alone are not universally accepted as a risk factor for coronary heart disease.

Checking Your Triglyceride Levels

Even with the lack of certainty that triglyceride level is an independent risk factor for heart disease, it's a good idea to have your own triglyceride level checked if:

■ Your parent, grandparent, or sibling died of or developed heart disease before age 50.

■ You have coronary heart disease.

■ You have multiple risk factors for coronary heart disease.

TABLE 15   *Triglyceride Level Guidelines*

Triglycerides		Therapy
(mg/dL)	*(mmol/L)*	
Less than 200	Less than 2.3	None required.
200–400	2.3–4.5	Dietary changes; drug therapy may be used.
400–1000	4.5–11.3	Dietary changes; drug therapy may be used.
Greater than 1000	Greater than 11.3	Immediate medical attention required.

- Your total blood cholesterol level is above 200 mg/dL (5.2 mmol/L).
- You have diabetes.

Triglyceride levels vary naturally throughout the day, and are generally higher with age. As a general rule, however, the guidelines in Table 15 provide a basic yardstick for measurements.

Most doctors consider triglyceride level as part of a package of factors that form a person's overall risk calculation. Clearly, high LDL and triglyceride levels together indicate increased risk of coronary heart disease, if only because of the LDL profile.

Since triglyceride levels rise after the consumption of fats and then stabilize, triglycerides should be measured only after 12 hours of fasting.

WHAT YOU CAN DO

Be sure to have your cholesterol and triglyceride levels checked regularly, and act to control them if they are elevated.

Control Your Cholesterol and Triglyceride Levels in a Drug-Free Way

If you have elevated blood levels of cholesterol or triglycerides, you may be able to control them through a program of a lipid-lowering diet, exercise, and, if you smoke, quitting cigarettes. As a bonus, losing weight if you need to, exercising regularly, and breaking the smoking habit will raise levels of HDL ("good") cholesterol. This same regimen is also helpful if you have high blood pressure or diabetes.

Watch Your Diet   A heart-healthy diet can reduce your cholesterol level by 5 to 10 percent. That's an average estimate; you may do better. The only way to discover how diet influences your particular situation is to alter your eating habits for 6 months and recheck your cholesterol levels.

The basic dietary guidelines for reducing cholesterol and triglyceride levels call for increasing your consumption of dietary fiber (rice, corn, oats, apples, dried beans) and decreasing your consumption of fat (especially saturated fat) and cholesterol (meats, dairy products, and oils). The fiber may help lower cholesterol levels in your blood and may boost your feeling of being full, which also helps you cut calories and lose weight. Reducing your intake of fat and cholesterol also works two ways: Not only will your cholesterol level drop, but since a gram of fat has 9 calories and a gram of carbohydrate or protein only 4 calories (less than half as many), you may lose weight as well.

See Part Six of this handbook for more information on a low-fat, low-cholesterol, high-fiber diet, along with delicious recipes for you to try.

**Drink in
Moderation**   Alcohol can apparently improve levels of HDL ("good") cholesterol. Moderate alcohol consumption has also been linked to lower coronary heart disease rates. The best advice concerning alcohol is that if you drink, do so moderately. If you don't drink, however, we don't recommend that you start, because alcohol consumption is associated with so many other health and social problems.

Exercise   Many studies show that exercise increases the level of HDL ("good") cholesterol and decreases the level of triglyceride in the blood. Among other benefits, exercise promotes weight loss and helps maintain weight at desired levels. See Part Five for a complete exercise program that can help.

Quit Smoking   Research demonstrates a connection between smoking and lower levels of HDL ("good") cholesterol. The chemicals in cigarette smoke adversely affect the various components that make up blood, and they increase the risk of clot formation—the final step in the biological process that leads to a heart attack. Moreover, studies have indicated that risk factors such as smoking can negate the heart-healthy benefits of lower cholesterol levels in the blood. See Part Five for a program to help you quit smoking.

Control Your Cholesterol and Triglyceride Levels Using Drug Therapy

If your doctor recommends drugs to lower your cholesterol or triglyceride levels, be sure you understand all the potential risks and side effects. No drug is without some degree of risk if taken for long periods of time. And cholesterol- and triglyceride-lowering medications will be your daily companions quite possibly for many years. Depending on your insurance coverage and finances, the cost of drug treatment might also be a factor. You should therefore make certain you have taken full advantage of the effects of proper diet and other lifestyle changes before pursuing drug therapy, although if your risk is very high, drug therapy may be necessary right away. Your doctor won't recommend such a course lightly, and you shouldn't undertake this course of action without full consideration.

When Should Drug Therapy Be Considered?

Your doctor may recommend medication to lower cholesterol and triglyceride levels if you have:

- Very high lipid levels.
- Coronary heart disease and an inability to maintain satisfactory cholesterol and triglyceride levels through proper diet and exercise.
- Any two coronary risk factors in addition to high cholesterol or triglyceride levels.
- High blood pressure.
- Diabetes.
- A family history of high cholesterol and/or triglyceride levels.

Postmenopausal women being considered for a cholesterol-lowering drug may find it more advantageous to take estrogens. Estrogen moderately lowers LDL cholesterol levels, moderately raises HDL cholesterol levels, and may cut the risk for heart disease by half. There may be, however, risks associated with estrogen (or hormone) replacement therapy, including an increased risk of breast cancer, so you should discuss the pros and cons of this therapy with your physician.

Keep Cholesterol in Perspective

Because high cholesterol is just one of several risk factors associated with atherosclerotic disease, reducing your cholesterol level does *not* offer complete protection against heart attacks, heart failure, or stroke. It is a prominent element, but not the only element, in a sound preventive program. However, maintaining a desirable cholesterol level is important for everyone—and especially important if you have an inherited predisposition toward high cholesterol or heart disease or already have coronary heart disease.

CHAPTER 10

Diabetes

WHAT YOU NEED TO KNOW

Diabetes, if detected in the early stages, can be successfully managed. If undetected, however, diabetes may result in fatal heart and kidney diseases, blindness, or serious circulatory ailments. That is why early detection and vigilant management of the condition are crucial to your health.

If you know that you have diabetes, you should already be under a doctor's care. If you suspect you may have it but aren't sure, see your doctor for tests. In either case, read this chapter to learn ways to manage your diabetes and protect your heart.

What Is Diabetes Mellitus?

Diabetes is an ancient Greek word meaning "siphon," which refers to one of the main symptoms of the illness—frequent and prolonged urination. *Mellitus*, another Greek word, meaning "honey sweet," refers to the body's inability to process sugar. Today, the word *diabetes* is frequently used alone, but it is accepted shorthand for the more complete name for the disorder, *diabetes mellitus*.

Best estimates are that approximately 14 million Americans have diabetes mellitus. Worldwide, according to data from the International Diabetes Federation, 100 million people, or about 6 percent of the adult population, have the disease.

People get diabetes when the pancreas fails to secrete enough of a hormone called *insulin* or when the body loses some of its ability to use insulin. Insulin controls the amount of a sugar (glucose) in the blood and is needed to transfer glucose from the bloodstream to the cells. When the regulation of glucose transfer breaks down, cells are damaged. They literally starve in a sea of nutrients. Since the cells can't take in glucose, the amount of glucose in the blood increases. In an effort to pass off the excess, the body allows glucose to spill into the urine. Noticeable symptoms of diabetes include greater frequency and volume of urination, increased thirst, weight loss despite increased appetite, and fatigue. Other warning signs are blurred vision, tingling or numbness in the hands and feet, and slow-to-heal infections.

Diabetes is a chronic illness. It will not disappear and cannot be cured. But if treated regularly, it can be controlled.

Just How Serious Is Diabetes?

Since early symptoms may be slight, many people are mildly diabetic and don't know it. Even at this level, the disease is serious. If untreated, diabetes can cause long-term damage to your heart, eyes, kidneys, and nerves. Diabetics have an increased risk of developing coronary artery disease and suffering a stroke, myocardial ischemia, or heart attack. Furthermore, because diabetes tends to mask symptoms of heart disease, diabetics are doubly at risk.

Diabetes can cause poor circulation to the feet and reduce foot sensitivity to pain. A stubbed toe, a cut, an abrasion, or another injury may go unnoticed, which can lead to severe complications. This risk is compounded for elderly people whose circulation in the extremities has declined.

If allowed to progress, diabetes can be fatal in and of itself. The body must be able to process sugar. The disease is, in fact, the seventh leading cause of death in the United States. Although diabetes cannot be cured, its effects can be controlled. As with so many illnesses and heart-threatening conditions, the keys are early detection; proper diet, exercise, and stress management; and judicious medication.

Who Can Get Diabetes?

Although anyone can acquire diabetes, most researchers have concluded that there is a definite hereditary tendency toward the illness. And since certain fats in the human body interfere with insulin-glucose activity, anyone who is obese is especially at risk. Damage to the pancreas, either through direct injury or from a disease such as mumps or measles, can also lead to diabetes. You do *not*, however, get diabetes from eating too much sugar.

Because of their genetic makeup, Native Americans, Blacks, and Hispanics are all at higher risk for diabetes than Whites. Women have the disease more frequently than men, and older adults are measurably more susceptible.

Types of Diabetes

There are two distinct types of diabetes.

▶ 1. *Insulin-dependent diabetes* (also called child-onset or Type I diabetes) usually begins before age 30. Most of the 1.4 million Americans with this form of the disease have had it since childhood. Type I diabetes is caused by severe insulin deficiency that results from problems with the insulin-producing cells in the pancreas. If a person with Type I diabetes does not receive the proper amount of manufactured insulin, he or she will go into a coma and will frequently suffer heart failure.

▶ 2. *Non-insulin-dependent diabetes* (also called adult-onset or Type II diabetes) usually occurs in people over 40 who become resistant to the insulin produced in their systems. Obese individuals are at special risk for this kind of diabetes: About 75 percent of all persons with Type II diabetes are overweight.

A form of Type II diabetes called *gestational diabetes* is seen in a few women who develop high glucose levels in their blood during pregnancy. Even though glucose levels usually return to normal after childbirth, there is some evidence that these women are at increased future risk of developing Type II diabetes.

How Can Diabetes Be Detected?

Your doctor can test you, or you can find reliable home-testing kits at many drugstores. If a home test indicates that you may have diabetes, you should seek a more specific diagnosis from a doctor. Everyone over the age of 40 should have a periodic laboratory check for diabetes, although how frequently depends on your doctor's analysis of your condition and family history.

Concentrations of sugar or glucose (measured on an empty stomach) that exceed 140 mg of glucose in every tenth of a liter (deciliter or dL) of blood indicate the disease. This concentration is about the same as dissolving three tiny grains of sugar in a large glass of water.

WHAT YOU CAN DO

The keys to handling diabetes are to find out if you have it, and then to monitor the condition vigilantly.

Test for Diabetes

Since early detection of diabetes is very important, you should be tested as part of your regular physical exam. You may want to be tested more frequently if you have a family history of this illness, or, of course, if you experience any symptoms. If you *don't* have diabetes, then following a heart-healthy lifestyle will increase the chances you'll never get it. If you *do* have diabetes, don't despair: The illness can be treated and its effects controlled.

Treat the Diabetes

The basic treatment strategy is to maintain good control over the amount of glucose in your blood. You can achieve this through medication, diet, exercise, and stress management, all under the care of a physician.

Medication for Diabetes

If you have Type I (child-onset) diabetes, you will require a regular dosage of the proper amount of insulin. (Some people who have Type II diabetes also benefit from this medication; ask your doctor.) Current thinking, based on a 1993 National Institute of Diabetes and Digestive and Kidney Diseases study, calls for up to four injections of insulin a day to maintain appropriate blood glucose levels. Subjects in the study also followed a recommended diet and exercise program. This regimen reduced the incidence of eye damage from diabetes by 69 percent, the incidence of nerve damage by 61 percent, and the incidence of clinically significant kidney damage by about 40 percent. Because the age range of the subjects was relatively young (13 to 39 years old), there was not much heart disease to monitor, but the regimen did reduce the risk of cardiovascular disease.

The study stressed, however, that frequent insulin injections must be carefully regulated by a physician because too much insulin can lead to *hypoglycemia*, or low blood glucose levels. This strict regimen is not recommended for children younger than 13; and you should consult your doctor for individual guidelines and monitoring.

Type II (adult-onset) diabetes can usually be adequately controlled with little or no medication, through diet, exercise, and stress management (which, in fact, are important to *all* diabetics). In individual cases, your doctor may recommend some oral medications to help your body produce greater amounts of insulin and maintain proper insulin balance.

The Diabetic's Diet

In general, if you are diabetic, your diet should be very low in fat and simple sugars. In a typical meal, 50 to 60 percent of the calories you consume should come from complex carbohydrates, as found in whole-grain breads, cereals, pasta, fruits, and vegetables. Less than 20 percent of the calories you consume should come from protein, and less than 30 percent from fats. Limiting your fat intake is important because high concentrations of fat in the bloodstream can reduce your body's ability to use insulin. And, obviously, you must avoid simple sugars because your body cannot process them. (In refined form, simple sugars are found in table sugar, syrup, and processed foods. That means you should avoid candy, cookies, and soft drinks.)

It's also important that you drink ample amounts of water—at least eight glasses a day. And since many studies show that a large number of diabetics have lower-than-normal amounts of vitamin B-6, magnesium, vitamin B-12, thiamine, and other essential elements in their systems, your ideal diet should be rich in these vitamins and minerals. Whole-grain breads, cereals, and pasta, and dried beans, peas, and other legumes are good sources for thiamine, magnesium, and vitamin B-6. Lean meat is rich in thiamine and vitamins B-6 and B-12. Milk and milk products and eggs are also abundant sources of vitamin B-12.

If you are diabetic, see your doctor or a qualified nutritionist to help you tailor a specific diet to fit your particular needs.

Also, for more detailed information on healthy eating, see Part Six of this handbook.

Exercise and Diabetics

If you are diabetic, exercise can help you in two major ways:

▶ 1. Exercise improves blood circulation throughout the body. This is important because diabetes can cause a decrease in circulation (especially to the hands, arms, legs, or feet) which often leads to complications.

▶ 2. Exercise decreases the concentration of sugars (glucose) in the blood by making cells throughout the body more sensitive to insulin. This increased sensitivity helps diabetics because it promotes a more efficient use of available insulin by the body.

Nationally established guidelines for exercise frequency and intensity, along with fundamental safety tips, are provided in chapter 2. See also Part Five of this handbook for a physical fitness program that you can adapt to your individual needs. Remember that everyone, especially those with diabetes, should stay within their personal limits when exercising.

Stress Management for Diabetics

The normal body response to stress produces sharp increases in the levels of blood glucose and blood pressure, both harmful for diabetics. Consequently, diabetics have extra motivation to learn to manage their stress. Understanding and using stress-management techniques, as well as getting regular exercise, will help keep your blood pressure and blood sugar levels under control. See chapter 18 for a further description of stress-management techniques.

Cope with Diabetes

If you have diabetes, you have an unusual responsibility for maintaining your own well-being. At times, managing the disease can seem difficult—especially if you view it as a lifetime of sacrifice. You can help yourself by establishing a healthy routine that fits the way you live and then living that routine one day at a time. Avoid needless worry about your condition. Instead, focus your attention on getting the most out of life.

Your medical advisor is committed to helping you in every possible way. And there are support groups available where you can meet others who are coping with diabetes and discuss common concerns. Ask your doctor for a list of local groups. You may find it helpful to share your thoughts and feelings with others. For additional information on support groups, see the listing under "Diabetes" in the "Resources" appendix.

Remember that you can successfully manage your diabetes and live a long, heart-healthy life. Millions are doing just that. You can, too.

PART FOUR

Risk Factors You Can't Change but Need to Assess

Gender

Age

Genetic Factors

CHAPTER 11

Gender

WHAT YOU NEED TO KNOW

As the self-test indicated, if you are a man, or a woman who has gone through menopause, that in itself is a risk factor. Read this chapter. You'll find that women have more gender-related choices for managing their risk (such as the decision to take estrogen after menopause), but the information presented here is important for both genders.

Your gender is important in determining your relative risk for heart disease. Men are at a higher risk than women throughout early and middle adulthood. For example, in 1991, of U.S. citizens aged 64 or under, twice as many men as women died of cardiovascular disease. With age, however, women's risk grows: Of persons between the ages of 65 and 84, the number of deaths from cardiovascular disease in the two genders was nearly equivalent, and of those 85 and over, the number of women who died was more than twice the number of men who died.

Women appear to be protected from cardiovascular disease by estrogen, whereas men are not. Because men do not have this gender-related protection, they should make a special effort to modify those behaviors that contribute to their cardiovascular risk. Of course, modifying risk-related behaviors is important for women, too, particularly because it can reduce their increased risk in the later years of life. Women do, however, have the option to take estrogen (or hormone) replacement therapy when their risk for heart disease increases after menopause.

Focus on Women (but Men Can Read This, Too)

Hormones, Menopause, and Heart Disease

Statistically, women tend to develop heart disease about a decade later than men. Among women under 40, heart disease is uncommon. Between ages 40 and 65, however, the chances that a woman will have a heart attack markedly increase. Among this age group, one in every three heart attack victims will be female. And from age 65 onward, women account for almost 50 percent of all heart attack victims.

Researchers have connected this pattern to decreases in the female hormone *estrogen* during menopause—a process that begins around age 50 and can continue for a few years.

Studies indicate that estrogen, which regulates menstruation, protects against heart attacks by increasing high-density lipoprotein (HDL) cholesterol levels in the blood. HDL cholesterol helps prevent the slow buildup of plaque in the arteries by carrying cholesterol away from the arteries and out of the body. Indeed, according to a report in the *American Journal of Cardiology,* HDL ("good") cholesterol levels are the most important predictor of an individual's cardiovascular health. The higher the HDL level, the lower the chance of having a heart attack or stroke. (For a full discussion of cholesterol, see chapter 9.)

Before menopause, women may also have two other hormone-based heart-health safeguards:

▶ 1. The uterine *prostaglandins,* hormones secreted by the uterus before menopause, may play a role in heart health, both by opening blood vessels and by preventing blood clots from forming.

▶ 2. A chemical compound called *tissue plasminogen activator (TPA),* a known clot-dissolving chemical, is also found in greater concentrations in women's blood than in men's. This chemical helps prevent heart disease by acting to dissolve the blood clots that do form. Estrogen is suspected of being one of the regulators that determine the concentration of this clot-buster in the bloodstream.

Body Weight

Research indicates that the relationship between body weight and heart disease is even stronger among women than men. For a woman, being even slightly overweight dramatically increases her risk. The distribution of fat on the body (discussed in detail in chapter 4) is also important. Women whose fat is retained around the waist (the male pattern) are at greater risk than women whose fat accumulates around the hips (the female pattern).

Pregnancy and Childbearing

Pregnancy places increased demands on a woman's cardiovascular system. Her blood volume increases, her circulation can be impaired by the enlarging uterus, and the growing fetus's demand for oxygen and nutrients is always increasing. These factors combine to cause significant additional work for the mother's heart. Even so, unless a woman has preexisting heart disease, in general, pregnancy won't affect her heart adversely.

However, pregnancy may trigger hypertension, especially during the final trimester. If hypertension does occur, it generally disappears after childbirth. Even so, it's a good idea for a woman to have her blood pressure checked during the weeks following childbirth to ensure a return to normal readings.

Your obstetrician has information on hypertension and other heart-related problems that may occur during pregnancy. Be sure to ask for it.

In the 1940s and 1950s, women with almost any form of heart disease were routinely advised to avoid getting pregnant. Thankfully, we now have a better understanding of the cardiovascular changes that occur in a woman's body during pregnancy. Today, only a limited number of cardiovascular problems cause a physician to counsel a woman to refrain from getting pregnant. And many of these conditions are correctable. However, if you do have heart problems and are contemplating becoming pregnant, you should consult with your doctor.

Women with heart problems who do become pregnant need the care of a cardiologist as well as an obstetrician, and the two physicians should work together as a team. These doctors can offer a clear understanding of the risks—both to mother *and* baby—and they can provide information on the hereditary nature of heart problems.

Another heart-health issue concerns the number of children a woman has. A study published in the *New England Journal of Medicine,* based on 4,890 women, indicated that women who bear more than six children are about 50 percent more likely to suffer a heart attack at some point in their lives than those who bear none. Age, weight, cholesterol level, and other factors were taken into consideration. This study, however, is not definitive and also showed no higher levels of risk among mothers of fewer than six children. To be safe, though, women with several children should pay even greater attention to living in a heart-healthy fashion.

Gender and Treatment Differences

Two recent studies, the results of which were published in the *New England Journal of Medicine,* provided evidence that gender bias definitely exists in the management of coronary heart disease. The findings showed that women who are hospitalized for coronary heart disease undergo fewer diagnostic procedures than men (although in part because some diagnostic tests are less accurate for women). Women were also less likely to undergo *balloon angioplasty* or *coronary artery bypass* to treat their disease. (See Part Seven of this handbook for explanations of these procedures.)

According to another published report, when women do receive treatment, they don't fare as well as men do. Mortality rates for those undergoing balloon angioplasty (the procedure that uses a small balloon inside an artery to open a clogged area) are around 2.3 percent greater for women than for men, and more women than men experience reclogging of the arteries involved.

Moreover, bypass surgery can be more dangerous for women than for men. Part of the reason for the added risk in these procedures is that by the time women undergo bypass surgery, they are generally older and sicker than the men who undergo these procedures. Also, research suggests that survival after bypass surgery is linked not to gender but to the size of the individual: Some speculate that it may be more difficult to operate on smaller arteries.

Most women do respond well to treatment, however. Studies indicate no significant gender differences in survival rates after the first critical year following treatment.

WHAT YOU CAN DO

Short of having a sex-change operation, you can't change your gender. So when it comes to heart health, gender differences must be respected. But if your gender, perhaps combined with your age, does put you at risk, there are important things to consider.

Pay Attention to Your Other Risk Factors

Both women and men need to incorporate heart-smart concepts into their lives at an early age. A healthy lifestyle is especially important for men under 50, but women aren't excluded from the need to start young.

Women's Options   Women also need to examine additional options and choices they may have, including those discussed below.

▶ **1.** *Estrogen (or Hormone) Replacement Therapy.* Women who are post-menopausal may benefit from estrogen (or hormone) replacement therapy. Analysis of the medical research indicates a 30 to 50 percent decrease in heart risk for women taking estrogen *orally.* The reason seems to be that estrogen increases HDL ("good") cholesterol levels in the blood. However, estrogen delivered through skin patches or creams bypasses the liver and so is less effective.

Why isn't estrogen replacement therapy recommended universally? Because research results have not been uniform and, more important, because estrogen has been associated with (although not necessarily a cause of) certain cancers.

For instance, some breast cancers are estrogen-dependent. That is, if a woman who has existing, undetected breast cancer takes estrogen, cancer growth *may* occur. But the level of the problem posed here is not clear. Many doctors believe that the benefits of estrogen replacement therapy are considerable and that the breast-cancer risk, which must be respected, is small unless the woman has a history of breast cancer in her family or is, for some other reason, at particular risk.

Estrogen used alone over a long period of time has also been associated with uterine cancer. To counter this effect, low-dose estrogen is used in combination with *progestin*, another female hormone. Progestin, however, may negate some of the cardiovascular benefits derived from estrogen replacement therapy by increasing LDL ("bad") cholesterol levels and decreasing HDL ("good") cholesterol levels.

So, if you're a postmenopausal woman, what should you do?

A woman who has normal blood pressure and cholesterol levels may have little reason for taking estrogen to prevent heart disease. And a woman who has family members with breast cancer or benign breast disease should be extremely cautious about taking estrogen.

On the other hand, for a woman who has a family history of heart disease and other risk factors that cannot be controlled through diet, exercise, and quitting smoking, estrogen replacement therapy may offer some protection. Heart disease is by far the biggest threat to the average woman's life. In fact, most researchers believe that protecting the heart will someday prove to be an overwhelming reason for recommending that most women take estrogen after menopause.

The best advice is to discuss estrogen replacement therapy with your physician. Together, the two of you must make the decision to begin therapy or not on an individual basis by considering your personal risk factors for both heart disease and cancer.

▶ **2.** *Oral Contraceptives.* A decade ago, studies revealed that oral contraceptives significantly raised a woman's risk of heart disease. The pills used at that time contained estrogen in levels high enough to raise blood pressure and increase the blood's tendency to clot. Oral contraceptives prescribed today, however, are considerably lower in estrogen and so don't have quite the same negative effect.

Nonetheless, we still don't have enough evidence to know whether oral contraceptives are entirely safe for women's heart health. Research has shown that the use of oral contraceptives does significantly increase heart disease in women who smoke cigarettes. Some studies have indicated that female smokers who use oral contraceptives are 39 times more likely to have a heart attack and 22 times more likely to have a stroke than women who neither smoke nor use oral contraceptives. For that reason, the American Heart Association suggests that women over 35 and younger women who have many risk factors for heart disease choose a different form of birth control. If you are already taking oral contraceptives or are thinking of starting, be sure to discuss these issues with your doctor or other health care provider.

▶ **3.** *Smoking.* Chemicals in cigarette smoke deprive the heart of oxygen, encourage the blood to clot, cause the arteries to spasm, and injure the lining of the coronary arteries. In women, smoking is particularly harmful because it also reduces the protective effects of estrogen.

The Nurses' Health Study, a Harvard survey of more than 117,000 female nurses, reported that women who quit smoking reduced their excess risk of coronary disease by one-third within 2 years. And, 10 to 14 years after quitting, their risk of coronary disease was the same as for women who had never smoked.

▶ **4.** *Alcohol.* Drinking a moderate amount of alcohol may help your heart health. According to guidelines established by the American Heart Association, a moderate amount is no more than 1 ounce (30 ml) of alcohol per day. One ounce of alcohol is contained in 24 ounces (720 ml) of beer, 8 ounces (240 ml) of wine, or 2 ounces (60 ml) of 100-proof liquor.

Please understand, we are *not* recommending that nondrinkers start. And the guidelines do *not* allow you to skip alcohol for several days during the week, then have six drinks on Saturday night. Indeed, heavy drinking can cause heart-related problems such as high blood pressure, stroke, arrhythmias, and cardiomyopathy.

Moreover, pregnant women and women with any condition that could make alcohol use harmful, including hypertension and diabetes, should, of course, not drink.

And don't forget that an average drink contains between 100 and 200 calories. Calories from alcohol often add fat to the body, which may contribute to the "apple" body shape that also increases the risk of heart disease.

▶ **5.** *Diabetes Mellitus.* Diabetes is more common in women than in men and poses a greater risk for women because it cancels the protective effects of estrogen. Indeed, women who have diabetes are much more likely to have cardiovascular disease than women who don't. Diabetes also increases the risk of second heart attacks in women who have already had one.

Proper management of diabetes is essential for heart health and requires consultation with a physician. See chapter 10 for a more detailed discussion of this disease.

A Last Word about Gender

When it comes to heart health, women clearly have more choices than men. So women must be aware of their health situations and follow appropriate medical guidelines—as we've tried to present. Having said all this, we still want to stress that, whether you're a woman or a man, you'll benefit most from following the basic guidelines of heart-healthy living—eliminating all the risk factors you can change, and carefully monitoring those you can control.

CHAPTER 12

Age

WHAT YOU NEED TO KNOW

If your self-test showed your age to be a risk factor, you obviously can't turn back the clock. But the question of age and the risk of heart disease is more complex than you might expect. Beyond a doubt, the older we get, the more susceptible we are to a variety of coronary diseases. Heart concerns, though, are not limited to the elderly. Babies are born with congenital heart defects, and teenagers establish habits they will carry through the rest of their lives. If some of those habits are heart-unhealthy, they may create problems in later life. However, for a better understanding of age and heart disease, it's best to start with the older heart.

The Older Heart

Older age is a risk factor for cardiovascular disease. In fact, heart disease is the leading cause of death among older Americans. However, many of the health problems associated with older age can be minimized by proper exercise, a healthy diet, and appropriate medical care. A recent study in the *New England Journal of Medicine* concluded that middle-aged and older men who begin exercising, quit smoking, maintain normal blood pressure, and avoid obesity, have lower rates of death from all causes, including heart disease. Several other studies have also suggested that you're never too old to improve your heart health.

Physiological Changes in the Aging Heart

As we grow older, our hearts tend to become less efficient. The heart walls may thicken, and the heart muscles may not relax as fully as they did in younger years. This is usually accompanied by a loss of flexibility, or stiffening of the arteries, and a decrease in the heart's ability to pump blood to muscles. As a result of these changes, the risk for men of developing cardiovascular disease increases steadily with age. The risk for women remains fairly low until menopause, and then increases so that women 65 and over have about the same risk of cardiovascular disease as men of equal age. This increase in risk is associated with a postmenopausal decrease in hormone levels and may be partially counteracted by hormone (estrogen) replacement therapy.

Common Cardiovascular Diseases of the Older Heart

Several cardiovascular diseases, such as coronary artery disease, hypertension, valve disorders, and arrhythmias, are more common among older people.

Hypertension, a condition which affects more than 60 percent of people over 65, is associated with increased risks of stroke and heart attack. Several studies have demonstrated that treating hypertension can drastically reduce cardiovascular death rates and the incidence of stroke in older men and women. Until age 55, men are at greater risk for hypertension than women; from 55 to 75, the risks for men and women are about equal; and after 75, women are at greater risk. Hypertension and its associated conditions can often be treated effectively with dietary changes, weight loss, exercise, and drugs. A recent study has suggested that postmenopausal hormone use contributes to a decreased risk of stroke in postmenopausal women.

Common valve disorders among the elderly include *aortic sclerosis* (a stiffening of the aortic valve) and *aortic stenosis* (a narrowing of the aortic valve). These conditions sometimes require surgical replacement of the diseased valve with a mechanical valve, a technique that is effective in both older and younger patients.

Arrhythmias, irregularities in the rhythm of the heart, also become increasingly common with age. Correcting an arrhythmia often requires that a pacemaker be implanted, but this operation has a low risk for patients of all ages. Pacemakers are particularly useful in treating slow arrhythmias and *heart block,* a condition in which the heart's electrical system fails to function properly. *Atrial fibrillation,* a fast arrhythmia, is also more common in the elderly, but can often be treated with medication.

Exercise

A recent study in *JAMA* (the *Journal of the American Medical Association*) found that older men who began exercising and became fit reduced their mortality rate by 44 percent compared to men who remained unfit. Similarly, a study of exercise in women 75 and over concluded that those women who were more active lived longer. The best reason to exercise, however, is to improve the quality of your life. Exercise not only increases life expectancy but also relieves stress and improves overall well-being. For more information on how to begin and maintain a healthy exercise program, please refer to chapter 15.

Diet

Diet is particularly important in combating coronary artery disease in older women. Studies suggest that 50 percent of women aged 55 to 74 would benefit from an improved diet that reduced blood cholesterol, body weight, and blood pressure. In fact, reducing the intake of fats and cholesterol and increasing consumption of fiber reduces mortality rates from heart disease in both men and women. In addition, decreasing sodium intake and increasing potassium consumption can aid in the treatment of hypertension.

Drug Treatment

Several changes that occur with age may affect how well some cardiovascular drugs work. These changes include a decrease in renin activity (an enzyme that plays a role in regulating blood pressure), a decrease in total body potassium, and a slower metabolic rate (the rate at which your body processes the chemicals in foods or drugs). As a result of these changes, older patients who are taking medications may experience more side effects and show greater sensitivity to many common medications, including vasodilators, anticoagulants, and nitroglycerine derivatives. Most drugs can still be used safely and effectively in older patients, but close attention should be given to dosage and possible complications.

Diagnosis and Treatment

Several recent studies suggest that older patients may sometimes receive inferior treatment for cardiovascular illnesses. For this reason, it is particularly important for older people to try to communicate effectively with their physicians. It is also important to discuss economic issues regarding treatment, which may be critical to older persons on a fixed income.

Today, many men and women are performing at higher physical levels in later life than was even imagined in previous generations. Controlling your other risk factors and obtaining regular, high-quality medical care are the keys to a long and heart-healthy life.

The Younger Heart

Although we usually think of a young heart as a healthy heart, addressing risk factors early on can do a great deal to minimize cardiovascular risk in later life.

Congenital Problems

Less than 1 percent of all newborn babies have a congenital heart disorder or a heart-related birth defect. Even so, medical science has devoted a vast amount of attention to these problems and, today, except for the most unusual conditions, treatments are available. See chapter 25 for a more detailed discussion of congenital heart disease.

The Crucial Teen Years

Few teenaged boys and girls have heart attacks. If a teenager does have a heart problem, it's usually the result of an inherited condition. Such problems are often virtually undetectable and only revealed during strenuous exercise. However, if a teen has a family history of sudden cardiac death, comprehensive screening by a pediatric cardiologist may be warranted. This is particularly true if the teen will be participating in competitive sports.

Although heart attacks in teenagers are rare, the teen years are important to future heart health for two main reasons:

▶ 1. Coronary artery disease is a progressive illness that begins in childhood.

▶ 2. Many adult habits are formed while we are teenagers.

So this is an excellent time for parents to instill heart-health consciousness and a basic understanding of cardiovascular risk factors in their teenagers.

Make sure you and your teenager are on the same wavelength concerning these seven critical heart-health issues.

▶ 1. *Smoking.* The lifelong habit of cigarette smoking or the use of other tobacco products tends to begin during the early teens. Peer pressure, a desire to appear older, and other factors combine to create too many teen smokers. But inhaling any smoke—whether from tobacco, marijuana, or another source—is harmful to the cardiovascular and respiratory systems. (See chapters 5 and 17 for more information and assistance on how to quit.)

▶ **2.** *Blood Pressure.* While considerably less than 3 percent of all children in this country under age 12 have high blood pressure, the condition becomes more common among teenagers. High blood pressure, or hypertension, is a serious condition because it can remain undetected for many years. And the longer elevated blood pressure continues untreated, the more damage is done to the body. All teens should have their blood pressure checked periodically, but checkups are essential for overweight teens and for those with a family history of high blood pressure, diabetes, or stroke.

▶ **3.** *Cholesterol.* Studies indicate that nearly 15 percent of all children in the United States have elevated cholesterol levels. (For children with no special risk factors, a total cholesterol reading of 190 mg/dL [4.9 mmol/L] or above is considered high. For children from high-risk families—those who have one parent whose total cholesterol is 240 mg/dL [6.2 mmol/L] or above, or those who have a parent or grandparent who was diagnosed with coronary artery disease before age 55—a total cholesterol reading of only 170 mg/dL [4.4 mmol/L] or above is considered high.) In less than 2 percent of this group, the cause is due to a genetic disease called *familial hypercholesterolemia.* For the rest, the problem most likely stems from too much fat in the diet. Teens should have their total cholesterol level checked if a parent has a total cholesterol level in excess of 240 mg/dL, or if the teenager smokes, is obese, has high blood pressure, or has a family history of heart disease.

▶ **4.** *Nutrition.* Eating the right foods for a healthy heart may be difficult for teens, and not just because of their desire for junk foods. A recent U.S. Department of Agriculture study showed that in 99 percent of the 545 schools participating, the average percentage of calories from fat in school lunches was 38 percent—as opposed to the recommended guideline of 30 percent or less.

As a parent, you have the right to request information about the nutritional policies in effect in your children's school. If necessary, solicit support from other parents in asking school administrators to meet acceptable dietary standards. You can contact the American Heart Association for clear recommendations for a heart-healthy school lunch program. (See "Cardiovascular Health" in the "Resource" appendix.)

You should also make your teenagers aware of what they eat, provide heart-healthy meals at home, and offer fruit as well as other low-fat snacks instead of the usual collection of commercially packaged products. (Again, see chapter 3 and Part Six for more practical guidelines on diet and healthy meals.) Since many food preferences are formed during the teen years, you can help your teenager establish heart-healthy eating habits now.

▶ **5.** *Obesity. Obesity,* defined as being 30 percent or more over your ideal body weight (according to the Metropolitan Height and Weight Tables—see Table 1 in chapter 1), is a serious condition that leads to cardiovascular and other health problems. Obesity in the teen years is of concern because an obese teenager is likely to become an obese adult. And overweight adults have higher rates of heart disease.

Teens who are overweight or obese should take steps to adjust their weight to fit within the appropriate range for their gender, height, and body frame size. A medical examination can indicate whether the overweight condition is due to diet or physical causes, and a doctor can assist in developing a plan to achieve necessary weight loss. (Parts Two and Five provide information and programs for fitness and weight control.)

▶ **6.** *Diabetes Mellitus.* Special care must be taken with teens who have developed Type I or child-onset, diabetes mellitus. Growth and drastic alterations in body chemistry present one set of challenges; changes in diet and tastes for certain foods may provide another. Please see chapter 10 for a more complete discussion of diabetes.

▶ **7.** *The Importance of Medical Examinations.* Teenagers need annual medical examinations. As teens gain more freedom than they had in childhood, they may have less time and desire for physical examinations. Nonetheless, teenagers should be taught to manage their time to allow for annual checkups. It's another habit that will help extend their lives.

WHAT YOU CAN DO

Remember that it's never too late—or too early—to begin improving your heart health.

Promote Heart Health in Your Later Years

First and foremost, eliminate any risk factors (such as smoking) that you *can* change and properly manage any risk factors (such as diabetes) that you can't control. That's good advice for any age, but it has special meaning in the later years when people are more vulnerable to heart disease.

As simple as it sounds, paying attention to diet and engaging in regular exercise can return high health dividends to older people. If you are over 50 and have not exercised in the past, be sure to consult with your physician before beginning any exercise routine or engaging in any level of sustained fitness training. In addition, the best heart-related counsel is to listen to your body, go at your own pace, and seek medical attention when you sense something is amiss.

Develop Heart-Healthy Habits in Your Teens

Teens have a chance to establish habits that can produce untold benefits in the future. This five-point checklist sets the basics:

▶ 1. Don't start smoking.

▶ 2. Check for high blood pressure.

▶ 3. Develop positive nutritional habits.

▶ 4. Learn the basic risk factors for heart disease.

▶ 5. Begin an exercise/fitness program.

The teen years can be trying times for both teens and their families. Yet teenagers need help in developing heart-healthy habits and encouragement to grow into health-conscious adults. Detecting problems early and becoming aware at an early age of the main cardiovascular risk factors can significantly improve your health and increase your longevity.

CHAPTER 13

Genetic Factors

WHAT YOU NEED TO KNOW

Although you cannot change your family history of heart disease or your race, it is important that you understand how each may affect your heart health. Since you cannot alter your basic genetic characteristics, you have to accept them. But understanding them can help you see the importance of reducing other risk factors.

Family History and Your Heart

For literally hundreds of years, the medical profession has recognized that certain types of illness seemed to "run in the family." It hasn't been until the last few decades, however, that a better understanding of genetics and new research data, including better health records, have enabled physicians and scientists to convincingly document these hereditary relationships.

For example, we now know that if any of your grandparents, parents, or siblings had a heart or circulatory ailment *before age 55,* then you are at greater risk for heart disease than someone who doesn't have that family history.

The *early* occurrence of heart disease in a direct blood relation is the factor that increases your risk. If a grandparent, parent, or sibling developed any form of heart disease *after* age 55, you need to consider that relative's age at time of death. If the relative died of heart failure at age 75, for instance, your own risk is substantially less than if he or she died at a younger age—say, 60.

We should also note, though, that there are limitations to our present knowledge of the role of genetic factors in heart disease. As with racial influences, it is difficult to obtain a clear, precise separation between hereditary influences and environmental factors. Although genes are inherited, family attitudes toward nutrition, smoking, alcohol, and exercise are learned. In many cases, the early occurrence of cardiovascular disease in a relative may have been precipitated by these environmental risk factors, *not* genetic influences.

Nonetheless, if there is a history of the early occurrence of heart or circulatory disease in your immediate family, you should consider yourself at greater risk. Moreover, if the early occurrence of heart disease has been pervasive in your family, affecting both a grandparent and a parent, for example, your risk is even more pronounced. You should also note, however, that an inherited predisposition does *not* mean that you will *definitely* suffer heart failure, heart attack, or stroke. A family history of heart disease merely means that you are *more likely* to develop heart disease than someone of your same age and background who has no such hereditary links.

Race and Cardiovascular Disease

For years, researchers and heart specialists have noticed that some forms of cardiovascular disease are more common among certain racial and ethnic groups. Although doctors and medical researchers have been highly motivated to clarify how race and ethnicity create a predisposition toward certain diseases, they have had difficulty conducting accurate studies. The main problem is that in the real world, race and ethnicity are not isolated factors. Socioeconomic forces, learned customs, and higher or lower concentrations of certain illnesses in various geographic locations are just three of the variables that combine to make research difficult. Nonetheless, the government tries.

A U.S. Department of Health and Human Services bulletin on Minority Health Care lists one majority and six distinct minority groups in the United States. The majority of the U.S. population is classified as White, and the minority groups include Blacks, Hispanics, Asians, Pacific Islanders, Alaskan Natives, and American Indians. While heart-health studies have been made within each minority group, the lion's share of minority-oriented cardiovascular research has focused on the two biggest minority groups: Blacks and Hispanics. The larger White population has been used as a baseline for comparison.

Such categorization is useful, even necessary, for statistical generalizations, of course. But wide racial and ethnic variances inside each classification complicate matters. There are also differences in income, education, behaviors, beliefs, and other cultural considerations both within and among different minority groups. Because of this, it's difficult to state conclusively that a higher or lower incidence of a particular trait or disease within one of these minority groups is solely racially based.

Keeping all that in mind, increasing attention to racial influences has offered insights into racial predispositions. And we *can* make some clear statistical statements concerning cardiovascular disease in certain groups.

Blacks and Heart Disease

Life expectancy for an average member of the total U.S. population is about 75 years, whereas life expectancy for an average Black is slightly less than 70 years. Yet the leading chronic diseases that cause deaths among Black Americans are the same as those for the general population.

Probably the most important heart-health difference between Blacks and Whites is a considerably higher incidence of high blood pressure, or hypertension, among Blacks. A little more than 70 percent of Blacks have hypertension, compared to 60 percent of Whites. The higher incidence of hypertension helps explain why the incidence of deaths from strokes is almost twice as high among Blacks as it is among Whites (Blacks are also at greater risk than Whites for nonfatal strokes).

Moreover, Blacks have shown more marked abnormalities in readouts from their electrocardiograms; Black men have slightly higher levels of coronary heart disease than White men; and Black women show significantly higher levels of coronary heart disease than White women. Death rates from heart disease are clearly higher for Blacks than for any other segment of the population. Again, however, no research has conclusively shown a racial explanation for these facts.

On the other hand, in a recent study of 428,300 male veterans treated for heart disease or chest pain at Veterans Administration hospitals, Whites were twice as likely as Blacks to have undergone heart bypass surgery, and one-and-a-half times more likely to have had their narrowed arteries unblocked through balloon angioplasty. This study is especially interesting in that all patients received free medical care, and the findings could be adjusted for age, marital status, geographic region, and other health problems. The researchers have suggested that the disparities in treatments received may be attributable to racial differences in the severity of heart disease, cultural differences in attitudes toward medical care, differences in access to care, racial bias, or a combination of those factors.

Other long-term studies have indicated that differences in the incidence of heart disease do *not* seem related to HDL ("good") cholesterol and total cholesterol levels: the levels for Blacks and Whites are about the same. Similarly, the heart attack risk factors for Black Americans are consistent with the rest of the population.

The differences between Blacks and Whites in the incidences of hypertension and coronary disease may be associated with differences in seven factors related to heart health.

▶ **1.** *Diet.* Diet has a direct influence on blood pressure. For instance, excessive sodium (salt) intake increases blood pressure in some people. Although some studies indicate that Blacks appear to consume about as much sodium as Whites, there are regional variations. Also, other research suggests that Blacks may be more likely to retain sodium in their bodies, a condition known to elevate blood pressure. Too much saturated fat in the diet also creates a risk for heart disease. And cooking with saturated fats such as lard seems to be higher among Blacks, especially in some geographic regions.

▶ **2.** *Stress.* Stress is a recognized risk factor for hypertension. Because stress causes temporary increases in blood pressure, some researchers propose that constant stress and tension—created by living in a dangerous, high-crime area, for example—can, over time, create consistently high blood pressure. Other stress-related causes might be rooted in the psychological responses to the unfair treatment Blacks still receive in a White-dominated society—suppressed hostility, or constant unexpressed anger. Research is continuing in this field.

▶ **3.** *Response to Medications.* Blacks and Whites exhibit observably different physiological responses to many of the medications used to treat hypertension. For example, the beta-blocker drugs have more effect on Whites than Blacks. On the other hand, Blacks appear to respond better to diuretics than Whites do.

▶ **4.** *Diabetes.* Diabetes is one-third more common among Blacks than Whites. Black women, especially those who are overweight, have the highest incidence of this illness (which may at least partially account for the higher incidence of heart disease among Black women than among White women). Furthermore, complications from diabetes—such as heart disease, stroke, kidney failure, and blindness—are more prevalent among Black diabetics than among White diabetics. Since diabetes is known to be an inherited disease, there appears to be a strong argument for racial predisposition toward this illness. But other factors, including diet and greater access to health care, must also have some influence.

▶ **5.** *Smoking.* The Centers for Disease Control and Prevention reported that, in 1992, 23.9 percent of Black women smoked, compared with 25.7 percent of White women. However, 32 percent of Black men smoked, compared with 28 percent of White men.

▶ **6.** *Body Weight.* Obesity (defined as being 30 percent or more over your ideal body weight) is more common among middle-aged and older Black women than among the rest of the population, and this may be one of the reasons for the prevalence of hypertension in this subgroup. Obesity is a known risk factor for heart disease and diabetes.

▶ **7.** *Alcohol.* Research indicates that Blacks are more likely than Whites to be either heavy drinkers or total abstainers. Excessive consumption of alcohol can contribute to heart disease, while moderate consumption (for example, two 12-ounce [355-ml] glasses of beer per day) may have some benefit. Abstinence is fine; binge drinking *isn't*.

Hispanics and Heart Disease

Hispanics or Latinos are a highly diverse ethnic group (a collection of many different ethnic groups, really), making it difficult to tie general health differences to racial causes. Mexican Americans, for example, have much lower stroke rates than Puerto Ricans living in New York.

Such variations aside, among U.S. residents, the incidences of deaths from cardiovascular diseases are 35 percent lower among Hispanic men and 20 percent lower among Hispanic women than among their non-Hispanic counterparts.

Age may partially explain these favorable statistics. The median age for Hispanic Americans is 26, while the median age for the entire U.S. population is 33. Approximately 38 percent of all Hispanic Americans are under the age of 19. The six factors influencing the heart health of Hispanics in America as compared to Whites are described below.

▶ **1.** *Diet.* Many of the cuisines popular among Hispanics use large amounts of fats and oils, which we would expect to increase their incidence of heart disease. However, since Hispanics have fewer deaths due to heart disease, other factors must be offsetting their high-fat diets. Sodium consumption among Hispanics also appears to be above that of Whites. We are forced to speculate that the youth of the Hispanic American population is the mitigating force. If so, as this population ages, we can, sadly, expect sizable increases in heart-related deaths.

▶ **2.** *Stress.* We have seen no evidence that stress is more or less prevalent or severe for Hispanic Americans than for White Americans.

▶ **3.** *Response to Medications.* No differences in reactions to drugs for treating hypertension or heart disease have been noted among Hispanic Americans; however, many Hispanics have a greater sensitivity to several antidepressants.

▶ **4.** *Diabetes.* The incidences of deaths from diabetes are 1.9 percent higher among Hispanic American men than among the general U.S. male population, and 2.4 percent higher among Hispanic American women than among the general U.S. female population. Hispanics should thus pay particular attention to risk factors (such as excess weight) for diabetes.

▶ **5.** *Smoking.* There is some indication that the incidence of cigarette smoking among Hispanic Americans is lower than among the general population. And those Hispanic Americans who do smoke report smoking fewer cigarettes per day.

▶ **6.** *Body Weight.* Although other cardiovascular risk factors are about the same for Hispanics as for the population as a whole, weight control may become important for the Hispanic American population (on account of its high-fat diet) as this relatively youthful population ages.

WHAT YOU CAN DO

From the perspective of heart health, each of us, no matter what our race or family heritage, will be better served by viewing ourselves as a unique individual rather than part of a loosely defined group. The same cardiovascular risk factors apply to all; while your individual family history of illness and your race are important, you can still increase your chances for better heart health by modifying the risk factors you do control.

Find Out about Your Family's Medical History

If you are unsure whether you are at risk because of hereditary predispositions toward heart disease, take the time to uncover your family's history of cardiovascular problems. Compiling your family's medical history can be an interesting and rewarding experience. Children and teenagers should be encouraged to participate. You can use the Family Medical History Questionnaire to help you collect the needed information. Sources for gathering information about your family's health history might include other relations, old family friends, past medical records, newspaper obituaries, and death certificates.

FAMILY MEDICAL HISTORY QUESTIONNAIRE

Check the appropriate response as to whether any member of your immediate biological family (including any one of your grandparents, parents, or siblings) has ever had the diseases or conditions listed.

	Yes	No
Heart disease		
Coronary heart disease	☐	☐
Congestive heart failure	☐	☐
Cardiomyopathy	☐	☐
Rheumatic heart disease	☐	☐
Arrhythmias	☐	☐
Sudden death	☐	☐
Vascular disease	☐	☐
Diabetes	☐	☐
High blood pressure	☐	☐
Stroke	☐	☐

Also indicate which member of your family had the disease, the age of the individual when the disease was discovered, and any other details about the condition you were able to learn.

Relation	*Age*	*Details*
_____	_____	_____
_____	_____	_____
_____	_____	_____
_____	_____	_____
_____	_____	_____
_____	_____	_____

If your family medical history or your race indicates a predisposition for coronary or vascular disease, you can use that information to design a healthier lifestyle for yourself. For example, a family history of heart disease makes it essential for you to eliminate or control all of the other heart-health risks you can. Part Five of this book provides detailed action plans and programs to assist you toward your goal of a healthier life, and Part Six gives recipes that can help your whole family eat more healthily.

CHAPTER 14

Getting Your Program Started and Keeping Yourself Going

WHAT YOU NEED TO KNOW

Now that you understand your personal heart-health risk factors, you're ready to begin the journey toward living a heart-healthy life. The programs and recipes described in the next six chapters will help you do just that. But before you turn to them, please read the information here about the three "tasks" that we believe will help you get your heart-smart program(s) started properly—and, just as important, help you maintain them for life.

Task #1: Define Your Goal(s)

Define your heart-health goals in terms of changes to your habits or behavior patterns. Think of adding healthy practices or subtracting unhealthy ones from your daily life. If at all possible, include a positive benefit in the definition of your goals. And don't worry about your goal sounding trivial to anyone else: You're doing this for yourself and the people who care about you, not for the approval of others. Finally, establish a deadline as part of your goal definition.

Here are three examples of heart-healthy goals:

▶ 1. On June 30, when I have taken cigarettes out of my life, I'll have whiter teeth and avoid those smoke wrinkles around my mouth and frown lines around my eyes. I'll also feel better, do my heart a favor, and be healthier.

▶ 2. On my birthday, when I am able to deal better with the stress in my life, I'll enjoy my kids and husband more. I'll also improve how I feel at the end of the day.

▶ 3. By adding exercise to my life *now,* I'll soon begin to look better, feel better, and have more energy. I'll be back in shape by my class reunion.

Before you begin your heart-smart journey, it's also useful to analyze where you are now and how you got that way. That is, before undertaking a behavioral change, assess how long you've been doing what you want to change and how the current behavior fits into your life. By understanding how you reinforce the bad habit, you'll have a better chance of replacing it with a healthy one.

For example, a middle-aged man who needs to start exercising regularly and lose some weight might describe his situation this way: "I started adding 3 or 4 extra pounds [1.4 or 1.8 extra kilograms] a year after I got out of school, and now I'm 50 pounds [23 kilograms] overweight. I enjoy eating and can't pass up a dessert. And I haven't seen the inside of a gym in several years." To begin his analysis, this man should recognize that he won't be able to regain his adolescent physique with just a few sit-ups (if ever). It might not take as long for him to lose the weight as it took to gain it, but he'd better be prepared for a long-term commitment to physical fitness and weight control. As for that dessert habit, it might be a good idea for him to come up with some new activity or routine to replace it—that would be a worthy companion to his new exercise program.

Task #2: Make an Action Plan and Commit to It

The programs in this part of the book offer detailed action plans. You can use them as they are or modify them as needed to fit your individual needs and meet your personal goals. Whatever you do, however, it's important that you choose a plan that defines specific actions to help keep you focused, and specific measures so you can see what progress you're making and how far you still have to go.

An effective action plan replaces an unhealthy habit with a healthy one. Habits thrive on repetition and diminish when neglected. The longer you do something, the harder it is to stop. So the longer you can do without (or with something else), the easier it will be to stay away. The overweight man in the example above may come up with an action plan that includes substituting an after-dinner walk for that hard-to-resist dessert. Perhaps later in the evening he can reward himself with a glass of juice or other nonfat treat. In any case, the more he continues to exercise even moderately instead of finishing off dinner with cake and ice cream, the easier that healthy routine will become. He'll have a new habit he won't want to break.

In time, the new behavior will be its own reward.

Remember also that you can't break all your bad habits overnight. Changes are made one habit at a time. Yet each new healthy habit pushes you closer to your overall goal of a heart-healthy life. Changes are also made one day at a time. Each day that our dessert-loving friend substitutes exercise for his cake and ice cream will take him one more step on his journey toward a heart-healthy life. Of course, he might wish to reward himself occasionally with a piece of that cake as he makes progress on his overall journey!

Task #3: Maintain Your Motivation

If you're like most people, you'll begin your heart-health improvement program with a burst of enthusiasm. And you'll find renewed commitment each time you succeed in overcoming unexpected challenges. The time will come, however, when your resolution will falter, the lure of your old habits will beckon, and your new routine suddenly just won't seem worth the effort.

Don't panic. And don't give up. It's simply time to reenergize yourself by rediscovering the motivation that inspired you to make the change in the first place.

In this regard, honesty is essential, for motivation is very personal. You must look inside yourself and try objectively to analyze what motivates you. You may rationalize your desire to exercise, lose weight, stop smoking, and/or reduce your stress along these lines: "I resolve to live a healthier, more productive life for my family and my company." And there may be some truth to that. But you may also be driven by vanity and a craving for attention: "I'll show that darn Marie," or "Wait 'til the boys see me next summer!"

We all have a right to be human. The point is, don't back away from what drives you to succeed. Generating motivation should never cause you embarrassment; the only mistake is not developing enough incentive to see you through to your goal. Besides, no one but you need ever know what keeps you going. Remember, in the heart-healthy motivation game, the end certainly justifies the means.

Begin your search for self-motivation with the basics. Following the programs described in this book will improve your odds of (1) avoiding heart disease and many other illnesses, (2) living longer, (3) looking better, (4) feeling physically fit, (5) having more energy, (6) being less stressed out, (7) enjoying life more, and (8) viewing yourself as a more worthwhile person.

If those reasons for change are too general for you, go back to the self-test in chapter 1 and review your individual risk factors. Then pick one and reread the appropriate chapter on it. Select one poor habit you feel the greatest need to change, and get started on an action plan. Perhaps the program looks too formidable, or maybe you're not ready to give up that bad habit just yet. If that's the case, try working on something you *can* give up, even if it isn't your most important bad habit or risk factor. Get started, or restarted, and find some success you can build on.

Let's suppose, though, that the day comes when you feel your motivation slipping away, or that you know even before you start that you'll need help staying on the program. You might want to follow some or all of the suggestions described below.

▶ **1.** *Chart Your Progress.* Keep a logbook and/or a progress chart on a wall in your home or office, and record any information that will help you measure your progress. You might, for instance, keep track of your weight, cholesterol level, and blood pressure; or you could write down what exercises you did each day; or even tabulate how many grams of fat you ate. Be as detailed or as schematic as you think you need to be. You could simply put a red check for completed exercises and a blue one for skipped desserts on a kitchen wall calendar used just for that purpose. However you chart your progress, these records will demonstrate that you're getting the job done and help you visualize how much you've accomplished.

▶ **2.** *Vary Your Routine.* While following a routine helps to establish new, healthy habits, introducing some variety can keep your program fresh and interesting. You might try changing the time of your workouts and/or alternating between different forms of exercises you enjoy.

▶ **3.** *Talk to Someone.* Tell a family member, friend, or coworker about your heart-healthy commitment and the problems (and successes) you're having. It's surprising how much your motivation can be recharged during a short conversation—especially if the person you're talking with is supportive. In fact, if that person has similar goals and is as committed as you are, try working together in a "buddy system."

▶ **4.** *Identify Your Most Frequent Temptations.* Think about the forces that are most likely to drive you off your program, and search for ways to avoid or overcome them. Maybe you overeat every time you visit a particular restaurant that you patronize often on business. If you can't arrange to go elsewhere, gear up your resolution ahead of time and vow to order something less caloric. Or perhaps you can enlist the support of your colleagues in changing your habits there.

▶ **5.** *Check That First Urge to Break the New Routine.* Win the critical initial skirmish. Each time you overcome the urge to give in to temptation, your ability to resist future temptations will strengthen.

Begin Your Heart-Healthy Lifestyle with Physical Fitness

Physical fitness is the foundation not only for good heart health but for good overall health as well. Recent research indicates that even moderate physical activity cuts the risk of heart disease in half. Regular participation in a fitness program benefits people with diabetes, hypertension, and high cholesterol levels. Physically active people find it easier to stop smoking, control their weight, manage their stress, and free themselves from alcohol and drug habits. So regardless of which cardiovascular risk factor you've decided to eliminate or control, you can begin by committing to a physical fitness/exercise program.

Turn to the next chapter for all the information you'll need to do so. Bon voyage!

CHAPTER 15

Achieving Physical Fitness

In order for the physical fitness program described in this chapter to work, you have to be willing to invest two things: time and effort. But how much of each? Not as much as you might think.

Your Time Investment

There is no such thing as instant fitness. To become fit, you have to invest some of your time. The question is, How much time does it take to get fit?

The answer is, It's pretty much up to you.

At the beginning, our program requires about 15 minutes a day, 5 days a week. As your fitness builds, additional elements are added that will require slightly more time. Even so, around 50 minutes a day, 5 days a week is all that our program will ever require. Sound, basic muscular strength, endurance, flexibility, and cardiorespiratory conditioning (conditioning of the heart and lungs) can all be developed in that length of time.

It makes no difference when you schedule those minutes. You can do it in the morning, afternoon, or evening. And there's no reason to do it at the same time each day, if that doesn't work for you. Most people find, though, that setting aside the same daily block of time helps them stick to the program. The only time constraint has to do with eating: Wait about an hour after a meal (the more you eat, the longer you should wait) before exercising; then wait 20 minutes or so to eat after exercising. But drink all the water you need when you need it. (Also note that in some parts of the country during certain seasons, it might be better for you to pick a morning or evening hour to exercise—when it's cooler.)

Naturally, you're free to add more time to your program if you like and feel up to it—or add more days, or both. As strange as it may seem if you've never been on a fitness plan, the odds are excellent that once you begin, you'll want to increase the duration of your workouts. *Up to a point* (which we'll discuss later), the more time you put in, the more fitness you can take out.

Your Effort Investment

The old "no-pain, no-gain" philosophy has no place in the average person's exercise program. In fact, pain of any kind should be taken as a warning: It indicates either that you're doing something incorrectly or that you have a problem. Either way, the only thing to gain from pain is the message that you should stop.

That said, you must also understand that there is no such thing as effortless fitness. To become fit, you have to invest some effort. The question is, How much effort does it take to get fit?

The answer is, Not as much as you might think.

You need to do enough to raise your heart rate and then hold it at that increased level for a brief period of time. As your fitness increases, the effort required to elevate your pulse will also increase. So your workout routine must take this into account.

Here are three ways to check your effort levels during sustained aerobic exercise.

▶ 1. *Heart Rate.* Keep your heart rate in your Fitness Zone, which is 50 to 75 percent of your maximum heart rate. (This range is also referred to as your target heart rate.) Maximum heart rate declines as we grow older, so the exact parameters of your Fitness Zone depend on your age. (See also chapter 2, especially Table 3, which lists the Fitness Zones for persons of different ages.)

To determine your individual Fitness Zone, first calculate your maximum heart rate (in beats per minute) by subtracting your age from 220, then multiply that number by 50 and 75 percent to determine the lower and upper boundaries, respectively, of your target heart rate.

For a 40-year-old, the calculations work out as follows: $(220 - 40) \times 0.50 = 90$ beats per minute, which is the lower limit; and $(220 - 40) \times 0.75$

= 135 beats per minute, which is the upper limit. So this person would exercise at an increasing intensity until attaining a heart rate of at least 90 and, if possible, close to 135 beats per minute, then try to keep his or her heart rate between those levels for 10 to 12 minutes. That, plus an additional 3 to 5 minutes for warm-up and cool-down, is all the time that's necessary for cardiorespiratory fitness.

Using your heart rate to monitor the intensity of your workout is a good technique if you've never exercised regularly (or have not done so recently) and are just beginning a fitness program.

▶ **2.** *MET Levels.* A MET (short for *metabolic equivalent*) is a measure of oxygen consumption per minute. The greater the volume of oxygen your body uses, the more energy you're using. One MET is the energy required by your body during one minute at rest. A sustained activity level at a rate of 3 to 6 METs is sufficient to develop cardiorespiratory conditioning in the majority of people.

The MET level is a good measuring tool once you've gained some degree of fitness and want some variety in your exercise program. Table 16 shows the MET levels for different activities. The heart benefits are best when you choose an activity that uses oxygen at a rate of 3 to 6 METs. If you are in reasonable condition, working below that level provides no heart-health advantages. Working above that level burns more calories (per minute or hour) but isn't necessary for improving your heart health.

TABLE 16 *MET Levels for Various Activities*

Activity	MET Level	Activity	MET Level
Walking (2 mph [3.2 km/h])	2.5	Dancing	
Dancing, ballroom (slow)	2.9	Ballroom (fast) or square	5.5
Sailing	3.0	Aerobic or ballet	6.0
Croquet	3.0	Ice-skating	5.5
Walking (3 mph [4.8 km/h])	3.3	Tennis (doubles)	6.0
Cycling (leisurely)	3.5	Karate or judo	6.5
Gardening (no lifting)	4.4	Roller-skating	6.5
Swimming (slowly)	4.5	Skiing (water or downhill)	6.8
Walking (4 mph [6.4 km/h])	4.5	Climbing hills	
Badminton	5.5	With no load	6.9
		With an 11-lb (5-kg) load	7.4
		Swimming (fast)	7.0
		Jogging (6 mph [9.7 km/h])	10.2

▶ **3.** *Casual Conversation.* This final measurement is useful because it requires no memory, math, or tables: When you reach the point where you feel you are working your body but can still carry on a normal conversation without *excessive* breathlessness, you are in the conditioning mode. Runners and walkers commonly use this guideline when exercising together.

If you are working out alone, you can use this test: Count to 15 out loud, saying each number. If you have to take more than two or three breaths during this count, you are exercising too hard. (On the other hand, if you can *sing* it, maybe you're not working hard enough.)

What You Should Do before Beginning

▶ **1.** *Check with your physician if:*

- You're taking a prescription medication.
- You've ever had any kind of heart problem, especially a heart attack.
- You have diabetes.
- You have bone or joint difficulties.
- You have uncontrolled high blood pressure.
- You have a family history of heart disease.
- You are a man over 45 or a woman over 50, if you are not accustomed to even moderate levels of exercise.
- You smoke.
- You're significantly overweight (10 percent to 20 percent above the maximum weight in your healthy weight range).

▶ **2.** *Check your motivation* and build more if you need it. (See chapter 14 for suggestions.)

▶ **3.** *Schedule exercise time in advance* in a personal daybook, calendar, or exercise logbook—at least a full week ahead.

▶ **4.** *Set your own pace.* Remember that this is not a competition; it's a conditioning process.

▶ **5.** *Dress suitably for the climate and conditions.* Comfortable, appropriate footwear and loose, soft clothing that doesn't bind or chafe your legs and arms while they're in motion are a must. Running shoes are especially suitable for walking, jogging, and running.

▶ **6.** *Time your workouts.* You'll need a watch. It doesn't have to be a stopwatch, although that capability is handy. If you use a regular watch, a sweep-second hand is ideal. Set the minute hand on 12 when you begin, so it will be easy to tell how many minutes have elapsed.

▶ **7.** *Check your heart rate.* This may take a bit more time during the early sessions because you must track your heart rate to set your personal baseline. Also, expect a new routine to add a couple of minutes to your session as you learn each exercise. Once you have the patterns well in mind, you'll work faster. (See Figure 1 and the accompanying discussion of how to check your heart rate in chapter 2.)

▶ **8.** *Breathe while exercising.* This advice may sound strange, but many people beginning an exercise program concentrate so hard on getting the exercise just right that they forget to breathe! But breathing is essential during exercise. This is an aerobic activity; you need all the air you can get.

▶ **9.** *Never exercise when ill.* If you have a fever or an infection or are sick—even with a cold—don't exercise without your doctor's permission.

▶ **10.** *Use common sense.* People sometimes get carried away with following their exercise program. Enthusiasm is fine, but use good sense. If you're overly tired, under tremendous stress, or are just feeling odd or out-of-sorts, lay off and try again the next day.

Starting Your Plan

When you're ready to begin, record your first week's schedule on a calendar or exercise logbook—a spiral-bound notebook like the ones you used in school will do fine. If you're using a logbook, write in the days and times you'll exercise in a tabular format, like this:

Sun	Mon	Tue	Wed	Thur	Fri	Sat
5:00 P.M.	5:30 P.M.		5:30 P.M.	5:30 P.M.		7:30 A.M.

Your minimum schedule would have only 4 days. Your maximum schedule would have 7 days. In the beginning, schedule 5 days. (You can skip a day occasionally without sacrificing your level of fitness.)

At the very bottom of the logbook or calendar page, in a small space, figure your maximum and target heart rates in beats per minute. (Recall that 220 – your age = your maximum heart rate, while your target heart rate is 50 to 75 percent of that maximum.) Write both your maximum heart rate and the range for your target heart rate somewhere on the page where you can find those numbers quickly if you need a reminder.

Our exercise program here is made up of three units. Each is beneficial, but we'll present them to you in the order of their importance to your heart, starting with aerobic conditioning, then, when you're ready, moving to flexibility, and finally, to muscle conditioning.

Now you are ready to literally take your first step toward physical fitness.

The Aerobic Unit

Get your watch and go for a walk. Walk briskly, with your shoulders back and head up. Breathe a bit deeper than usual, but comfortably. Most people seem to enjoy walking outside, but it's also possible to walk indoors— even in place. In any case, swing your arms a little more and lift your knees a little higher than you normally would.

Try to walk for 6 minutes, then stop and take your pulse. If you were able to walk comfortably for 6 minutes without your heart rate exceeding your target range, you should move on to Phase 2. If, on the other hand, you find that you can't walk for 6 minutes, then stop when you feel that you've exerted yourself as much as you can. You need to exercise at the Phase-1 level.

Phase 1:
Under 6 Minutes
(Building to
12 Minutes)

For that first session, record the time walked and your pulse rate at the end in your logbook or on your calendar. (From here on, we'll just say "log" for your written record.) If your pulse rate at the end of your walk was *above* your target heart range, then for the next session, walk 60 seconds, take your pulse, and note what it is. If it is at or above the upper boundary of your target range, stop. Enter the length of time you walked and your heart rate in your log. That's your base conditioning measurement: 1 minute. That's how long you'll want to walk on your exercise days for the remainder of your first week. Continue to record each day's walk time and your heart rate at the end.

If, however, after 1 minute your heart rate is at or *below* the lower boundary of your target range, walk another minute and take your pulse again. Continue until your heart rate rises to within your target range. Enter the length of time you walked and your heart rate in your log: That's your base conditioning measurement. That's how many minutes you'll want to walk on your exercise days for the remainder of your first week. Continue to record each day's walk time and your heart rate at the end.

For your second week, add 10 percent to your walking time. (The easiest way to do this is to calculate your walking time in seconds, then add 10 percent, then convert it back to minutes.) Log your walk time and heart rate at the end for every session.

Each week add another 10 percent, and log your walk time and heart rate.

Continue adding 10 percent each week until you succeed in walking for 6 minutes with your heart rate within or below your target range. Don't worry about how many weeks it takes you to do this. You're walking to improve your fitness—and that's *exactly* what you're accomplishing.

You may be tempted to add *more* than 10 percent to your walk time each week. Don't. It's not necessary. You're doing fine.

Once you can walk for 6 minutes with your heart rate within or near your target range, continue to increase your walk time by 10 percent each week until you can walk for a full 12 minutes with your heart rate remaining within or near your range.

If, as you build toward 12 minutes, your heart rate rises substantially above your target range, stop and rest. Take this as a sign that you're trying to do too much too soon. Let your body guide you. Return to the previous week's walk time, and skip the 10 percent increase until your heart rate is under control. Then proceed.

Once you reach 12 minutes, you'll be exercising at the exertion level and duration required for cardiorespiratory conditioning. Adding more time will burn more calories, but will not significantly increase the cardiovascular benefits. Your goal now will be to increase your exertion level so that you'll reach your target heart rate sooner, so you can stay there for a longer part of the 12 minutes.

After attaining the 12-minute level, continue stopping after 6 minutes to check your heart rate. At some point you'll find that your pulse has remained below your target range—which means you'll have to walk faster to get it there. Take this as a sign that you're ready to advance to Phase 3. So skip Phase 2.

Phase 2:
12 Minutes

Start here if you were able to go the full 6 minutes on your first walk without your heart rate exceeding your target range.

If your heart rate at the end of 6 minutes is within your target range, slow your walking pace slightly and try to keep it there. Check your pulse each minute until you have completed 12 minutes of walking.

If your heart rate is *significantly above* your target range at your first 6-minute check, or goes above the upper limit of that range as you continue toward the 12-minute mark, then your walking time to the minute *before* the heart-rate increase will be your base conditioning measurement. Note that time in your log, and follow the instructions from Phase 1 about increasing that time by 10 percent each day until you can make the full 12 minutes and remain within your target range.

If your heart rate remains *below* your target range after 6 minutes of walking, continue walking for 3 more minutes, then check it again. If it's still below your target range, complete the full 12 minutes.

In any case, when you can walk for the full 12 minutes with your heart rate within or near your target range, then you're ready for Phase 3.

Even if you make the 12 minutes in good shape the first time you try it, be sure to enter your heart rate and walk time in your log.

Phase 3:
16 (2 + 12 + 2)
Minutes

Take this final phase of the aerobic unit at your own pace.

Your goal now is twofold:

▶ 1. To gradually increase your heart rate over a 2-minute period at the start of your walk until it reaches your target range, to hold it there for 12 minutes, and then to walk more slowly for 2 minutes to let your heart rate fall again.

▶ 2. To add the flexibility unit to your exercise session.

To do this, you will embark on a 16-minute aerobic workout followed by a 2-minute stretching activity.

For the aerobic portion, you may need to experiment a little so that you can increase your workload to match your improving fitness.

A reasonable beginning test would be as follows:

▶ a. Walk 1 minute, then jog slowly for 30 seconds.

▶ b. Check your pulse.

If your heart rate is below your target range, jog another minute. Then check your pulse again. If it's still too low, jog another minute. Continue in this manner until your target is reached and 12 minutes have elapsed. Log your length of jogging time and the highest heart rate you reached for use the next time you work out.

If your heart rate is too high after the 30-second jog, then walk until it is within your target range, jog slowly for 15 seconds, then check it again. Repeat this until your target is reached. Make note of your jogging time and the highest heart rate you reached.

Continue the walking-jogging-walking routine until you can maintain your target heart rate for the 12-minute period. Now your entire exercise time is 16 minutes, which allows for a 2-minute walking warm-up, a 12-minute walk-jog within your Fitness Zone, and a 2-minute slow-down, cool-off walk.

Please understand that jogging is *not* the important factor here. The exercise load placed on your respiratory and circulatory systems is what counts. Your goal is to raise your heart rate to your target range, keep it there, and then allow yourself to taper back to a normal number of beats per minute. You may be able to do this by walking fast or striding. Jog only when that's the amount of exertion you need to hold your pulse within or near your target range.

If you wish to walk-jog longer than the 12 minutes, that's fine. According to the latest findings, though, cardiovascular conditioning is *not* greatly improved by more than 30 minutes of daily exercise. A 45-minute period is a reasonable goal, therefore, and should consist of 2 or 3 minutes of stretching, 7 minutes to warm up and reach your target heart rate, no more than 30 minutes within or near your target range, and 5 minutes to cool down while continuing your activity at a reduced pace. With sufficient training, any person in normal health, with no muscular or skeletal problems, should be able to perform this 45-minute routine. If you feel like it, then do so. If not, stay with the 16-minute plan.

Please recall the restrictions and warnings listed earlier in this chapter concerning age and preexisting conditions. You can work with your doctor to modify this program if necessary.

Note that walking is used as the basic exercise for the aerobic component of this plan because the activity requires no special equipment, can be done indoors or outdoors, and is well within the capabilities of the vast majority of people. So begin with walking; then, after a few months, if you wish to do some cross-training, switch to another form of aerobic exercise. You can substitute any activity with a MET level between 3 and 6 (see Table 16).

As soon as you can go the full 12 minutes with your heart rate within or near your target range, you should add the flexibility unit to your session. If you have opted for a longer walk-jog session, the flexibility series is even more important. The added demands on your heart are low, and the payoff may be greater than you'd imagine.

The Flexibility Unit

This unit works your major joints and stretches your muscles. Here are the important things to remember.

▶ **1.** *Stretch Slowly.* Make no sudden or swift movements. Take your time.

▶ **2.** *Avoid Pain.* If something hurts, stop doing it and don't do it again until you find out why. Skip that part.

▶ **3.** *Don't Strain.* Everyone has his or her flexibility limits: Don't go beyond yours. When you feel the slightest strain against the stretch, that's more than enough.

▶ **4.** *Repeat Often.* The benefits come from stretching over and over—*not* from stretching the farthest or the hardest.

▶ **5.** *Flow with Your Routine.* The various stretches are designed to follow one another and almost become a sort of dance. Try to glide slowly and smoothly from one to another. This will be difficult at first, because you won't know the routine. With practice, however, you'll be able to flow from one to the next, and completing all 10 stretches will take a total of only 2 minutes or so.

STARTING POSITION	**SLOW SHOULDER ROLLS**

Stand in a relaxed manner, feet about shoulder-width apart, arms hanging loosely at your sides. Look straight ahead. Breathe normally.

Slowly begin shrugging and rolling your shoulders, both at the same time, circling them forward and upward toward your ears, then back around and down to the starting position. You'll feel your shoulders rotate in a full circle.

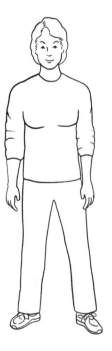

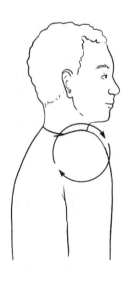

Roll them twice, starting the circle by lifting and moving your shoulders forward. Then repeat the same circular movement by pressing your shoulders backward then upward through the circle for 2 more repetitions.

FULL ARM SWINGS

From the starting position, keep your right arm relaxed and slowly bring it up in front of you, past your head, then back around to its starting point in a giant circle, as if you were doing the backstroke in a swimming pool. Your feet and body should remain in their starting positions.

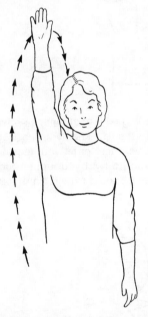

Circle the right arm twice. Then do the left arm twice, the same way.

Go back to the right arm again, and repeat the circle in the opposite direction, by moving your relaxed arm to the rear, then up and around as if you were swimming freestyle. Do 2 reps in this manner with the right arm, then 2 more with the left arm.

Remember: S-l-o-w and easy.

ARM DANGLES

Dangle your relaxed arms at your sides. Now gently shake them, allowing your hands to flap. The key here is to let your arms feel as limp as possible.

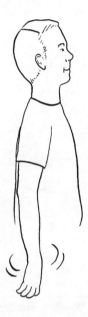

UPPER BODY STRETCH

From the starting position, with your arms at your sides, slowly press both arms straight back behind you, reaching up as far as you can without feeling pain.

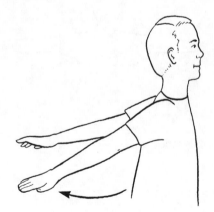

When you reach your maximum extension, bring your arms back down and forward, bend your elbows, and bring your hands up and around to touch the tops of your shoulders. Right fingers touch right shoulder, left fingers touch left shoulder. This should leave your upper arms parallel to the ground.

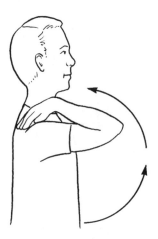

Now rotate your shoulders, straighten your elbows, and extend your arms out to your sides so that your body makes a large "T." Then lower your arms and hands to your sides to return to the starting position.

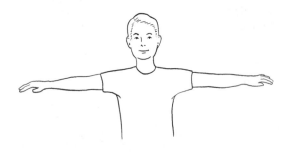

Do this series twice.

TORSO TWISTERS

From the starting position, raise both arms out in front of you until they are parallel to the ground, with your fingers pointing straight ahead.

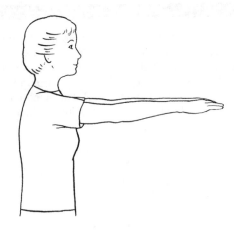

Now, leading with your chin, s-l-o-w-l-y twist your torso to the left. Keep your back straight. Don't move your feet or let your legs or hips twist: You want to twist your upper body only. The movement should extend from your head to your waist.

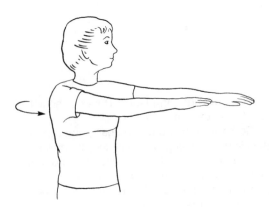

Twist as far as you can to your left, then, without pausing, swing back to the right. Don't stop at the straight-ahead position. Instead, swing slowly through center and continue to the right until you reach your limit on that side. Don't overdo the stretch. Go only as far as you comfortably can.

When you hit your limit, return to the left—but again, don't stop in the middle. When you reach your maximum left extension, turn back to the right again. Go as far right as possible, then return to the straight-ahead position and lower your arms to your sides.

Two complete left-right swings are enough. (Some people find this stretch easier to do properly if they stand with their toes pointed slightly inward as opposed to straight ahead or turned out: this helps them keep their hips stationary.)

NECK TWISTERS

From the starting position, keep your back straight and your arms at your sides, relaxed. *Do this stretch slowly and gently.*

Without moving your shoulders or torso, turn your entire head to the left as far as you can, then return to the starting position.

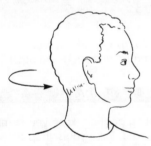

Now turn your head to the right as far as you can, then return.

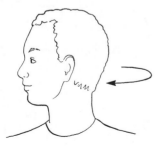

Next, slowly let your head slump forward, bringing your chin toward your chest. Then lift your head back up to return to the starting position.

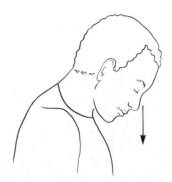

Move slowly and deliberately. Don't jerk or thrust your head forcefully. Gradually, under full control of your muscles, turn it left, right, down, and back up. The goal here is to stretch your neck lightly.

REACH FOR THE SKY

From the starting position, lift both hands to your breastbone and intertwine your fingers so that your hands are clasped palm to palm.

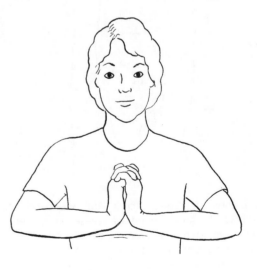

Keeping your hands together like this, slowly raise them straight up in the air, reaching toward the sky (or ceiling) as far as you comfortably can.

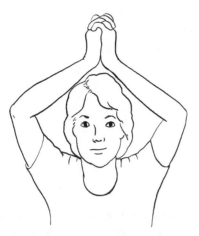

Then, without untwining your fingers, roll your palms outward and continue rotating your wrists and forearms until your palms face upward.

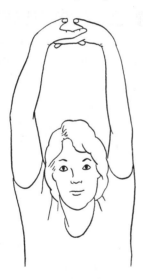

You should feel the stretch in your wrists and forearms. Hold this position for a few seconds, then rotate your wrists and forearms back and lower your arms to your breastbone again.

Do this series twice.

LEG SHAKEDOWN

From the starting position, let your arms relax and dangle. Standing on one foot, raise the other foot off the ground and *gently* shake it, letting the whole leg go limp.

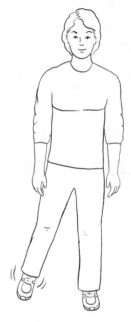

After a few seconds of shaking, return to the starting position and lift and shake the other leg.

BOUNCERS

From the starting position, keep your arms at your sides, relaxed. Raise yourself up on your toes as far as you can, then lower yourself back down onto your heels. Then lift your toes up off the ground.

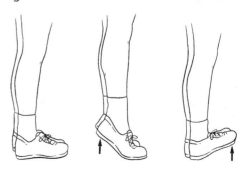

Start on your hands and knees with your back parallel to the floor. Gently lower your head and arch your back upward, like a cat stretching.

Then return your head and back to their original positions. Repeat once.

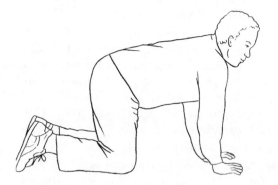
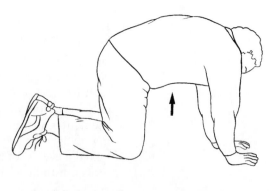

That's the flexibility routine. It's quick, easy, and effective.

The number of repetitions we suggest should be enough for most people, but if you feel like doing more, go for it. But go slowly, move smoothly, and stay relaxed. You defeat the purpose of stretching if you tighten up or get jerky.

You've now added the flexibility unit to your 16-minute walk-jog session. Each time you complete the walk-jog, perform the flexibility exercises as well. Keep track of your progress in your logbook. After you've done the walk-jog and flexibility series for 2 weeks, it will be time to add the third and final unit to your fitness regimen.

The Muscle-Conditioning Unit

It's now time to bring your major muscle groups up to the same level of tune as your cardiorespiratory organs. To reap the most benefit from this program, perform your muscle-conditioning exercises first (approximately 5 minutes), then your walk-jog or other aerobic exercise (up to 45 minutes, including stretching, warming up, and cooling down), and, to finish the session, a little more stretching (5 to 10 minutes).

Before You Begin   Walking exercises the legs and, to a lesser degree, the buttocks and belly, but does little for the upper body. This unit focuses on the muscles in your upper body. Here is some information you'll need before you begin:

- The total time required to perform this series of exercises is about 5 minutes. This allows for ample breathers between exercises.

- Our program offers two sets of exercise variations: the first for *beginning* muscle conditioning, and the second for *maintaining* it. Within each exercise, there are six different intensity levels for your workout. Everyone should begin at Level 1 of the first variation, and then, after an appropriate number of sessions (which varies depending on age; see below), progress to the next level. Once you've completed Level 6 of the first variation of exercises, you're ready to move on to Level 1 of the second variation.

- Do each exercise slowly. Be controlled in your movements. Don't fling your arms, for instance. Move deliberately at a comfortable rate.

- As with the flexibility unit, if something you do as part of this unit hurts, stop immediately. And don't perform that exercise again until you know why it hurt. When in doubt, check with your physician.

- Remember that exercising is a time for you to work your own muscles, at your own pace, to improve your own physical fitness. You are not in competition with anyone.

Repetitions and Your Age   This unit consists of two variations of five exercises each, suitable for both men and women. Each exercise is to be repeated a certain number of times per session (see Table 17). The number of sessions to be completed before proceeding to the next level depends on your age.

- If you're under 30, remain at the first and each subsequent level for at least three sessions and then, if you're comfortable, progress to the next level.

- If you're between 30 and 50, remain at the first and each subsequent level for at least five sessions and then, if you're comfortable, progress to the next level.

- If you're over 50, remain at the first and each subsequent level for at least ten sessions and then, if you're comfortable, progress to the next level.

TABLE 17	*Recommended Number of Repetitions for Muscle-Conditioning Exercises*						
First-Variation Exercises	*Second-Variation Exercises*	*Level 1*	*Level 2*	*Level 3*	*Level 4*	*Level 5*	*Level 6*
Reaches	Extended Reaches	4	5	8	10	14	18
Curl-Ups	Extended Curl-Ups	3	4	5	8	12	16
Push-Offs	Push-Offs/Push-Ups	5	6	8	10	12	15
Side Swipers	Trunk Twisters	6	7	8	10	12	14
Knee Benders	Arches	2	3	4	6	8	12

How to Progress

Everyone should begin at Level 1 of the first variation of exercises, for *beginning* muscle conditioning, and progress through the various levels. Once you've completed Level 6 of the first variation, you're ready to move on to Level 1 of the *second* variation of exercises, for *maintaining* muscle conditioning.

Although the number of repetitions at each level remains the same, the second-variation exercises are more challenging than those in the first variation.

You progress through the various levels of the second variation the same way you did through those of the first: by performing the stated number of repetitions for the appropriate number of sessions for your age. Once you've reached Level 6 of the second variation, you should stay there to maintain good muscle conditioning and strength.

Although the various exercises appear to be easy to perform, that may be deceptive: Everyone should begin at Level 1 of the first variation and do the number of repetitions indicated for each exercise. You may find that you are able to handle them with ease. Nevertheless, *don't* give in to the temptation to increase your reps or to jump to the second variation, for part of the goal here is to condition your muscles *without* pain, strain, or soreness.

On the other hand, if you can't at first perform the number of repetitions indicated for Level 1, then do only as many as you can, and gradually try to work up to the number of reps indicated. This will be just like building up to a 12-minute walk-jog: Don't overdo it, but work to the comfortable limit of your ability. That's how you'll improve.

Similarly, you may find that you've reached your "personal best" for a particular exercise at a number of repetitions *below* that indicated for

Level 6. That's all right. It's even okay if you find yourself able to do *more* than the indicated number of repetitions for some of the exercises and *less* for others. This is *your* program. *You* set the pace and exertion level.

Scheduling

Our program assumes five exercise sessions a week. If you're only walk-jogging three times a week, do the muscle conditioning exercises for five sessions for at least the first 6 weeks. And remember to do the flexibility unit after each muscle-conditioning session, whether you also walk-jog or not.

There is no double-up-and-catch-up here. If you miss a session for any reason, continue doing the same number of repetitions until you've completed the specified number of sessions at that level for a person of your age. *Then* proceed to the next level.

You might want to copy Table 17 into your log (or tape down a photocopy). It tells you the number of repetitions you will do for each exercise at each level. You could also post a photocopy of this table near where you'll actually be doing the exercises.

If you find that you can't perform the indicated number of repetitions, drop back to the previous level, stay there for about five more sessions, then try moving up again. Don't hurry, and don't be concerned. Proceed at your own pace.

Many people find it helpful to schedule each exercise session in their log. Then, after completing that session, cross it off as another motivation-reinforcing action. You can also, of course, track your progress on a wall chart. Use whatever organizational tool helps you stay on track and on schedule.

The First Variation

Before beginning the first exercise, walk around a bit, gently shaking your arms, rolling your shoulders, and turning your head from side to side. After slowly loosening up like this for a minute or two, you'll be ready to start. Perform each exercise deliberately and slowly, with controlled movements. Do not thrust or jerk your limbs, torso, or head. Instead, try to flow into each movement.

REACHES

Sit with your right leg extended slightly away from center, dig the heel of your right foot into the floor, and draw the sole of your left foot in against the extended leg. Turn your torso to face the extended leg.

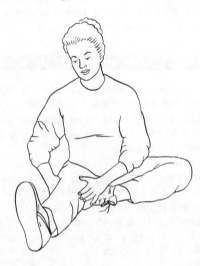

Bend forward from the hip over the extended leg, and take the calf in your hands; but do *not* lock your knee.

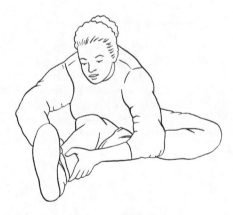

Repeat the exercise on your left side.
   One repetition includes both sides. Level 1 calls for 4 reps, working up to 18 at Level 6.

CURL-UPS

Lie on your back with your arms lifted slightly off the floor at your sides, your knees up, your feet together, your heels on the floor, and your toes lifted.

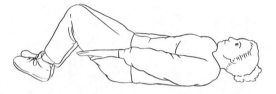

Using the muscles in your abdomen, raise your head and shoulders until your shoulders are about 4 to 6 inches (10 to 15 cm) up off the floor.

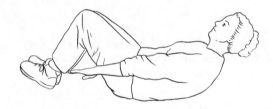

Then lower your head and shoulders back down to the floor. You want to curl up slowly, then roll back down.
   One repetition includes lifting your head and shoulders up and lowering them back down to the floor. You'll do 3 reps to start, and eventually reach 16 at Level 6.

PUSH-OFFS

Stand 2 to 3 feet (60 to 90 cm) in front of a wall and brace your hands against the wall at shoulder height.

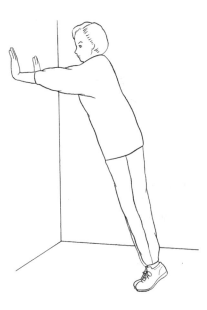

Keeping your back and legs straight and in line, bend your elbows to lower yourself forward until your nose touches the wall.

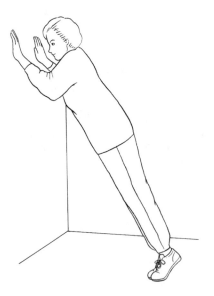

Then, by straightening your arms, push yourself back to your starting position.

One repetition is down to touch your nose and back to the starting position. Level 1 calls for 5 push-offs; by Level 6, you'll be doing 15.

(Note: If this exercise is too easy for you, try bracing your hands against a lower support, such as a waist-high table or chair, or lie face-down on the floor and do a traditional push-up.)

SIDE SWIPER

Stand with your feet shoulder-width apart. Place your hands behind your head and interlace your fingers. Check your posture to be sure your back is straight, head erect, and elbows back. This is the proper starting position.

Without moving your feet and looking straight ahead, bend your torso over and down to the right side as far as you can, stop for an instant when you reach your limit, then return to the starting position. Then bend your torso over and down to the left side, stop for an instant, then return to the starting position.

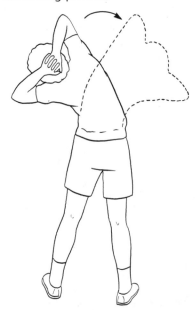

One repetition includes bending over to both sides and returning to the starting position. Do 6 reps for Level 1, and 14 for Level 6.

KNEE BENDERS

Stand with your feet about a foot apart. Looking straight ahead, bend your knees slightly, and place your hands on your thighs. This is the starting position.

they appear directly above your toes (you'll need to look down to check). Then straighten up again as if getting up out of that imaginary chair, and return to a standing position.

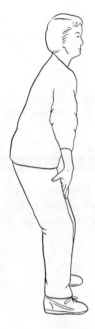

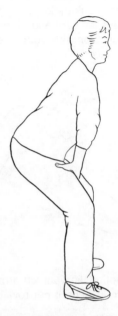

Keeping your back straight, head up, and hands on your thighs, slowly bend your knees as if to sit in a chair. Bend your knees only until

One repetition includes bending down and straightening up. Level 1 calls for only 2 reps; Level 6 has you working up to 12.

When you've completed the fifth exercise, you're done. Take another minute to walk around a bit and shake out your limbs and joints. That's it! You've finished your muscle-conditioning exercises. Now do your walk-jog, end with your stretching exercises, then call it a day.

The Second Variation

Begin by gently shaking yourself loose. As always, perform the exercises slowly and deliberately. Don't try to thrust or force yourself into position: This is usually a sign that you're attempting to do too much.

EXTENDED REACHES

Sit with your right leg extended as far away from center as you can comfortably put it, and draw the sole of your left foot in against the extended leg. Your left hand should hold your left knee. Bend gently toward the floor and place your right arm, palm up, alongside your extended leg. Do not lock your knee.

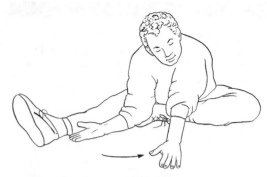

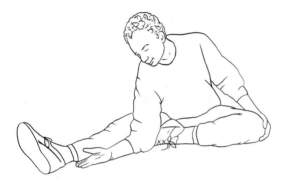

In a slow, fluid motion, lift your left arm up and over your head and extend it out toward the toe of your right foot.

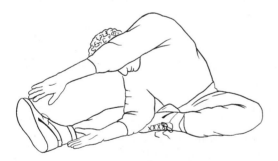

Finally, sweep your left arm along the floor from right to left, leaning and reaching forward slightly as you do so, then sit back upright and return your left hand to your left knee. Switch the positions of your legs, and repeat the exercise on your left side.

One repetition includes both sides. Back at Level 1 again, you'll do 4 reps, while Level 6 calls for 18 reps.

EXTENDED CURL-UPS

The starting position is lying flat on your back with your feet raised up and placed together against the wall so that your legs form a 90° angle at the knees.

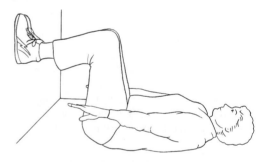

Keep your arms at your sides, raised slightly above the floor. Using the muscles in your abdomen, curl your head and shoulders up from the floor.

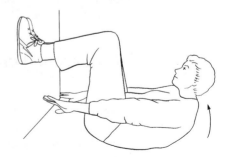

When your shoulders are about 8 to 10 inches (20 to 25 cm) off the floor, slowly roll yourself back down to the starting position.

One repetition includes raising your head and shoulders up and lowering them back down. You'll do 3 reps at Level 1 and 16 reps at Level 6.

PUSH-OFFS/PUSH-UPS

Stand about 2 feet (60 cm) in front of a waist-high table, window ledge, countertop, large chair back, or other solid structure. Bend forward from the waist, and place both your hands on the structure. Your hands should be about shoulder-width apart. Next, set your feet back about 2 more feet (another 60 cm) and lean into the structure so that your full weight is supported by your hands and feet approximately equally. This is the starting position.

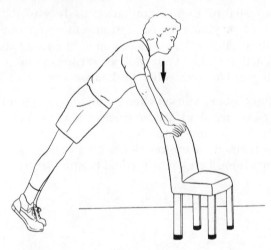

Keeping your back straight and your head up, bend your arms at the elbow and lower your chest until your breastbone touches the support. Then, by straightening your arms, push yourself back up to the starting position.

One repetition is down and back up again. Level 1 calls for 5 push-offs; by Level 6, you'll be doing 15.

(Note: You have to adjust this exercise based on what you did in the first variation of exercises. If you did push-offs against a wall then, for this second variation, try pushing off a waist-high sup-port or doing full push-ups off the floor. And if a push-off is too easy but a traditional push-up too hard, then allow your feet and knees to remain in contact with the floor, and push up just your head, shoulders, and chest.)

TRUNK TWISTERS

Lie on your back with your knees up, your feet to-gether, your heels on the floor, and your toes lifted. Place your fingertips against the back of your head, then curl your head and shoulders up and to the left. (Move your right elbow toward your left knee.) Roll back down, then curl up and to the right, then roll back down again. That whole series is one repetition.

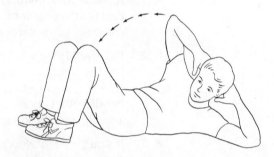

Do 6 reps at Level 1, working up to 14 reps at Level 6.

ARCHES

For the starting position, lie on your back with your arms at your sides. Keeping your knees to-gether, bend them in such a way that your heels remain on the floor, slightly forward of your knees, toes lifted. Then slowly arch your hips up-ward, keeping your waist, shoulders, and feet on the floor.

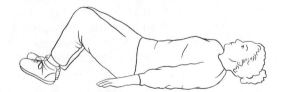

Hold this position for a couple of seconds, then return to the starting position.

One repetition includes arching your hips up and lowering them back down. You'll need to do 2 reps at Level 1, and 12 at Level 6.

After doing these arches, stand up and shake your arms, legs, head, and body loose. That's it! You're done with the second variation of muscle-conditioning exercises.

Maintaining Your Enthusiasm

After several weeks of doing the same routine, you may find your workout getting stale, that it's no longer challenging or enjoyable. Here are three ideas on how to refresh your enthusiasm.

▶ 1. If you want to skip a day now and then, you can do so without significantly affecting your degree of fitness. Use this leeway to vary your exercise schedule somewhat.

▶ 2. Use the MET levels table (Table 16) to find alternatives to the walk-jog for the aerobic component of your exercise session. Once you can walk-jog at your target heart rate for 12 minutes, you're fit enough to handle other sports and activities. Cut your walk-jog sessions to twice a week, and do something else for your other workouts.

▶ 3. If you've been working out alone, join an exercise or aerobics group and interact with other people. Share your experiences with them, and they will most likely do the same with you. Conversely, if you've been working out with others, try a session alone. It's a change, and change creates a different atmosphere—which could be stimulating in and of itself.

Going on from Here

When you reach Level 6 of the second variation of the muscle conditioning exercises, you'll be doing those exercises *plus no more* than 30 minutes of walk-jogging (or some other aerobic activity) plus the flexibility routine in a continuous workout that can range from 23 to 60 minutes.

Try to have a good time with fitness. If it helps you, continue to use your logbook to track your progress, and concentrate on making the workout sessions part of your everyday life.

Now you're ready to move on to the other programs in this part of the book. Good luck!

CHAPTER 16

Controlling Your Weight

The weight-control program presented here has been developed for adult men and women who are in normal health and wish to minimize or eliminate the heart-health risk factor of being overweight. You should consult with your doctor before beginning this or any other weight-control plan if you are:

- Receiving treatment for or recovering from any form of heart ailment.
- Suffering from any disease.
- Pregnant.
- Over 40.
- Inactive.
- A cigarette smoker.
- More than 20 percent above your healthy weight range (see Table 1 in chapter 1).

Why You Gain or Lose Weight

The basics of why you gain or lose weight are well understood. The food you eat supplies the energy your body needs to carry out your daily activities. That energy is measured in calories. If your food intake provides more calories than you use, the excess is stored as fat. For each 3,600 calories you don't burn, you gain 1 pound (0.5 kg).

Yet the converse is also true: Each time you expend 3,600 more calories than you take in, you lose 1 pound (0.5 kg). If you want to lose weight, you must use more calories than you consume.

Age and Weight Gain

The basic caloric-intake/expenditure equation has some interesting implications for older people. As you age, the rate at which your body uses calories slows. And because most people tend to become less active as they grow older, the disparity between calories consumed and calories used is compounded. So if you eat the same way at 55 as you did at 25, you're going to add pounds (kilograms)—which explains, to a great degree, why middle-age spread is common enough to be taken for granted.

Fortunately, this problem has a simple—and surprisingly easy—solution. All you need to do is eat sensibly for your age and maintain a reasonable level of physical activity.

Exercise and Weight Loss

Exercise, while very important, often burns far fewer calories than most people believe. A ditch digger using a shovel would have to dig steadily *for 9 solid hours* in order to burn 3,600 calories or 1 pound (0.5 kg) of fat. A runner would have to run 6-minute miles (3-minute kilometers) *for 4 hours without stopping* to have the same effect. (Both the ditch digger and the runner would also lose several pounds [kilograms] of water weight, which they would quickly regain.)

Exercise, though, can be effective in a weight-loss effort over a period of time. If you add 15 minutes a day of walking at a pace that will cover 3.25 miles (5.2 kilometers) in an hour, and you do that every day for a year, you'll expend 27,000 calories, the equivalent of 7.5 pounds (3.5 kg). Now, if that walking was over and above your normal activity pattern and you did not change your eating habits during the year, those extra 27,000 calories that you burned would result in either a slower weight gain or a weight loss. In addition, exercise can help your weight-reduction program because it tends to suppress appetite. If you exercise regularly, you are likely to consume fewer calories.

So even though it may take time, exercise can play a vital part in controlling your weight.

Why Diets Aren't the Right Answer

It would seem that if you have to use more calories than you consume in order to lose weight, then drastically cutting your intake of calories ought to really drop off those unwanted pounds. That sounds logical, but it doesn't usually work.

With traditional diets, we try to shed pounds by totally altering our eating habits overnight, and we expect immediate results. Do we lose weight? Certainly. Does the weight stay off? In the majority of cases, no. Because the moment most of us reach our desired weight level, we leave the diet behind and revert to our old, familiar, and beloved eating habits—precisely the behaviors that created the overweight condition in the first place.

Another key element in the body's response to dieting also works against it as an effective means of weight loss. Your body reacts to a sudden, abrupt drop in caloric intake by changing the rate at which you burn calories, even at rest, in an effort to preserve your sharply reduced supplies of energy. The body's natural response means you use fewer calories during your daily routine. Then, when you return to more normal eating patterns (or lose control and binge), your body stores every extra calorie it can as body fat to stock up energy for the next "famine" period. As a result, the modern cultural phenomenon of "dieting" (by which we mean suddenly eating much less of what we want and more of what we don't) becomes, for most of us, a self-defeating process of weight fluctuation rather than permanent weight loss.

Your Weight-Control Program

The best method for ending a weight problem is a sustained weight-control program.

Weight control entails changing both your eating habits *and* your activity patterns just enough to help you lose pounds *slowly*. Your weight is reduced gradually because you have lowered (reasonably) your caloric intake and raised (safely) your caloric expenditure. And because you make long-term changes in your habits, the effects are *not* temporary; indeed, the benefits can stay with you for life.

The weight-control program that we present here includes a commitment to physical fitness and the gradual substitution of new eating and exercise habits for your current ones. We have broken the program down into six distinct steps. For detailed descriptions of each, read on.

Step 1: Committing to Physical Fitness

If you have not already done so, begin the physical fitness program described in chapter 15.

Fitness is an important component of weight control for three reasons:

▶ 1. A regular fitness program will help speed your weight loss by burning more calories.

▶ 2. A regular fitness routine will help you to use some of your stored body fat and to build muscle mass.

▶ 3. Regular workouts can allow you to directly offset the number of calories you consume. For example, if you choose a rich dessert such as cheesecake instead of a fruit plate, you can add 15 minutes of walking *each evening for a week* to burn off the additional calories.

Take the first step in controlling your weight: Begin the fitness program and make it a regular part of your life.

Step 2: Motivating Yourself

If you're in a normal state of health and are truly committed to losing weight, you can. If you aren't committed, chances are you won't. Your personal motivation, as with all behavior modification, is critical.

Popular culture sends us many conflicting messages about beauty. Fashion magazines idolize the young, the tall, and the thin, while encouraging their readers to pursue individuality and to appreciate inner beauty. Although most people realize that having a trendy body type (for example, the waif look in female fashion models) isn't necessarily healthy, it's easy to admire such an image of beauty and compare ourselves to it. The key to a healthy body image is to focus not on how you *look*, but on how you *feel*. If those extra pounds keep you from participating in activities you enjoy, then that should be your motivation to lose them. If you lose weight, you'll feel better physically—and you'll probably feel better emotionally as well. Don't try to measure up to an image you can never reach. By focusing on total health instead of appearance, you'll take an important step toward physical and emotional well-being.

Be positive. If you've tried dieting before and failed, forget it. Let your positive feelings grow as you set your goals and discover how easy it is to lose weight *gradually*.

Step 3:
Defining Your
Eating Habits

Most of us would assume, if we ever gave it much thought, that we had a pretty good idea of what, how much, and when we ate. However, most of us would be surprised to find that our knowledge of our own eating habits was far from precise. Nevertheless, knowing your eating habits in detail is critical for success in weight control. It's important to know not only what you eat, but also where you eat, when you eat, how you eat, and in many cases, why you eat, because these factors also affect your daily caloric intake.

Sounds tedious and daunting, yes. But by examining and understanding all these factors, you'll gain the ability to make small modifications in your diet that will substantially alter your caloric intake. And better—you may be able to do so without making major changes in your basic eating habits.

Here's how to define your eating habits. Keep a notebook that lists *every* item of food you eat for at least a week. Add notes indicating what time you ate, how hungry you were, what you were doing, and if you were with anyone. Be sure to note when you eat out of boredom or in response to emotional stress. Take time to write down *everything* you eat. Be thorough, and make your notes as soon after eating as possible. Also, don't forget snacks. If you eat it or drink it, list it, and list all of it. A notation of "1 cup of coffee," for example, may not be the whole story if that cup of coffee contained 2 spoonfuls of sugar and a packet of nondairy creamer.

Remember, your goal is to examine your eating habits to identify small changes that can make big differences in the number of calories you consume. You'll have to take detailed notes on what you eat for at least a week, or until you feel you have chronicled your typical eating habits. This information is vital to the final steps in the program.

Step 4:
Establishing
Your Weight-
Loss Goal

While tracking your eating habits, determine what your healthy weight should be. The weight tables in chapter 1 and pinch-an-inch tests in chapter 4 can help. By subtracting the midpoint of your healthy weight range from your present weight, you find the number of pounds (kilograms) you need to lose. This is your goal.

In the notebook where you've detailed your eating habits, or in your exercise logbook, write your present weight, your ideal weight, and the difference, which is your weight-loss goal (the number of pounds [kilograms] you need to lose). Leave space to write in a deadline for reaching your goal.

Step 5:
Determining the
Degree of
Change You
Need to Make

Now you need to decide how long it will take to reach your weight-loss goal, and what changes will get you there.

First, figure out how many pounds you want to lose per month (see guidelines below). Next, convert that number of pounds (kilograms) to calories by multiplying by 3,600 (8,000 for kilograms). Now decide what dietary and exercise changes are necessary so that you burn off that many calories more than you consume each month.

If you are already losing weight, just continue your current eating habits and activity levels. You are already accomplishing your goal. If you are gaining weight, multiply your monthly weight gain in pounds by 3,600 (or in kilograms by 8,000) to determine the number of calories you must eliminate or burn off each month just to stabilize your weight at your present level. Enter your monthly weight gain and the corresponding number of calories in your log. You'll need that information shortly.

If you haven't been monitoring your weight recently, you'll have to start. Record your weight in your exercise logbook each week. This information will help you adjust your weight-control program as you go.

Now consider this: The more time you're willing to take to lose your excess weight, the less you'll have to modify your present diet and activity levels. It's up to you to decide how quickly you want to attain your goal.

Understand, though, that in most cases it's more effective to lose weight gradually, so that once you attain your ideal weight, only a few dietary and exercise adjustments will be necessary to keep you there.

Here are some suggested minimum time frames:

▶ 1. For losing 10 pounds (4.5 kg) or less, allow 5 months. That's at most 2 pounds (1 kg) per month, or 7,200 calories.

▶ 2. For losing 10 to 20 pounds (4.5 to 9 kg), allow 10 months. That's between 1 and 2 pounds (0.45 and 1 kg) per month, or 3,600 to 7,200 calories.

▶ 3. For losing over 20 pounds (9 kg), allow 12 months minimum, and keep the needed calorie deduction between 7,200 and 10,800 per month.

In any case, do not attempt to lose weight faster than 1 percent of your body weight each week. For those with average activity levels, that rate would require a daily intake of only about 1,200 calories, which for most people would amount to a drastic change along the lines of traditional dieting. It would be very difficult to make the changes needed to reduce your caloric intake by this much, and harder still to incorporate those changes into your daily life.

Once you've decided on the length of time you require to reach your ideal weight, perform the following calculations:

▶ 1. Multiply your weight-loss goal in pounds by 3,600 (in kilograms by 8,000) to find the number of calories you need to eliminate in order to reach your healthy weight. Divide that number of calories by the number of months you have selected as your weight adjustment period.

Example: Your weight-loss goal is 12 pounds (5.4 kilograms). 12 × 3,600 calories/pound (or 5.4 × 8,000 calories/kilogram) = 43,200 calories total. 43,200 calories ÷ 8 months = 5,400 calories/month, which is how much you'll have to expend *in excess* of what you consume during the 8-month period.

Note: These calculations are sufficient only if your weight has been stable recently. If after monitoring your weight for a few weeks, you're still gaining, add the results of the next two calculations.

▶ 2. Multiply your monthly weight *gain* in pounds by 3,600 (or kilograms by 8,000) to define the number of calories you must eliminate in order to stabilize your weight at your present level.

Example: You gain weight at the rate of 1 pound (0.45 kilograms) per month. 1 × 3,600 (or 0.45 × 8,000) = 3,600 calories/month, which is how much less you'll have to consume and/or more you'll have to expend just to hold your weight where it is today.

▶ 3. Add the number of calories you have to eliminate each month just to stabilize your weight and the number of calories you have to eliminate each month in order to reduce your weight to your healthy weight, and the sum is the number of calories you must eliminate each month in order to attain your healthy weight in the time frame you've selected.

Example: 5,400 calories/month from calculation (1) + 3,600 calories/month from calculation (2) = 9,000 calories/month, which is how much less you'll have to consume and/or more you'll have to expend for 8 months to attain your ideal weight.

Don't let the total number of calories per month deter you. Your weight didn't get where it is overnight, and you won't correct it in a week. Remember, weight control isn't dieting: It's a long-term effort to reach your healthy weight.

If the total number of calories you must eliminate each month seems daunting, lengthen your time frame. In the example provided above, increasing the length of time to 10 months (instead of 8) would lower the total number of calories you must eliminate each month to 7,920.

Enter the number of calories you're going to eliminate each month and the number of months you've established as your weight-loss time frame into your logbook, on your calendar, or wherever you're keeping records.

Step 6:
Substituting
New Habits for
the Old Ones

To begin eliminating those calories, you must first focus on what, how much, when, and how you eat.

Use the information you gathered in Step 3 to answer these six questions:

▶ 1. Did you eat when you weren't really hungry? If you did, maybe to be polite or out of boredom, you've located a problem habit. Confront and overcome it, and you'll lower your caloric intake.

▶ 2. Do you frequently eat high-calorie foods? These include rich desserts and snacks, rich dishes, potatoes smothered in butter and sour cream, and so on. A slight change in this habit can make a big difference over time.

▶ 3. Is a lot of your eating done away from the table? Maybe you consistently eat in your car or at your desk, or you grab a bite as you pass through the kitchen. It takes well over 15 minutes for your stomach to tell you that you're full. Eating slowly while seated at a table may be a way for you to reduce your caloric intake.

▶ 4. Do you skip meals, then try to make up for the missed meal later, or eat at irregular hours? If you do, chances are you're taking in excess calories. Try to eat at regular times.

▶ 5. Are you always through eating before anyone else at the table? Do you gobble your food so as to make time for something else? If you slow down, you'll most likely feel full sooner and eat less.

▶ 6. When do you eat the greatest amount? You should eat the most when you're most active, and the least when you're relaxed and sedentary. For most people, this means having 75 percent of your food intake during the day, before your evening meal. Moreover, eating a large meal late in the day and going to bed on a full stomach can make you gain weight.

Search for habits such as these, and change what you can. Use the detailed notes on your eating habits to find slight changes in what you eat that you can make without much difficulty. For example, switching from eating a 400-calorie piece of cake after dinner to some apple slices and celery sticks saves you 350 calories and lowers your fat consumption at the same time. That's a healthy exchange.

Remember that small changes add up. Cutting out one pat of butter a day will cover a third of the needed 9,000-calorie reduction in the example presented earlier. Little things truly mean a lot over time.

Copy a list of caloric values for a variety of foods from a diet book at the library, or make a small investment and buy a pocketbook that lists the caloric values for a large number of foods. As an alternative, you can use the "nutrition facts" label on most foods you purchase at the grocery store to determine their caloric content. Then check your eating habits and see how many small, 100-calorie changes you can make without drastically affecting your current habits.

Some sample changes might include replacing one soft drink a day with an artificially sweetened drink (about 100 fewer calories), substituting 2 tablespoons (30 ml) of an oil-and-vinegar dressing for 2 tablespoons (30 ml) of a Russian or Roquefort dressing once a day (about 80 fewer calories), or having a sliced turkey sandwich for lunch in place of a club sandwich (about 300 fewer calories). Those three alterations alone, done over a month, would eliminate more than 14,000 calories! (And you'd lose about 4 pounds [2 kg].)

Your object is to find substitutions you can make that appeal to you, that reduce your caloric intake, and that lower your consumption of fats. It's small things, like eating a handful of pretzels as opposed to a handful of peanuts (about 200 fewer calories), that will reduce your calorie and fat consumption.

Be imaginative. And remember, it's not only what you eat and how much you eat that's important: Where and when you eat make a difference, too. So avoid the mall, with its tempting "food court," when you have an empty stomach, and try to skip that fattening late-night snack. On the other hand, the list of what you *can* do is almost endless. Try the recipes provided in Part Six of this handbook. These aren't starvation rations: They're low-fat, low-calorie dishes and meals that are nutritious, can make you feel full, and can help you control your weight.

Remember, too, that reducing the calories you consume is only one part of the weight-control program; increasing the calories you expend is the other part.

Bicycling at 6 miles per hour (10 kilometers per hour), walking at 2 miles per hour (3 kilometers per hour), gardening, and mowing the lawn with a push mower are all activities that burn about 120 calories every half hour. Playing tennis, bicycling at 12 miles per hour (19 kilometers per hour), and walking at 3 miles per hour (5 kilometers per hour) all burn more than 150 calories every half hour.

If you had not been exercising regularly, you'll burn over 35,000 additional calories per year by following the fitness program described in the previous chapter. That's the equivalent of almost 10 pounds (4.5 kg) of body weight. Combine that with reducing your daily caloric intake by 100 calories per day, and you'll lose 20 pounds (9 kg) in a year.

Six Rules for Effective, Long-Term Weight Control

▶ 1. *Start and Stick with Your Fitness Program.* During your weight-loss period, build yourself up to a half hour of any aerobic activity you select, and enjoy that activity at least five times a week.

▶ 2. *Don't Make Too Many Changes at Once.* And the bigger the change, the longer you should wait before changing something else. Be deliberate, but don't be hasty.

▶ 3. *Follow the Recipes in This Book.* Set aside two or three meals each week to try one of them. Find three or four you especially like, and serve them often. You'll cut both calories and your fat consumption.

▶ 4. *Drink Six to Eight Glasses of Water Each Day.* This is especially important during your weight-loss period.

▶ 5. *Consider a Two-Stage Program.* If you need to lose a large number of pounds (kilograms), but still less than 20 percent of your body weight, consider doing it in two stages. First, shed half the needed pounds (kilograms) and stabilize yourself at that point for several weeks until your new eating and activity patterns become fixed. Second, begin to lose weight again until you reach your healthy weight. This two-stage approach will allow for a more gradual adjustment in your eating and exercise behaviors.

▶ 6. *Keep the Faith.* Just because this program is simple and gives you maximum choice, don't think it's not effective. It is, and if you follow it, you can minimize or eliminate the heart-health risk of being overweight for years to come. We're asking you to believe not only in the program, but also in yourself.

When You Reach Your Healthy Weight

First of all, congratulate yourself. You did it! And you should be proud.

Maintaining your healthy weight is a matter of trial and error. The new eating habits you've adopted will help. Continue with your fitness program, along with the adjustments you've made to your diet, and keep track of your weight. If you keep losing pounds (kilograms) beyond your target, add a few calories to find the proper balance of calorie intake and expenditure. But when you add those calories, pay special attention to your total-body exercise routine, because you'd rather put on weight as muscle than flab.

Check your weight every couple of weeks at least, so that you can spot gains (or losses) and correct them before they become bigger fluctuations. And each time you step on the scale, remind yourself that you were successful.

CHAPTER 17

Quitting Smoking

How do you make the next cigarette you light the last one you'll ever smoke? For some people, it's relatively easy. For others, it's more difficult. But anyone can do it. All it takes is some understanding, a bit of self-motivation, and a program. The following program can help you quit, but if it doesn't, or if it doesn't seem quite right for you, please don't give up! Try a different program. For example, your doctor may want to prescribe nicotine chewing gum or patches to help you get through the difficulties of withdrawing from nicotine. See the "Smoking" section in the "Resources" appendix for the names, addresses, and phone numbers of sources for other programs to help you quit.

What You Need to Do to Stop Smoking

To stop smoking, you need to:

- Decide for yourself that you really want to quit. The right attitude is critical; you must think of stopping as a positive choice.
- Use that decision to help you follow a simple program. You need more than an act of will: You must systematically change ingrained behaviors.

■ Understand that the act of stopping is not the final goal. Anyone can quit; nearly all smokers do at some point. The real goal is not beginning again.

Your First Steps   Think about why you started smoking and why you have continued to smoke. Write these things down if doing so helps you to focus. Next, write down your commitment to stop smoking, in the form of a promise, and sign it. Leave space underneath your promise so you can list at least ten benefits you'll gain from quitting. Finally, post this declaration where you'll see it often.

Here's a sample promise to give you an idea of the form it might take.

I, _____ , promise myself that I am going to stop smoking cigarettes. And after I stop, I'm not going to start again. Signed: _____ Here are the benefits I'll gain from quitting:

Don't try to set a quitting date or any other deadline. Also, don't list any of the benefits yet. Just write the promise and post it. Then reread it the next day. And the day after that. If, on the third day, you still agree that you want to quit, you've already started to do so.

In conjunction with quitting smoking, you should begin a physical fitness program like the one described in chapter 15. By starting an exercise routine, you'll be adding a new activity to your life that is *not* compatible with smoking.

In fact, if you're out of shape and believe that you can handle only one major habit change in your life, you should begin by starting a fitness program. When that is well established, *then* try to quit smoking.

If you already exercise regularly, proceed to the 10-day countdown below, and discover how much quitting smoking will do for your exercise stamina.

The 10-Day Countdown to Q-Day

The basic program to help you quit smoking takes 10 days. If you want to do it faster, that's fine. It's your plan. The 10 days, however, give you enough time to bring about a gradual change of habit.

For some, the timing of *Q-Day,* the day you'll actually quit smoking, can be critical. If you smoke at work, set Q-Day during your vacation or on a weekend, when your routine is changed anyway. Or make Q-Day fall on your birthday, anniversary, or even a holiday. You don't have to set Q-Day on a special occasion or other day when your routine changes, but doing so might give you added incentive.

Day 1
Reread your promise to quit smoking and ask yourself if you really want to stop. Then ask yourself if now is the right time. Be positive. Don't remind yourself of the difficulties. You'll be able to take those in stride if you really want to quit.

If you still have some mental hesitation about stopping, try to figure out why and think of reasons to quit (phrased in the form of benefits you'll gain) that will help you get motivated. Don't let fear of failure hold you back. You can succeed with this program. Also, avoid falling into the thought process that you'll live to be 70 if you smoke or 73 if you don't, and you'd rather smoke now and forget those extra years later. It's a trap, because there's more at stake than 36 months: Quitting now will improve the *quality* of your later life as well as the duration.

When you can honestly tell yourself you want to quit, then you're ready for Day 1. During this first day in the countdown to quitting, do the following things (if it helps you to remember them, write each one in a logbook or on a card you can carry with you).

- Talk to at least one other person about smoking and quitting smoking cigarettes.
- Notice how nonsmokers react to smokers, and remind yourself that nonsmokers are the majority.
- If you can find an ex-smoker, ask that person how he or she quit.
- Write your target date for stopping next to your promise. Your target date is 10 days from today.
- Below your promise, write two benefits you'll gain from quitting. Make them as personal as possible and honestly important to you. Such benefits might include proving to yourself that you can, smelling better to your spouse, and so on. The two benefits you list in writing don't necessarily have to be the most important you can come up with, but they must mean something to you personally.

■ Continue to smoke as you usually do, unless you feel like smoking less. Do what feels natural. Don't attempt to force yourself into any action.

■ Continue your fitness program. In fact, if it's not a strain, exercise for a minute or so longer than usual.

■ Just before you go to bed, tell yourself you're going to quit smoking in 9 more days.

Day 2

■ Continue your fitness routine. Add another minute to your workout if doing so is comfortable.

■ Add one more benefit to the list below your promise.

■ Start your smoking record, which is a sheet of ruled paper that you'll wrap around your open pack of cigarettes so that you can't take one out without removing the paper. Hold the smoking record in place with rubber bands, and each time you feel the urge to smoke, unwrap the smoking record to take out a cigarette. Before lighting that cigarette, though, jot down the time of day on the record and *replace it around the pack*. The smoking record will be important later, because it will reveal your smoking patterns. Keeping the record around the pack of cigarettes helps ensure that you write down the time of each smoke. Adding a brief note on what you were doing when you wanted to smoke is also helpful. Wrapping the smoking record around the pack in such a way that it must be removed everytime you want a cigarette also makes you think about your smoking each time.

■ Smoke one less cigarette today. Once during the day, at a time when you wanted to and otherwise would have lit up, don't. Skip it.

■ Just before you go to bed, congratulate yourself. You're making progress.

Days 3, 4, and 5

■ Continue your fitness routine. Add another minute to your workout if doing so is comfortable.

■ Each day, add one more benefit to be gained from quitting to your list.

■ Change the brand of cigarette you smoke. Switch to a low-tar, low-nicotine cigarette, but make sure you do *not* inhale any deeper.

■ Continue to wrap the package with your smoking record.

■ Smoke at least one less cigarette each day—more if you can.

■ Study your smoking record, and identify any patterns you find. Write those patterns in your log.

Days 6, 7, and 8

■ Continue your fitness routine. Add another minute to your workout if doing so is comfortable.

■ As soon as you finish one pack of one brand of cigarettes, change brands. Don't go back to your favorite brand. Stay with the low-tar, low-nicotine varieties, but smoke them the same way you smoked your original brand. This will help reduce your physical dependence on nicotine.

■ Continue to smoke at least one less cigarette each day.

■ Continue to use your smoking record.

■ Postpone each cigarette for a while. When you feel the urge to smoke, put it off for a few minutes.

■ If possible, brush your teeth five times a day to keep your mouth fresh.

Day 9

■ Continue your fitness routine. Add another minute to your workout.

■ Continue postponing each cigarette for a few minutes.

■ Continue brushing your teeth about five times a day.

■ Review your smoking record, and enter into your log the times you tend to smoke.

■ Try to identify which cigarettes you're going to miss most—in other words, which activities or times of day most strongly trigger your desire to smoke. These might be during your mid-morning coffee break, right after lunch, at the end of a tense meeting, or on the drive home from work. Whatever they are for you, write them down.

Day 10

■ Tell yourself that tomorrow, for one day only, you're not going to smoke.

■ Continue your fitness routine. Add another minute to your workout.

■ Review your smoking record and list of triggers.

■ Continue postponing each cigarette by a few minutes.

■ Continue brushing your teeth about five times a day.

■ After your final cigarette of the day at your office or workplace, discard all remaining cigarettes and matches that you have there. Also, remove or hide all lighters and ashtrays. Don't give the cigarettes to someone; throw them away. If you normally carry cigarettes on your person, you may continue to do so. But have none in your workplace that belong to you.

- After your last smoke of the day at home, do the same thing you did in your workplace: Get rid of all cigarettes and matches. Remove or hide all lighters and ashtrays. And don't forget your car. Empty and clean the ashtrays there, and make sure there are no cigarettes left in the vehicle.
- Before going to bed, renew your promise not to smoke the next day.

Q-Day

- When you awaken, remind yourself that for this day only, you're not going to smoke.
- Plan to stay busy. Go to a movie. Keep occupied. This is a good time to send all your clothes to the cleaners or laundry to remove the odor of cigarette smoke. It's also an ideal day to have your teeth cleaned. In any case, brush them frequently.
- Drink large amounts of juice or water.
- If one of the activities that triggered your desire to smoke was drinking coffee or an alcoholic beverage, be especially careful if you do either of these things.
- Use your insight into your smoking patterns to be watchful during times when you tended to smoke. If you can, change your routine for a couple of days to avoid doing the same things at the same times you're accustomed to doing them.
- If one of the benefits you'll gain from quitting is the money you'll save, make a list of gifts you'd like to give yourself or a family member or friend. Then estimate how many packs of cigarettes you'd have to not buy in order to afford those things. You can take this incentive another step by opening a special bank account and depositing the money you've saved by not buying cigarettes. When you've saved enough, go out and treat yourself (and/or your family member or friend) to those gifts.

After you've managed to avoid cigarettes for the first day, take each of the next days one at a time. Avoid "forever" thinking. Just focus on not smoking for one day. Then do it again and again.

Your Critical Period: The First Week

The first few smokeless days are important because your body is adjusting to new conditions. Some people who have stopped smoking report a sense of edginess and short temper. Recognize that it's possible to have physical withdrawal symptoms—after all, nicotine is an addictive drug. You might, for instance, experience irregular bowel movements, temporary weight gain due to retained fluids, and sore gums or tongue. These conditions are not abnormal. View them as side effects of the treatment and thus as signs that you're recovering.

Each day you refrain from smoking you weaken the habit. Get through a smoke-free week, and you'll have crossed a major threshold. You can do it, one day at a time. Here are a dozen proven ideas to help you:

► 1. If you feel the urge to smoke, talk to someone—not necessarily about smoking. Any subject will help take your mind off cigarettes.

► 2. If you miss the sensation of having a cigarette in your mouth, use a pencil or fake cigarette. The same holds true if you're bothered by not having a cigarette in your hand.

► 3. This is a good time to change your pace for the weekend. Go on a short getaway, increase your exercising, clean house, garden, or do something active.

► 4. If finishing a meal was one of the activities that triggered your desire to smoke, temporarily change your pattern. Leave the table when you're through eating and go brush your teeth.

► 5. Places where smoking is not permitted can be havens. Libraries, theaters, stores, churches, and museums all fall into this category. Use and enjoy them.

► 6. Maintain a clean taste in your mouth by brushing your teeth or using mouthwash frequently.

► 7. Since it's difficult to smoke and wash dishes, dish washing is a good antidote to a craving for cigarettes.

► 8. Combat the urge to light up by using one of the relaxation techniques discussed in chapter 18 on managing stress.

► 9. If you have to go to a cocktail party, dinner party, or other social event where it will be more difficult to keep from smoking, try to stay with a nonsmoking group.

► 10. Tell your friends you're quitting and need all the assistance they can give you. Friends will help.

► 11. Smoking and water don't mix well. So take a shower or bath to combat the need for a cigarette. Swimming is a good idea, too, because you can make it part of your fitness routine.

► 12. It helps many people to use their hands. So knitting, typing, cooking, or any activity that is hand-intensive can be a great help.

The Second Week

Continue using your notes to remind yourself of the benefits you'll gain from quitting. Notice how good food tastes when your taste buds aren't dulled by the taste of smoke. Treat yourself to some special pleasure (such as a new hairdo, a manicure, or a massage) as a reward for remaining off cigarettes for a week.

During the second week, especially if you've been relying on snacks or candy to help satisfy your cravings for cigarettes, you may begin to add a little weight. Don't concern yourself about this now. Keep your attention on not smoking. Concentrate on the one-day-at-a-time thought process. Also, your fitness program is very important at this juncture: Stick with it.

After the Second Week

After 2 cigarette-free weeks, you have your new habit well in hand.

This is a good time to begin weighing yourself every day and noting your weight in a logbook or calendar, if you haven't already been doing so as part of your fitness program. Don't worry if you're adding a few pounds, because many people do. Check yourself, though, to determine whether or not you're eating more at meals. If that's the reason for your weight gain, level out your food intake a little. Your exercise routine will also help you hold your weight in check.

If you've turned to small snacks or sweets to satisfy your cravings for cigarettes *and you're now gaining weight,* start substituting carrot sticks, celery slices, or other low-fat, low-calorie items. Also, Part Six of this handbook offers a number of heart-healthy and interesting recipes that should help you lose weight: Try a few of them.

Continue to find motivation for not smoking where you can. Also, be aware that stress, anger, frustration, anxiety, depression, and even relaxation can all place you at high risk of breaking your promise to not smoke. Deal with these emotions and states as they come, one at a time. And just for today, avoid cigarettes.

After the First Month

Congratulate yourself. A cigarette-free month is a notable achievement. You will have unwound much of your tobacco habit and are well on the road to kicking the habit for good.

However, don't panic if you've broken down and smoked a cigarette. This doesn't mean you've failed. Feeling guilty will only make things worse. Instead, try to understand why you smoked, so you can possibly avoid a similar temptation later. And understand that occasional relapses are part of the recovery process. More than anything else, though, realize that you are no longer a smoker. You quit the habit.

Use your understanding of your personal triggers to develop ways to avoid or deal with each one. People who use effective coping skills are more likely to remain nonsmokers.

You *can* remove the cigarette habit from your life. And the sooner you do so, the better off you'll be. Perhaps that advice is something like the Surgeon General's warning on cigarette advertising and packaging—something you've been told so often it no longer registers. Well, it's the truth, and you can believe it with all your heart.

CHAPTER 18

Managing Stress

Since stress is an unavoidable part of your life, you must learn not only how to live with it but how to manage it as best you can. In fact, you probably have devised several techniques for dealing with stress already—some more effective and some healthier than others. But chances are, you feel you could do better. What you need is a stress-management program.

Managing Your Stress

Since reaction to stress is highly personal, no single stress-management strategy works equally well for everyone. We have, therefore, provided a number of relaxation techniques that have proven successful for a variety of people. By trying several and selecting the ones that work best for you, you'll be designing your own personal stress-management program.

Because this program involves exercise, you may need to check with your physician before following the suggestions offered here. See the opening section of chapter 16 for a list of characteristics that would require you to visit your doctor before beginning any exercise program.

Principles of Stress Management

To manage stress effectively, you must be able to:

▶ 1. Recognize when you're feeling overstressed.

▶ 2. Identify the causes of stress in your life, change those you can, and learn to live with those you can't.

▶ 3. Minimize the effects of stress on your body and mind.

Those three tasks are also the three steps in our basic stress-management program.

Step 1: Recognizing When You're Feeling Overstressed

The key to interrupting the negative cycle of stress is simply recognizing that it's occurring. However, this may not be as easy as it sounds. When you're confronted with one crisis or conflict after another, you may not notice the strain until you feel physical symptoms.

The first step is to learn the mental and physical signs of being stressed, which are listed in Table 18. You can then check yourself for those signs from time to time during the day, and if you find you frequently have several of them, you can either try to avoid the causes or use relaxation techniques. However, try not to become so preoccupied with monitoring yourself that the very process becomes stressful. Also, please recognize that any of these signs may be the result of conditions other than stress. When in doubt, consult your doctor.

Step 2: Identifying the Causes of Stress in Your Life

Once you can recognize that you're under stress, you can begin to keep a record of when and why you feel stressed, to see if there are any patterns. By analyzing your records, you will then be able to identify the causes of stress in your life.

Your Stress Diary

In a special notebook (or using about 10 or 12 pages of your exercise logbook), write your stress-management pledge. Make this a simple statement of your commitment to control the stress in your life, and be sure to in-

TABLE 18   *Symptoms of Stress*

Sudden heart pounding	Headaches	Overreaction to what happens around you
Cold, clammy hands	Upset stomach or heartburn	Irritability
Drumming fingers or tapping foot	Sudden anger	Impatience
Nervous coughing	A constant feeling that there isn't enough time	Grinding teeth
A general feeling of fatigue	Sudden tears for no apparent reason	Binge drinking
Dry mouth		Binge eating
Difficulty breathing	Sudden sense of impending bad news or doom	Chain-smoking
Muscle aches		Nail biting
Clenched jaws or other tight facial muscles	Frustration	Constant picking at fingernails or face
Stiff neck	Depression	Trying to do two or three things at once
Tics at the mouth or eyebrows	Anxiety or anxiousness	
Sudden sweating	Talking too much	Fiddling with, twisting, or pulling out hair
Turning red-faced	A sudden inability to express yourself	

clude the benefits you'll gain by doing so. This is the most important part of your stress diary.

Several times each day for a week, check yourself for signs of stress and note the time and cause of each episode in your stress diary. Add any comments that might be helpful later in identifying stress patterns.

Stressful happenings might include annoyance over being kept waiting an appointment, sudden anger over a trivial matter such as the car ahead of you waiting too long to move after the light has turned green, or a tense exchange with a family member.

Each time you find yourself tense, try to understand why. If it's just the general pressure of the day rather than a specific event, note that. It's not uncommon for people who work under constant pressure to feel their stress level rise as they approach their workplace. If you feel this way, record that, too.

As the week progresses, you'll become more adept at recognizing the triggers of stress in your life. Try to analyze those triggers to see if there's a common core reason. Maybe you hate meeting with a particular person at work, and every time you do, you grow tense. Ask yourself why you dislike meetings with this person: Is he or she overbearing? Intimidating? Are the meetings personally frustrating or threatening? If so, why?

You need not record names in your stress diary (code names or a simple X will do). Your purpose is to note the presence of stress, the time you experience it, and its source.

Use your stress diary in this manner for a week. Each evening, sit quietly for a short while and review the day's stress points. Try to discover any relationships or patterns that might exist between and among the different incidents. There may be none. Then again, there may be a clear link.

Also check the flow of your stress. Your stress during the day may recede and return—that is, build from a low point to a high point, then fall back to a low level before rising again. If so, you probably have good control over the stress you're experiencing. On the other hand, your stress may build and build: rising, then falling only a little, rising even higher, then dropping back only a bit before climbing higher still. In that case, you're most likely operating in a condition of potentially harmful stress.

After a few days, you'll have formed a good idea about what stresses you and what your daily stress patterns are. And don't be discouraged if some of the causes of your stress remain unspecified. A daylong accumulation of minor irritations and frustrations, each relatively unimportant in itself, can combine to cause stress that seems to have no detectable basis.

Also, consider that a major stressor, such as being laid off or ending a significant relationship, can produce depression, which changes the character of normally nonstressful, routine events. Recognize, too, that even positive changes in our lives, such as an impending marriage, a new car, the birth of a baby, or a job promotion, can make for more stress during a period of adjustment.

The stress diary can also be revealing in another way. Many people find themselves so overwhelmed by their stress that a sense of hopelessness and an inability to cope almost immobilizes them. For someone in this condition, keeping a stress diary could be a difficult if not taxing chore. If you rule out keeping a stress diary because you think that nothing will help your situation or that things are just too much out of control, then you should consider consulting a health professional. Your physician can determine if there are any physical reasons for your condition and, if so, care for them. If there are no physical reasons, some form of counseling might help you. Be assured that, no matter how powerless you might feel, help *is* available.

Even if patterns emerge in the causes of your stress after your first week of keeping the stress diary, continue for another 7 days. After 2 weeks, you should have some clear insights into the nature and strength of your stress triggers. And once you've defined the causes of stress in your life, you're in a position to deal with them.

Changing What You Can and Learning to Live with What You Can't

To deal with stress, first modify as many of the situations that create the stress in your daily life as possible. Then start to rethink your mental attitude toward those conditions you can't alter.

As an example, if you're late for an appointment because you're stuck in traffic, you may feel your stress building even though there's nothing you can do to change the situation. What you *can* change is how that traffic jam affects you, how you *choose* to respond to it. Follow the four steps described below.

▶ **1.** *Recognize your Limitations.* Tell yourself that you won't reach your destination any sooner by agonizing over the situation or becoming angry.

▶ **2.** *Relax.* Use one of the relaxation techniques offered later in this chapter to unwind for a moment. If you're alone in the car, scream or yell, if that makes you feel better. But you have to scream or yell forcefully, so that it takes physical effort. That way, when you're through, there's some physical relaxation.

▶ **3.** *Try to Understand Why the Situation Is so Distressing.* Is it just being late for your appointment? Or is it also that you hate having your path blocked by others? Or are you perhaps mad at yourself for not having allowed more time? Understanding the underlying reason(s) for our response often makes us less emotional about the specific situation at hand.

▶ **4.** *Think about Ways You Can Keep Yourself from Having This Experience Again.* The act of deliberating solutions tilts your focus away from the problem and can thus help you relax. You can't solve a chronic traffic problem, but you might not have to drive in it. Maybe you can join a car pool or change your schedule so you're not on the roads during rush hour. If you can't avoid the traffic, then either allow yourself more time to keep from being late or buy a car phone so you can call ahead and inform those involved that you're stuck in traffic but doing your best to get there. Be inventive. Find interesting solutions.

Step 3: Minimizing the Effects of Stress on Your Body and Mind

Exercise has proven to be one of the most effective means of moderating stress and thus lessening the impact of stress on your body. So a regular exercise program will help your stress-management efforts.

The fitness program described in chapter 15 is an organized, effective, well-rounded approach to exercise. If you're not currently following a fitness regimen, start today. If you do have a plan, be sure you're getting enough aerobic exercise to benefit your heart, and also be sure to include stretching, because most people who are experiencing stress notice that their muscles tend to tense and stiffen: Slow stretching combats muscle tightness and promotes relaxation.

In addition to exercise, the critical factor in minimizing the effects of stress on your mind and body is the ability to relax.

As odd as it may seem to someone who has a problem relaxing under the best of conditions, it is possible to relax in the most stressful and distracting situations. One easy relaxation technique uses controlled breathing.

Breath-Control Stress-Buster

Sitting with your back straight, inhale slowly through your nose. Check to be sure your stomach is doing some of the expanding as your lungs fill. (Some people tense their stomach muscles while taking a breath; keep your abdomen relaxed.)

When you think you have a full breath, try to take in a little bit more air.

Hold your breath.

After 3 or 4 seconds, expel the air slowly through your mouth. Your lips should be pursed as if to whistle. Use your stomach muscles and diaphragm to squeeze out all the air you can. Then try to squeeze out just a little bit more.

Pause for a second with your lungs as empty as you can get them, then begin inhaling once more. Repeat the cycle of inhalation and exhalation three times.

Do this deep-breathing exercise four or five times a day, when you're feeling stressed.

Another relaxation technique depends on mental focus. The process takes a bit longer, but you may find it very effective.

Mind and Body Stress-Buster

Pick a number, a name you like, or a simple word. Lean back in a chair, stretch out on a bed, or lie on the floor. Make yourself comfortable, and close your eyes.

Relax your muscles. Start with your toes: Ask yourself if all ten are relaxed. Then proceed upward, checking the muscles of your feet, ankles, shins, knees, thighs, hips, stomach, back, chest, shoulders, neck, and face. When you reach your scalp, begin silently repeating to yourself the word you selected. Do not speak out loud; just say it over and over in your mind.

If another thought breaks into your repetition of the word, stop, check your relaxation from toe to head again, and go back to repeating your word. If you focus on the word, you will relax.

This technique is easier to master than it seems. By practicing it a couple of times a day, you can easily master it in a week. And the benefits are worth the time and effort you'll invest.

A Smorgasbord of Relaxation Techniques

Here are ten other things you can do to reduce the level of stress in your life:

▶ 1. Reduce your intake of caffeine. Research shows that people who drink coffee or other beverages containing caffeine while they're working experience intensified stress.

▶ 2. Avoid alcohol and drugs. They're not stress relievers; they're actually stress *intensifiers*.

▶ 3. Take a warm bath.

▶ 4. Reduce your intake of sugar, too much of which can increase your stress.

▶ 5. If you're angry with someone, write them a letter. Make it as nasty and mean as you like. Read it, then tear it up. Write *but don't send* it.

▶ 6. Smile. If that sounds too elementary, try it. Not a grimace—a smile.

▶ 7. When you work on a task, try to concentrate completely on only what you are doing. (Forget the boss or why you got the assignment.) Your work and your stress level will improve.

▶ 8. Cry. Crying can release anxiety, so don't be afraid to just let yourself go now and then.

▶ 9. Take time out every day to have at least a few minutes of fun. If you can't bring yourself to "play," at least try to find pleasure in something between the time you wake up in the morning and the time you go to sleep at night.

▶ 10. Understand that not every task can or needs to be done perfectly. Striving for unattainable perfection is a common stress producer.

Stress under Control

The rewards of bringing your stress under control are many, varied, and go far beyond the important benefit of removing a risk factor for heart disease from your life. Stress management is the key to improving your outlook on life and to forging closer relations with associates, friends, and loved ones. Do your heart and yourself a favor by learning to manage your stress.

PART SIX

Heart-Smart Cooking

Basic Tips

Heart-Healthy Recipes

CHAPTER 19

Basic Tips

Good nutrition and a balanced diet are simple and very effective means of reducing your risks of heart disease, many types of cancer, and other health problems.

You achieve good nutrition by eating a variety of foods (see the Food Guide Pyramid in chapter 3), moderating your intake of certain kinds of foods, and controlling the amount of food and calories you consume. For some people, that means an extensive dietary overhaul. You may, however, be pleasantly surprised to find that sensible eating habits require only small changes—and that good nutrition includes some very tasty dishes.

Three Fundamental Rules

Your key to heart-smart cooking entails following three simple rules:

▶ 1. Shake less salt.

▶ 2. Carve away fats.

▶ 3. Cook with the right oils.

By sticking to these, you can continue to enjoy many of your favorite meals without putting a strain on your cardiovascular health. (You'll also want to consult chapter 3 of this handbook for more detailed information on diet and nutrition.)

Shaking Less Salt   As noted in chapter 3, you should limit your daily intake of salt to no more than 6 grams (g), roughly a teaspoon, which contains 2,400 milligrams (mg) of sodium, an element that is a major regulator of fluid volume in your body. And if you have high blood pressure or another cardiovascular disease, your doctor may recommend an even lower sodium consumption level. You can take several steps to reduce your sodium intake:

- Taste before you shake—maybe you don't need the salt after all.
- Switch to one of the salt-free seasonings. Reduced-sodium, low-salt, or salt-free products are now available and can be substituted in your recipes. Although several of these items still contain some salt, the amount is reduced. (For example, low-sodium canned soups are now readily available.)
- Use herbs and spices or lemon juice as a flavor enhancer in place of salt.
- Use half the salt recommended in standard cookbook recipes. You'll find that it's not uncommon for a recipe to call for too much salt, and the reduction actually improves the flavor of the food.
- Cook with no salt and let diners add their own from a shaker at the table. Some evidence suggests people may use only a fraction of the amount indicated in the original recipe.
- When dining out, don't hesitate to ask if a recipe can be prepared using less salt or even no salt at all. And remember: Monosodium glutamate and many meat tenderizers contain sodium.
- Read the labels on packaged foods. Nearly half the sodium we consume comes from salt or sodium compounds added to foods during processing. Salt appears unexpectedly and can be "hidden." Tomato and vegetable juice cocktails, for instance, contain large amounts of sodium. And sodium can appear under other names, including *monosodium glutamate* (often used as a flavor enhancer in Chinese foods), *sodium benzoate* (a preservative), *sodium citrate* (which controls acidity), and *sodium propionate* (a mold inhibitor). Also, don't forget to check your water supply. Many bottled waters are high in sodium, as is drinking water passed through a water softener.
- Avoid or limit your consumption of snack and convenience foods. Chips, lunch meat, and junk food often contain large amounts of both salt and fat. So do meats such as ham, bacon, sausage, and hot dogs.

For many people, salt is a condiment for which their tolerance increases: The more salt they shake on their food, the more they need to shake in order to get the salty taste they seek. When you reduce salt in your diet, the taste will be missing for a while. Then, suddenly, it's as if your ability to taste salt has returned, and foods you thought were fine will suddenly have a very salty taste. When that happens, you'll know you're on your way to a lower-salt diet.

Carving away Fats

Reducing the amount of dietary fat and cholesterol you consume isn't as hard to do as you might think. You may simply need to make changes such as the following in your eating habits:

- Avoid fried foods. You can eat roasted, baked, grilled, steamed, and broiled foods, but you should avoid eating fried foods. When a food is fried, fat is added during the cooking process.

- Find alternatives to breaded meats and vegetables, which are fried. However, you can enjoy many of these foods by "oven-frying" them: Place the food on a nonstick cookie sheet, and bake it at 400°F, turning it as necessary for even browning.

- Buy only lean cuts of beef, lamb, veal, and pork, then pare away as much visible fat as possible before cooking. Serve portions that are about the size of a deck of playing cards (around 3 ounces) when cooked.

- Eliminate from your diet liver, kidney, sweetbreads, and brains, which are all heavy in cholesterol. Be aware that bacon, sausage, hot dogs, bologna, salami, and other processed meats may also be cholesterol-laden as well as high in fat and sodium content.

- Choose chicken and turkey, but remove the skin before cooking. Leaving the skin doubles the fat content. Other fowl, like ducks and geese, are higher in fat than chicken or turkey. Ground chicken and ground turkey can be substituted for ground beef in many recipes, but be sure you're using a lean version: Some commercially available ground turkey contains skin and organ meats; purchasing skinless turkey breast and having the butcher grind it to your specifications is probably best.

- Turn to fish, another fine replacement for beef, pork, lamb, and veal. Fish can be either fatty or lean. Fatty fish (for example, salmon or mackerel) come from the deep sea and contain high amounts of omega-3 fatty acids, which have been credited in some studies with helping reduce plaque buildup in blood vessels. Lean fish, from fresh or salt water, have little or no omega-3 fatty acids. Fish isn't free of cholesterol but is very low in saturated fat. If you use canned fish, like tuna, salmon, or sardines, buy those packed in water. Then drain the fish carefully to remove the water and any oils, add water to the can, and drain it again to rinse the fish before use. Shellfish are also very low in fat. Shrimp and lobster, though, contain a bit more cholesterol than fish, lean red meat, or poultry. So choose these shellfish less often.

■ Because dairy products are another source of fats and cholesterol, use the lowest fat forms. Gradually work your way from whole milk to 2 percent to 1 percent to skim (nonfat) milk. When baking, replace whole milk called for in a recipe with skim milk. Evaporated skim milk can be substituted for cream. Many cream sauces can also be made using skim milk. Use other low-fat dairy products like low-fat or fat-free margarine, yogurt, and cheeses. (Low-fat cheeses, however, are usually high in sodium.)

Aged cheeses, including cheddar and American varieties, have a high fat content. In recipes, replace them with low-fat varieties, like ricotta, part-skim mozzarella, or low-fat cottage cheese. A low-fat cheese should have no more than 6 grams of fat per serving. This information is found on the label. Always make cheese sauces with low-fat cheese, and use them sparingly.

Low-fat as well as fat-free varieties of sour cream are also available. Then again, yogurt may be successfully substituted for sour cream in most recipes. "Mock" sour cream can also be made by blending 16 ounces of nonfat cottage cheese with 2 tablespoons of lemon juice and 2 tablespoons of plain, nonfat yogurt.

One egg yolk contains 213 milligrams of cholesterol, so the recommended limit is four yolks per week, including those used in cooking. Egg whites, on the other hand, contain no cholesterol and are good protein sources. For cooking, two egg whites may be substituted for one whole egg, and three egg whites will replace two whole eggs. Also, low-fat, low-cholesterol egg substitutes are now available in the frozen and refrigerated foods sections of most supermarkets.

Ice cream, a festive food, should be saved for festive occasions. Made from eggs, sugar, and cream, the dessert contains high concentrations of fat and cholesterol. Sherbet, fruit ices, frozen fat-free yogurt, and fat-free ice milk are great substitutes.

■ Although nuts and seeds deliver protein, they're high in fat and calories. When baking, reduce the quantity of nuts called for, or substitute a hard, crunchy cereal.

■ Use unsweetened plain cocoa powder in place of baking chocolate when making desserts.

*Cooking with
the Right Oils*

Butter is a great flavor enhancer; it is also mostly saturated fat. Unfortunately, its longtime substitute, margarine, contains *trans* fatty acids, which have recently also been associated with coronary artery disease. Both butter and margarine, then, should be used as little as possible. (All fats should make up no more than 30 percent of your daily calories.)

Current evidence indicates that oils with a high percentage of monounsaturated fat, such as olive, canola, or peanut oils, are not harmful and might actually be beneficial to your heart health. So, if you're cooking with oil, try to use one of these three.

To reduce the amount of oil in cooking, use nonstick pans or buy nonstick vegetable oil sprays to replace the oil used to coat cooking surfaces. Also, both chicken and fish may be cooked in a microwave oven without fat of any kind.

In recipes for baked goods, try replacing the suggested amount of oil with an equal quantity of applesauce. If the recipe's only liquid is oil, use one-half applesauce and one-half skim milk to ensure moistness.

Small amounts of sherry, wine, lemon juice, or low-fat chicken broth can replace oil or margarine when sauteing vegetables or browning meats. However, it's best to use a lower than normal heat setting when sauteing or browning without oil.

And for salad dressings, skip the oil and use wine or herb vinegar, or make your own oil-and-vinegar dressing so you can control the amount of oil in the finished product. Although you can purchase nonfat salad dressings, they're almost always high in sodium and therefore not recommended.

How to Start Cooking the Heart-Smart Way

A good first step toward heart-smart cooking is to clean out your pantry and refrigerator. Read the food labels to decide which products you want to keep and which ones you'll need to toss after finding healthier substitutes.

Once that's done, begin reducing your consumption of those fats that are easiest to refuse, including butter, fried foods, commercially bottled salad dressings, and fatty (and salty) meats like bacon, sausage, hot dogs, and luncheon meats. And limit your use of potato chips, as well as other chip-type products, ice cream, chocolate, candy bars, and peanut butter. Notice the key words here are "reducing consumption," and "limit use." Cut back on these foods slowly, possibly focusing on only one at a time. And as you deal with each one, find a heart-smart replacement.

Make the switch from whole milk to 2 percent milk. Buy low-sodium soups and no-salt canned vegetables. Or, even better, start using fresh or frozen vegetables and make your own soups.

One final tip: Pleasing the eye as well as the palate adds to the enjoyment of any meal. A few sprigs of parsley, several thin slices of sweet red bell pepper or twists of lemon peel, or any other appropriate garnish can dress up the plate and add appeal to the meal. It only takes a moment, and can make a great dish even more memorable.

Heart-smart eating is a habit. By taking your present taste preferences and slowly modifying those that need changing, you can gain a new perspective on food—and enjoy the benefits of a healthier diet.

CHAPTER 20

Heart-Healthy Recipes

Breakfast Dishes

Fiesta Egg Scramble

Serves 4 (¾ cup per serving)

Vegetable cooking spray
⅓ cup chopped sweet red pepper
3 tablespoons chopped green onions
2 tablespoons chopped green chiles, drained
1¼ cups frozen egg substitute with cheese,
   thawed
3 tablespoons skim milk
¼ cup (1 ounce) shredded reduced-fat
   Monterey Jack cheese
½ cup low-sodium picante sauce

Coat a large nonstick skillet with cooking spray; place over medium-high heat until hot. Add sweet red pepper, green onions, and chiles; saute until vegetables are tender. Combine egg substitute and milk; stir well. Pour over pepper mixture in skillet, and cook over medium heat, stirring frequently, until egg substitute mixture is firm but still moist.

Remove from heat. Sprinkle cheese over eggs, cover and let stand 1 minute. Divide eggs evenly among 4 plates. Spoon 2 tablespoons picante sauce over each serving.

■ Per serving: Calories 123; Fat 5.5 g; Cholesterol 8 mg; Sodium 387 mg.

From *Cooking Light 1992*® © 1991. Published by Oxmoor House®, P.O. Box 2463, Birmingham, AL 35201.

Maple-Cinnamon French Toast

Serves 4 (2 1-inch slices per serving)

1 loaf (about 12 oz.) crusty French or Italian
   bread, preferably whole wheat

¾ cup thawed, fat-free egg substitute, or 1
  large egg plus 4 egg whites
1¼ cups skim milk
¾ teaspoon vanilla
¾ cup plus 1 tablespoon pure maple syrup,
  preferably dark amber
½ teaspoon ground cinnamon
Vegetable cooking spray, preferably
  butter-flavored

Cut bread diagonally into 1-inch slices and arrange in a single layer in a large baking pan or
casserole dish; set aside. In a small bowl, whisk
together egg substitute, milk, vanilla, ¼ cup
plus 1 tablespoon maple syrup and ¼ teaspoon cinnamon. Pour mixture over bread,
cover, refrigerate and let soak about 25 minutes or overnight, turning slices over after 15
minutes.

Preheat oven to 475°F. Transfer bread into another large baking pan generously coated with
cooking spray, and arrange in a single layer.
Bake 8 minutes, then turn bread over and bake
until golden brown and crisp, 7 to 8 minutes
longer. Meanwhile, in a small saucepan whisk
together remaining maple syrup and cinnamon. Bring mixture to a simmer over low heat
and keep warm until needed.

To serve, arrange French toast on plates and
drizzle with warmed syrup.

■ Per serving: Calories 450; Fat 4 g; Cholesterol 1 mg; Sodium 688 mg.

Reprinted from *American Health Magazine*, September
1993.

Turkey Sausage Casserole

Serves 6 (¾ cup per serving)

Vegetable cooking spray
½ pound ground turkey sausage
3 tablespoons chopped green onions
3 cups cubed French bread
1 cup (4 ounces) shredded 40% less-fat mild
  Cheddar cheese
1⅓ cups skim milk
¾ cup frozen egg substitute, thawed
1 teaspoon prepared mustard
¼ teaspoon pepper

Coat a large nonstick skillet with cooking
spray; place over medium-high heat until hot.
Add sausage and green onions; cook over medium heat until meat is browned, stirring to
crumble. Drain and pat dry with paper towel.
Set aside.

Place bread cubes in an 8-inch square baking
dish coated with cooking spray. Layer sausage
mixture and cheese over bread. Combine milk
and remaining ingredients; stir well. Pour over
sausage and cheese. Cover and refrigerate at
least 8 hours. Bake, covered, at 350°F for 30
minutes. Uncover and bake an additional 15
to 20 minutes or until set. Let stand 5 minutes
before serving.

■ Per serving: Calories 201; Fat 7 g; Cholesterol 33 mg; Sodium 494 mg.

From *Cooking Light 1993*® © 1992. Published by
Oxmoor House®, P.O. Box 2463, Birmingham, AL
35201.

Soups and Salads

Cream of Asparagus and Leek Soup

Serves 4 (¾ cup per serving)

1 bunch of asparagus spears (about 8)
4 teaspoons margarine
1½ cups chopped leeks (white portion only)

1 tablespoon all-purpose flour
2 cups low-salt, low-fat chicken broth
½ cup evaporated skim milk
⅛ teaspoon white pepper
Pinch of nutmeg

Trim bottoms from asparagus. Steam asparagus until cooked, about 5 minutes. Cut off and reserve tips. Puree stems in blender or food processor until smooth.

Melt margarine in saucepan; add leeks. Saute over medium-high heat until soft, about 8 minutes. Whisk in flour; gradually stir in broth. Add pureed asparagus and simmer 10 minutes; then add milk, asparagus tips, and seasonings. Heat soup through, but do not boil, and serve.

■ Per serving: Calories 108; Fat 6 g; Cholesterol 1 mg; Sodium 89 mg.

Reprinted from *Eat Smart for a Healthy Heart* © 1987 by Denton A. Cooley, M.D., and Carolyn Moore, Ph.D., R.D. Permission granted by Barron's Educational Series, Inc., Hauppauge, NY 11788.

Herbed Broccoli Bisque

Serves 5 (¾ cup per serving)

3 medium leeks
1 minced garlic clove
2 teaspoons reduced-fat margarine
3 cups defatted chicken broth
4 cups small broccoli florets
1 pound peeled and ¾-inch cubed boiling
    potatoes (about 4 medium)
1 teaspoon dried basil leaves
1 teaspoon dried thyme leaves
¼ teaspoon ground white pepper
1½ cups of 2% fat milk
1 teaspoon lemon juice
½ teaspoon salt, or to taste
Tiny blanched broccoli florets or fresh broccoli
    leaves (garnish)

Clean leeks by trimming off the root ends and all but about 1 inch of the green tops; discard. Peel off and discard 1 or 2 layers of the tough outer leaves. Then, beginning at the green end, slice down about 1 inch into the leeks. Put the leeks in a colander. Wash them thoroughly under cool running water.

Wash again to remove all traces of dirt. Set them aside until well drained. Cut into ½-inch pieces.

In a Dutch oven, combine the leeks, garlic, margarine, and 3 tablespoons of the broth. Cook over medium heat, stirring frequently, for 10 minutes, or until the leeks are tender, but not browned. (Add a bit more broth if liquid evaporates.) Add the broccoli florets, potatoes, basil, thyme, pepper, and remaining broth. Bring to a boil.

Cover, reduce the heat, and simmer for 11 to 14 minutes, or until the potatoes and broccoli are tender. Remove from the heat and let cool slightly.

Working in batches, puree the mixture in a blender on low speed for 10 seconds. Raise the speed to high, and process until completely smooth. Return the puree to the pot. Add the milk, lemon juice, and salt. Mix well. Cook for an additional 4 to 5 minutes; do not boil.

Garnish individual servings with the blanched florets or leaves.

Editor's Note: You can substantially reduce the sodium content of this recipe by using low-salt, low-fat chicken broth.

■ Per serving: Calories 207; Fat 3.5 g; Cholesterol 5 mg; Sodium 774 mg.

Reprinted from *100% Pleasure* © 1994 by Nancy Baggett and Ruth Glick. Permission granted by Rodale Press, Inc.; Emmaus, PA 18098.

Vegetable Minestrone

Serves 5 (¾ cup per serving)

1 large chopped onion
1 thinly sliced celery stalk
1 minced garlic clove
2 teaspoons olive oil
5 cups of defatted chicken broth, divided
2 cups coarsely shredded cabbage

1 cup sliced zucchini and/or yellow squash
1 peeled and thinly sliced carrot
1 bay leaf
1 teaspoon dried thyme leaves
1 teaspoon dried basil leaves
½ teaspoon dried oregano leaves
⅛ teaspoon ground black pepper
Dash of ground celery seeds
1 can (19 ounces) cannellini beans or 1 can
   (16 ounces) kidney beans, rinsed and drained
½ cup radiatore (pinwheel-shaped pasta)
1 can (8 ounces) tomato sauce

In a Dutch oven, combine the onions, celery, garlic, oil, and 3 tablespoons of the broth. Cook over medium heat, stirring frequently, for 5 to 6 minutes, or until the onions are soft. Add the cabbage, zucchini and/or squash, carrots, bay leaf, thyme, basil, oregano, pepper, celery seeds, and the remaining broth. Bring to a boil.

Cover, reduce the heat, and simmer for 15 minutes, or until the vegetables are almost tender. Add the beans and pasta. Simmer for 8 to 11 minutes, or until the pasta is tender. Remove and discard the bay leaf. Stir in the tomato sauce and serve.

Editor's Note: You can substantially reduce the sodium content of this recipe if you use low-salt, low-fat chicken broth and no-salt tomato sauce.

■ Per serving: Calories 200; Fat 3 g; Cholesterol 0 mg; Sodium 1349 mg.

Reprinted from *100% Pleasure* © 1994 by Nancy Baggett and Ruth Glick. Permission granted by Rodale Press, Inc.; Emmaus, PA 18098.

California Cucumber Salad

Serves 4 (½ cup per serving)

2 cucumbers, scrubbed, not peeled
⅓ cup raisins
¼ cup chopped unsalted dry-roasted walnuts

1 tablespoon chopped fresh dill
½ teaspoon minced garlic
2 tablespoons chopped green onion
⅛ teaspoon white pepper
¼ cup plain nonfat yogurt
4 romaine lettuce leaves

Remove seeds from cucumbers, shred, and drain. Place in a bowl and add remaining ingredients. Toss to mix well.

Serve on lettuce-lined salad plates.

■ Per serving: Calories 109; Fat 5 g; Cholesterol 0 mg; Sodium 18 mg.

From *The American Heart Association Cookbook, 5th Edition* by Ruth Eshelman © 1993 by The American Heart Association. Reprinted by permission of Times Books, a division of Random House, Inc.

Savory Cabbage Slaw

Serves 6 (1 cup per serving)

⅓ cup apple cider vinegar
2 tablespoons chopped fresh chives or
   1 tablespoon dried chives
1 tablespoon granulated sugar
1½ teaspoons canola or safflower oil
½ teaspoon Dijon mustard
¼ teaspoon mustard seeds (optional)
¼ teaspoon celery seeds
¼ teaspoon celery salt
¼ teaspoon ground black pepper
5 cups lightly packed shredded green cabbage
2 medium carrots, peeled and shredded
¼ cup finely chopped sweet red peppers
¼ cup finely chopped celery

In a large nonreactive bowl, combine the vinegar, chives, sugar, oil, mustard, mustard seeds (if using), celery seeds, celery salt, and black pepper until well blended. Stir in the cabbage, carrots, red peppers, and celery. Mix well. Cover and refrigerate for at least 15 minutes (preferably 1 hour). Toss briefly before serving.

■ Per serving: Calories 48; Fat 1.4 g; Cholesterol 0 mg.

Reprinted from *100% Pleasure* © 1994 by Nancy Baggett and Ruth Glick. Permission granted by Rodale Press, Inc.; Emmaus, PA 18098.

Summer Couscous Salad

Serves 4 (1 cup per serving)

1 cup plus 2 tablespoons water
¾ cup couscous, uncooked
6 ounces fresh aparagus
½ cup diced sweet yellow pepper
½ cup cherry tomatoes, quartered and seeded
¼ cup thinly sliced green onions
1½ tablespoons canned no-salt-added chicken broth, undiluted
1 tablespoon frozen orange juice concentrate, thawed and undiluted
1 tablespoon balsamic vinegar
1 teaspoon grated orange rind
1½ teaspoons olive oil
½ teaspoon ground cumin
¼ teaspoon salt
4 romaine lettuce leaves

Bring water to a boil in a medium saucepan. Remove from heat.

Add couscous; cover and let stand 5 minutes or until couscous is tender and liquid is absorbed. Fluff couscous with a fork, and transfer to a serving bowl.

Snap off tough ends of asparagus. Remove scales from stalks with a knife or vegetable peeler, if desired. Cut spears into 1-inch pieces. Cook asparagus in boiling water 1 minute or until crisp-tender. Drain and rinse under cold water until cool; drain again. Add asparagus, yellow pepper, tomatoes, and green onions to couscous; toss gently.

Combine broth and next 6 ingredients in a small bowl, stirring well with a wire whisk. Pour over couscous mixture, and toss gently. Cover and chill at least 8 hours.

Spoon 1 cup of couscous mixture onto each individual lettuce-lined salad plate.

Editor's Note: Couscous (pronounced koos-koos) is a North African dish. The box of couscous sold in the United States is a pre-mixed and cooked substance, comparable to dried noodles. It is not a grain. Couscous is a great substitute for rice, noodles, or potatoes. It is excellent served as a base for vegetable stews.

■ Per serving: Calories 174; Fat 2 g; Cholesterol 0 mg; Sodium 9 mg.

From *Cooking Light 1995*® © 1994. Published by Oxmoor House®, P.O. Box 2463, Birmingham, AL 35201.

Meat and Poultry Entrees

Braised Sirloin Tips

Serves 8 (3 to 4 ounces per serving)

¼ teaspoon freshly ground black pepper
½ teaspoon unseasoned meat tenderizer
2 pounds beef sirloin tips, all visible fat removed, cut into cubes and drained on paper towels
2 cloves of garlic, finely minced
½ cup finely chopped onion
1¼ cups low-sodium beef broth
⅓ cup dry red wine
1 tablespoon low-sodium soy sauce
2 tablespoons cornstarch
¼ cup cold water
¼ cup minced fresh parsley

Place a large nonstick skillet over medium-high heat. Sprinkle pepper and meat tenderizer on meat. Brown meat on all sides, turning often, until well browned. Add garlic and onions and cook until onions are translucent.

Add broth, wine, and soy sauce and heat to boiling. Reduce heat, cover and simmer 1½ hours, or until meat is tender.

In a small bowl, blend cornstarch and water until smooth, then slowly pour mixture into skillet, stirring constantly. Continue to cook and stir until gravy thickens. Sprinkle parsley on top.

Serve with rice or wide noodles if desired.

■ Per serving: Calories 177; Fat 5 g; Cholesterol 67 mg; Sodium 244 mg.

From *The American Heart Association Cookbook, 5th Edition* by Ruth Eshelman © 1993 by The American Heart Association. Reprinted by permission of Times Books, a division of Random House, Inc.

Pork Chops with Maple-Pecan Sauce

Serves 4 (1 chop per serving)

4 4-ounce lean, boneless center-cut loin pork
  chops
2 teaspoons Dijon mustard
2 tablespoons all-purpose flour
½ teaspoon ground ginger
Vegetable cooking spray
2 teaspoons vegetable oil
2 tablespoons reduced-calorie maple syrup
1 tablespoon chopped toasted pecans
Celery leaves (optional)

Trim fat from chops. Place chops between 2 sheets of heavy-duty plastic wrap, and flatten to ¼-inch thickness, using a meat mallet or rolling pin. Spread mustard on both sides of chops. Combine flour and ginger; stir well. Dredge pork chops in flour mixture.

Coat a large nonstick skillet with cooking spray; add oil. Place over medium heat until hot. Add chops and cook 3 minutes on each side or until chops are browned. Combine maple syrup and pecans; add to pork chops, stirring to coat. Cover and simmer 4 minutes or until chops are tender, turning once.

Transfer chops to a large serving platter, and garnish with celery leaves, if desired.

■ Per serving: Calories 234; Fat 11.9 g; Cholesterol 71 mg; Sodium 151 mg.

From *Cooking Light 1992*® © 1991. Published by Oxmoor House®, P.O. Box 2463, Birmingham, AL 35201.

Grilled Chicken Breasts with Honey Mustard Glaze

Serves 2 (1 breast per serving)

1 whole chicken breast, about 12 ounces
2 teaspoons virgin olive oil

Honey Mustard Glaze

2½ tablespoons coarse-grained mustard
4 teaspoons Dijon-style mustard
2 teaspoons honey

Bone chicken breasts and lightly pound meat flat. Grill over charcoal fire for about 15 to 20 minutes, or broil in oven for about 15 minutes (begin cooking skin side down if grilling, skin side up if broiling). Prepare sauce by combining ingredients. When chicken is about half cooked, turn over and brush with sauce. Finish cooking and cut breast in half. Transfer to serving plates. Drizzle each serving with 1 teaspoon olive oil.

■ Per serving: Calories 326; Fat 18 g; Cholesterol 87 mg; Sodium 463 mg.

Reprinted from *Eat Smart for a Healthy Heart* © 1987 by Denton A. Cooley, M.D., and Carolyn Moore, Ph.D., R.D. Permission granted by Barron's Educational Series, Inc., Hauppauge, NY 11788.

Herbed Chicken Breasts with Lime and Tomatoes

Serves 4 (1 breast per serving)

¼ teaspoon finely grated lime zest
2 tablespoons lime juice
1 teaspoon chili powder
¼ teaspoon finely crumbled dried rosemary
¼ teaspoon salt
4 boneless, skinless chicken breast halves
   (4 ounces each)
1 teaspoon olive oil
½ cup defatted chicken broth
¾ cup peeled and diced tomatoes

In a glass or ceramic bowl, stir together the lime zest, lime juice, chili powder, rosemary, and salt to form a paste. Add the chicken and toss until the pieces are well coated. Cover

and refrigerate at least 20 minutes and up to 2 hours.

In a 12-inch nonstick skillet over medium-high heat, warm the oil until hot but not smoking. Add the chicken, reserving the leftover paste. Cook, turning the chicken occasionally, for 4 minutes, or until the pieces are lightly browned. If necessary, lower the heat slightly to prevent burning.

Add ½ cup broth to the bowl with the remaining paste and stir well. Pour the mixture over the chicken. Lower the heat and simmer for 9 minutes; add a bit more broth, if necessary, to prevent the pan from boiling dry.

Add the tomatoes and simmer for 2 to 3 minutes, or until the chicken is just cooked through.

Editor's Note: You can reduce the sodium content of this recipe if you use low-salt, low-fat chicken broth.

■ Per serving: Calories 101; Fat 4.1 g; Cholesterol 46 mg; Sodium 239 mg.

Reprinted from *100% Pleasure* © 1994 by Nancy Baggett and Ruth Glick. Permission granted by Rodale Press, Inc.; Emmaus, PA 18098.

Seafood Entrees

Fettuccine with Shrimp and Spinach

Serves 8 (1 cup per serving)

½ cup part-skim ricotta cheese
½ cup nonfat plain yogurt
¼ cup nonfat buttermilk
¼ cup grated Parmesan cheese
½ teaspoon chicken-flavored bouillon granules

¼ teaspoon garlic powder
¼ teaspoon salt
¼ teaspoon crushed red pepper
1 pound medium-sized fresh shrimp, peeled
   and deveined
10½ ounces fettuccine, uncooked
2 cups shredded fresh spinach

Combine first 8 ingredients in a medium bowl; stir well. Set aside.

Bring 1 quart of water to a boil in a large saucepan; add shrimp, and cook 3 to 5 minutes. Drain well; rinse with water, and drain again. Set shrimp aside.

Cook fettuccine in a Dutch oven, according to package directions, omitting salt and fat; drain. Immediately return fettuccine to pan; add spinach, and stir mixture well to combine. Cover and let stand 1 to 2 minutes or until spinach wilts. Add ricotta mixture and shrimp, stirring well to combine. Serve immediately.

■ Per serving: Calories 229; Fat 4.1 g; Cholesterol 67 mg; Sodium 315 mg.

From *Cooking Light 1992*® © 1991. Published by Oxmoor House®, P.O. Box 2463, Birmingham, AL 35201.

Oven-Fried Catfish Fillets

Serves 4 (1 fillet per serving)

⅓ cup corn flake crumbs
1½ tablespoons grated Parmesan cheese
1 tablespoon dried parsley flakes
4 4-ounce farm-raised catfish fillets
2 tablespoons reduced-calorie margarine, melted
Vegetable cooking spray

Combine corn flake crumbs, cheese, and parsley flakes in a small bowl; stir well. Brush fillets with melted margarine; dredge in crumb mixture.

Place fillets in an 11 × 7 × 2-inch baking dish coated with cooking spray. Bake, uncovered, at 400°F for 20 minutes or until fish flakes easily when tested with a fork. Transfer to a serving platter, and serve immediately.

■ Per serving: Calories 223; Fat 9.7 g; Cholesterol 69 mg; Sodium 305 mg.

From *Cooking Light 1992*® © 1991. Published by Oxmoor House®, P.O. Box 2463, Birmingham, AL 35201.

Trout Amandine

Serves 4 (1 fillet per serving)

½ teaspoon paprika
⅓ cup all-purpose flour
4 skinless trout fillets, 5 ounces each
4 teaspoons safflower oil
4 teaspoons reduced-fat margarine, melted
¼ cup dry sherry
Juice of 1 lemon
⅓ cup blanched sliced almonds, lightly toasted
¼ cup finely chopped fresh parsley

Combine paprika and flour. Dredge trout in flour mixture to coat lightly. Heat oil in a large nonstick skillet over medium-high heat; add trout, and saute until tender and flaky, about 10 minutes, turning at least once during cooking. Melt margarine in a small saucepan. Add sherry and lemon juice and heat thoroughly. Pour sherry sauce over trout, and let stand for 3 to 4 minutes. Remove trout from sauce. Transfer to a warm platter, sprinkle with almonds and parsley, and serve.

■ Per serving: Calories 447; Fat 31 g; Cholesterol 78 mg; Sodium 58 mg.

Reprinted from *Eat Smart for a Healthy Heart* © 1987 by Denton A. Cooley, M.D., and Carolyn Moore, Ph.D., R.D. Permission granted by Barron's Educational Series, Inc., Hauppauge, NY 11788.

Vegetables and Side Dishes

Cauliflower Pie

Serves 10

10 cups cauliflowerets (about 1 medium head)
Butter-flavored vegetable cooking spray
1 8-ounce container nonfat sour cream
  alternative
½ cup egg substitute
½ cup shredded reduced-fat Cheddar cheese
1 2-ounce jar diced pimiento, drained
¼ teaspoon salt
¼ teaspoon ground white pepper
⅓ cup soft whole wheat bread crumbs
¼ teaspoon paprika

Arrange cauliflower in a vegetable steamer over boiling water.

Cover and steam 8 minutes or until tender. Drain well. Arrange in a shallow 1½-quart round casserole coated with cooking spray.

Combine sour cream and next 5 ingredients in a bowl; stir well. Pour sour cream mixture over cauliflower. Combine bread crumbs and paprika; toss gently. Sprinkle over sour cream mixture. Coat bread crumb mixture with cooking spray. Bake, uncovered, at 375°F for 20 minutes or until hot and bubbly.

■ Per serving: Calories 66; Fat 1.4 g; Cholesterol 4 mg; Sodium 155 mg.

From *Cooking Light 1994*® © 1993. Published by Oxmoor House®, P.O. Box 2463, Birmingham, AL 35201.

Creamy Sliced Potatoes

Serves 8 (½ cup per serving)

1¼ pounds round red potatoes, cut into
  ¼-inch thick slices
1 tablespoon reduced-calorie margarine
1½ tablespoons all-purpose flour
1 cup skim milk
¼ teaspoon salt
¼ teaspoon dried whole dillweed
⅛ teaspoon pepper
¼ cup nonfat sour cream alternative

Cook potatoes in a large saucepan in boiling water to cover 10 or 15 minutes or until tender. Drain. Place in a medium bowl; set aside, and keep warm.

Melt margarine in a small saucepan over low heat; add flour, stirring until smooth. Cook 1 minute, stirring constantly with a wire whisk. Gradually add milk; cook over medium heat, stirring constantly, until mixture is thickened and bubbly. Stir in salt, dillweed, and pepper. Remove from heat, and stir in sour cream alternative. Add sour cream mixture to potatoes; toss gently. Serve warm.

■ Per serving: Calories 90; Fat 1.1 g; Cholesterol 1 mg; Sodium 111 mg.

From *Cooking Light 1994*® © 1993. Published by Oxmoor House®, P.O. Box 2463, Birmingham, AL 35201.

Eggplant Zucchini Casserole

Serves 8 (3¼ × 4½-inch slice per serving)

Vegetable oil spray
2 8-ounce cans no-salt-added tomato sauce
2 teaspoons Worcestershire sauce
Freshly ground black pepper to taste
1 teaspoon oregano
½ teaspoon basil
2 medium cloves garlic, crushed
1 medium eggplant, peeled and sliced
2 medium zucchini, sliced
1 cup uncooked spaghetti, broken in pieces
3 medium stalks of celery, chopped
1 medium onion, chopped
1 medium green bell pepper, chopped
8 ounces part-skim mozzarella cheese, cut into 18 small slices

Preheat oven to 350°F. Lightly spray a 9 × 13-inch casserole dish with vegetable oil.

In a bowl, combine tomato sauce, Worcestershire sauce, black pepper, herbs, and garlic. Mix well and set aside.

In prepared casserole dish, arrange half of the eggplant slices in a single layer. Top with half of each of the following: zucchini slices, spaghetti, celery, onion, and bell pepper. Next, arrange 9 slices of cheese over this, and spoon half of tomato mixture on top of cheese. Repeat layers.

Cover and bake about 1 hour, or until vegetables are tender.

■ Per serving: Calories 136; Fat 5 g; Cholesterol 15 mg; Sodium 194 mg.

From *The American Heart Association Cookbook, 5th Edition* by Ruth Eshelman © 1993 by The American Heart Association. Reprinted by permission of Times Books, a division of Random House, Inc.

Hay and Straw Noodle Toss

Serves 4 (½ cup per serving)

2 cups yellow summer squash, cut in narrow lengthwise strips
2 cups cooked spinach noodles
1 large tomato, diced
1 tablespoon olive oil or other acceptable vegetable oil
1 teaspoon basil
½ cup low-fat cottage cheese
Freshly ground black pepper to taste

Steam squash in a vegetable steamer over medium-high heat until tender.

Remove squash to a large bowl. Add remaining ingredients and toss gently. Serve hot or cold.

■ Per serving: Calories 180; Fat 5 g; Cholesterol 2 mg; Sodium 120 mg.

From *The American Heart Association Cookbook, 5th Edition* by Ruth Eshelman © 1993 by The American Heart Association. Reprinted by permission of Times Books, a division of Random House, Inc.

Louisiana Green Beans

Serves 8 (½ cup per serving)

1 pound fresh green beans, rinsed and trimmed, or 2 9-ounce packages frozen no-salt-added green beans
2 cups canned no-salt-added tomatoes
½ cup chopped celery
¼ cup chopped green bell pepper
½ teaspoon onion powder

Cook green beans until tender. Drain. In a skillet, combine green beans, tomatoes, celery, bell pepper, and onion powder. Cook over medium heat 15 minutes, or until thoroughly heated.

■ Per serving: Calories 26; Fat 0 g; Cholesterol 0 mg; Sodium 18 mg.

From *The American Heart Association Cookbook, 5th Edition* by Ruth Eshelman © 1993 by The American Heart Association. Reprinted by permission of Times Books, a division of Random House, Inc.

Savory Spinach

Serves 4 (½ cup per serving)

1 10-ounce package frozen no-salt-added leaf
  spinach, thawed
2 tablespoons prepared horseradish
2 tablespoons chopped, cooked Canadian
  bacon

Cook spinach in ¼ cup of water 4 to 5 minutes, or until tender. Drain spinach, mix in
horseradish and bacon, and serve.

■ Per serving: Calories 24; Fat 0 g; Cholesterol
  3 mg; Sodium 117 mg.

From *The American Heart Association Cookbook, 5th
Edition* by Ruth Eshelman © 1993 by The American
Heart Association. Reprinted by permission of Times
Books, a division of Random House, Inc.

Seasoned Black-Eyed Peas

Serves 16 (½ cup per serving)

1 pound dried black-eyed peas
Water
¼ pound Canadian bacon
2 medium onions, chopped
2 stalks celery, chopped
1 small bay leaf
1 clove garlic, chopped
¼ teaspoon cayenne pepper
1 6-ounce can no-salt-added tomato paste
Freshly ground black pepper to taste

Rinse peas and place them in a large saucepan.
Cover with water and let soak for 45 minutes.

Cook Canadian bacon until crisp in a skillet
over medium-high heat. Drain on paper towels. Chop and set aside.

Drain peas and return them to the large saucepan. Add just enough fresh water to cover. Add
bacon and remaining ingredients. Bring to a
boil over medium-high heat. Reduce heat,
cover, and simmer 3 hours or until tender.

■ Per serving: Calories 115; Fat 1 g; Cholesterol 3 g; Sodium 104 mg.

From *The American Heart Association Cookbook, 5th
Edition* by Ruth Eshelman © 1993 by The American
Heart Association. Reprinted by permission of Times
Books, a division of Random House, Inc.

Tortellini with Zucchini and Sun-Dried Tomatoes

Serves 4 (1 cup per serving)

¼ cup sun-dried tomatoes (without salt or oil)
½ cup hot water
Olive oil–flavored vegetable cooking spray
1 tablespoon olive oil
1 cup chopped zucchini
3 gloves garlic, minced
2 green onions, cut into 1-inch pieces
¼ cup chopped sweet red pepper
1 teaspoon dried whole oregano
1 (9-ounce) package fresh cheese tortellini

Combine tomatoes and water in a small bowl;
cover and let stand 15 minutes. Drain tomatoes and slice thinly; set aside.

Coat a large nonstick skillet with cooking
spray; add olive oil. Place over medium-high
heat until hot. Add zucchini and garlic; saute
2 minutes. Add green onions, sweet red pepper, and oregano; saute 1 minute. Stir in tomatoes. Remove from heat and keep warm.

Cook tortellini according to package directions,
omitting salt and fat; drain well. Place tortellini in a serving bowl. Add zucchini mixture;
toss gently. Serve immediately.

Editor's Note: Unless you *really* like garlic, we
suggest you use half the recommended amount.

■ Per serving: Calories 249; Fat 6.9 g; Cholesterol 30 mg; Sodium 384 mg.

From *Cooking Light 1993*® © 1992. Published by
Oxmoor House®, P.O. Box 2463, Birmingham, AL
35201.

Desserts

Strawberry-Banana Sorbet

Serves 6 (⅔ cup per serving)

1 medium fully ripe, but not overripe, banana
3 cups unsweetened frozen strawberries, cut
  into equal-size pieces
½ cup frozen cranberry juice cocktail
  concentrate
1–2 tablespoons light corn syrup or mild
  honey, such as clover

Peel the banana and wrap it in plastic. Freeze for at least 1½ hours, or until solid.

Place the strawberries in a food processor. Process with on/off pulses until finely chopped; stop several times to scrape down the sides of the container. Then process the mixture for about 1½ minutes, or until very smooth. Scrape down the sides of the container.

With the machine running, add the juice concentrate. Process for 1 minute, or until completely smooth.

Slice the frozen banana. With the machine running, slowly add the slices. Process for at least 1 minute, or until the mixture is completely smooth and creamy. Sweeten to taste with the corn syrup or honey; process briefly.

Serve immediately or transfer to a chilled storage container and freeze for 30 minutes.

■ Per serving: Calories 164; Fat 0.3 g; Cholesterol 0 mg.

Reprinted from *100% Pleasure* © 1994 by Nancy Baggett and Ruth Glick. Permission granted by Rodale Press, Inc.; Emmaus, PA 18098.

Butterscotch Brownies

Serves 32 (1 brownie per serving)

Vegetable oil spray
1 cup firmly packed dark brown sugar
¼ cup unsalted, low-fat soft margarine
Egg substitute equivalent to 1 egg
½ teaspoon imitation butter flavoring
½ teaspoon vanilla extract
¾ cup sifted all-purpose flour
1 teaspoon baking powder
½ cup unsalted dry-roasted chopped pecans

Preheat oven to 350°F. Lightly spray an 8-inch square baking pan with vegetable oil.

In a large mixing bowl, cream sugar and margarine together. Add egg substitute and extracts. Blend well.

In another bowl, sift flour and baking powder together. Add to margarine mixture and mix well. Stir in nuts.

Spread evenly into prepared pan. Bake 20 to 25 minutes. Cool slightly and cut into 32 bars.

■ Per serving: Calories 62; Fat 3 g; Cholesterol 0 mg; Sodium 32 mg.

From *The American Heart Association Cookbook, 5th Edition* by Ruth Eshelman © 1993 by The American Heart Association. Reprinted by permission of Times Books, a division of Random House, Inc.

Fresh Peach Crumble

Serves 4 (½ cup per serving)

Vegetable cooking spray
2 cups sliced peeled peaches
2 teaspoons lemon juice
½ teaspoon almond extract

2 tablespoons sugar
⅓ cup whole wheat flour
⅓ cup firmly packed brown sugar
2 teaspoons safflower oil
½ teaspoon ground cinnamon
2 tablespoons chopped blanched almonds

Preheat oven to 375°F. Mix peaches, lemon juice, almond extract, and sugar in a large bowl. Transfer to a 9 × 5-inch loaf pan lightly coated with nonstick spray. Bake 30 minutes.

Blend flour, brown sugar, oil, cinnamon, and almonds. Sprinkle over fruit and continue baking until topping is lightly browned, 15 to 20 minutes. Serve warm.

■ Per serving: Calories 191; Fat 5 g; Cholesterol 0 mg; Sodium 6 mg.

Reprinted from *Eat Smart for a Healthy Heart* © 1987 by Denton A. Cooley, M.D., and Carolyn Moore, Ph.D., R.D. Permission granted by Barron's Educational Series, Inc., Hauppauge, NY 11788.

Hong Kong Sundae

Serves 4 (½ cup ice milk with 2 tablespoons topping per serving)

Topping (makes 2½ cups)
1 11-ounce can mandarin oranges, in light syrup
1 tablespoon cornstarch
1 8½-ounce can crushed no-sugar-added pineapple, undrained
½ cup orange marmalade
½ teaspoon ground ginger
½ cup sliced preserved kumquats

Sundaes
½ cup topping recipe
2 cups vanilla ice milk

Drain oranges, reserving ¼ cup of syrup. Set oranges aside.

Combine orange syrup with cornstarch in a saucepan over medium heat. Stir until well blended. Stir in pineapple with its liquid, marmalade, and ginger. Cook, stirring, over medium heat until mixture thickens and bubbles.

Stir in oranges and kumquats.

Cover and refrigerate for later use, or serve warm.

For sundaes, place ½-cup scoop of vanilla ice milk in each bowl. Add 2 tablespoons of warm topping to each. Unused topping may be refrigerated for later use.

Editor's Note: If you want to offer your guest a dessert that tastes great and looks a bit exotic, try this recipe. The topping is easy to prepare and can be made 24 hours before to serving.

■ Per serving: Calories 178; Fat 3 g; Cholesterol 9 mg; Sodium 58 mg.

From *The American Heart Association Cookbook, 5th Edition* by Ruth Eshelman © 1993 by The American Heart Association. Reprinted by permission of Times Books, a division of Random House, Inc.

Hot Fudge Pudding Cake

Serves 16 (1 slice per serving, 16 slices per cake)

Vegetable cooking spray
1 cup self-rising flour
½ cup sugar
2 tablespoons cocoa
½ cup skim milk
2 tablespoons liquid Butter Buds
1 cup Grape-Nuts cereal
1 cup brown sugar (packed)
¼ cup cocoa
1¾ cups hot water

Heat oven to 350°F. Measure flour, granulated sugar, and 2 tablespoons cocoa into a bowl. Blend in milk and Butter Buds; stir in Grape-Nuts cereal. Pour into a square pan coated with cooking spray. Stir together brown sugar and ¼ cup cocoa; sprinkle over batter. Pour hot water over batter. Bake 45 minutes. While hot, cut into squares; invert onto a dessert plate and spoon sauce over each serving. Cake and sauce bake in the same pan.

Editor's Note: As this cake cools, the sauce becomes more like a pudding. It is good served either warm or cold.

- Per serving: Calories 137; Fat 0.5 g; Cholesterol 0 mg; Sodium 171 mg.

Reprinted from *Butter Busters: The Cookbook* © 1994 by Butter Busters Publishing, Inc. Permission granted by Warner Books, Inc., New York, NY 10020.

Norwegian Apple Pie

Serves 8 (1 slice per serving, 8 slices per pie)

Vegetable cooking spray
2 egg whites or egg substitute equivalent to
    1 egg
¾ cup sugar
1 teaspoon vanilla extract
1 teaspoon baking powder
½ cup all-purpose flour
½ cup unsalted dry-roasted chopped walnuts
1 cup diced apples

Preheat oven to 350°F. Lightly spray an 8-inch pie plate with vegetable oil.

Beat egg, sugar, vanilla extract, and baking powder in a large mixing bowl until smooth and fluffy. Beat in flour until smooth and well blended. Stir in walnuts and apples.

Turn into prepared pie plate and bake for 30 minutes. Pie will puff up as it cooks, then collapse as it cools. Serve warm.

- Per serving: Calories 154; Fat 5 g; Cholesterol 0 mg; Sodium 50 mg.

From *The American Heart Association Cookbook, 5th Edition* by Ruth Eshelman © 1993 by The American Heart Association. Reprinted by permission of Times Books, a division of Random House, Inc.

Savory Walnut Bread

Serves 16 (1 slice per serving, 16 slices per loaf)

Vegetable cooking spray
2 cups sifted all-purpose flour
2 teaspoons baking powder
¼ teaspoon baking soda
½ teaspoon salt
½ cup firmly packed light brown sugar
1 egg
1 cup skim milk
¾ cup unsalted dry-roasted finely chopped
    walnuts

Preheat oven to 350°F. Lightly spray an 8 × 4-inch loaf pan with vegetable oil.

In a large bowl, sift together flour, baking powder, baking soda, salt, and brown sugar. Set aside.

In a large bowl, beat egg until thick and lemon colored. Add milk and continue beating until well blended. Add sifted dry ingredients and walnuts, stirring until mixture is moist.

Turn mixture into prepared loaf pan. Bake 40 minutes, or until a cake tester or a wooden toothpick inserted in the center comes out clean. Loosen loaf from sides of pan with spatula. Turn out, right side up, on a wire rack to cool.

- Per serving: Calories 125; Fat 4 g; Cholesterol 17 mg; Sodium 131 mg.

From *The American Heart Association Cookbook, 5th Edition* by Ruth Eshelman © 1993 by The American Heart Association. Reprinted by permission of Times Books, a division of Random House, Inc.

PART SEVEN

When Something Goes Wrong

What to Do If You Think Someone Is Having a Heart Attack

How to Choose and Work with Your Doctor

The Cardiovascular System

The Symptoms of Heart Disease

Congenital Heart Disease

Diseases of the Heart Muscle

Arrhythmias

Diseases of the Heart Valves

Coronary Artery Disease, Angina, and Heart Attacks

Diseases of the Peripheral Arteries and Veins

Heart Failure

Diagnosing Heart Diseases

Heart Surgery

Recovering from Heart Surgery or Heart Disease

CHAPTER 21

What to Do If You Think Someone Is Having a Heart Attack

If you're with someone who's having a heart attack, or if you're the first person to arrive on the scene, what you do may mean the difference between life and death. When the heart suddenly stops, minutes make a big difference: In less than 120 seconds, the brain begins to be damaged irreversibly from the lack of oxygenated blood. So you owe it to yourself, your family, and your friends to be prepared in case of such an emergency.

Be Prepared

Know where to call for help. In many cities, you can call 911 for emergency help, and almost all pay telephones will allow you to reach an operator by dialing 0 without inserting a coin. Or carry an emergency assistance number with you, and also post it by your phone.

When calling for emergency medical aid, follow these steps:

▶ 1. State the problem clearly. Explain that you think someone is having a heart attack.

▶ 2. Explain where you are and where to send help. (Emergency callers often forget to provide the location.)

▶ 3.   Give the operator the number of the phone you're calling from.

▶ 4.   Answer all questions. If you don't know or aren't certain of the answer, say so.

▶ 5.   Wait for the emergency service operator to break the connection. Don't be the first to hang up.

If it's quicker to take the person to a hospital than to wait for an ambulance to arrive, go directly to the hospital.

If possible, call the hospital before transporting the person, explain the emergency, and tell them when you expect to arrive. If calling ahead isn't possible or if it will take a long time to do so, then take the patient without notifying the hospital. If others are helping you, have someone else call the hospital while you're en route. And remember to drive safely. An auto accident could injure you and might well be the difference between life and death for the person you're transporting.

Additional Safety Tips

▶ 1.   *Learn CPR.* With the right training, almost anyone can perform CPR properly, so *everyone* should learn how to do it. But remember that it is *extremely dangerous* to practice CPR on a healthy person.

Virtually every town in America has at least one organization that offers CPR training. The "Resources" appendix gives a telephone number for the American Heart Association, which can direct you to community hospitals or other local organizations in your area that offer CPR training, often at minimal or no charge. Don't put it off, because the life you save may be dear to you.

▶ 2.   *Record Emergency Numbers.* Take a few minutes to write down the following numbers to keep near your telephone. You may also want to carry them with you, and it's not a bad idea to make wallet-sized copies of this information for your family or friends to carry, too. Even if they're used only once, that's more than enough to justify the time spent preparing them.

■ Paramedic or ambulance phone number. If you live in a city where 911 or a similar number serves for *all* emergency calls, write it down anyway. In an emergency, you can temporarily forget even well-known information.

■ Your physician's name, address, and phone number.

- Hospital name, address, and phone number. This may be a hospital near your home or work, a hospital selected by your physician, or a hospital with a 24-hour emergency care center.
- Other physicians' names and phone numbers. These could be physicians who are caring for your family, friends, or coworkers (especially those with known heart problems).

▶ **3.** *Use the Numbers.* If you live by yourself, keep your emergency number (911 or its equivalent in your town) on or near your telephone. If you experience any of the warning signs of a heart attack listed below, don't wait to see what happens next: Go to your telephone, and call the emergency number.

How to Tell If Someone Is Having a Heart Attack

The symptoms of heart attack can range from an uncomfortable sensation in the chest to a sudden loss of consciousness. The most common symptoms are:

- A tightness or feeling of being squeezed in the chest area.
- A sudden shortness of breath.
- A sharp, unrelenting pain in the chest.
- Pain originating at the base of the neck, in the jaw, or shooting down the left arm.
- Clammy, cold, sweaty skin.
- Nausea, from mild to intense.
- Dizziness, unsteadiness, or an inability to stand.
- Loss of consciousness.
- A wild, erratic heartbeat or pulse.
- The absence of any heartbeat.

If you're with someone who falls unconscious or experiences any of these symptoms, or if you even suspect a heart attack, you should assume that the person *is* having a heart attack. Do *not* hesitate, because time is of the essence. If you're wrong, nobody will be hurt; but if you're right, you may save that person's life.

Even though you may feel unsure about calling for an ambulance or yelling for help, don't let your inhibitions or emotions delay you. Act first and worry about other people's reactions later.

What to Do in a Heart Emergency

If you think someone is having a heart attack, you should do three things as quickly as possible. If someone else is with you, the two of you can do all three at the same time.

▶ 1.   Stay calm.

▶ 2.   Get help.

▶ 3.   Attend to the afflicted person.

▶ 4.   If necessary, attempt CPR.

Stay Calm

Try to stay calm. Remember that someone's life may depend on your ability to think and act.

Get Help

If there are other people around, point to a particular person and say, "You, go get help." This will avoid confusion and ensure that someone will get help. If you're alone with the afflicted person, yell for help or go to the nearest telephone and call for help.

Attend to the Afflicted Person

As soon as you know that help is on the way, turn your attention to the afflicted person. Do not intervene unless you're sure the person is unconscious. Gently shake the person and ask, "Are you okay?" to confirm whether the person is unconscious. The combination of touching and asking aloud is important in case the person has a hearing disability. If you get no response, try to find out if the person is breathing and has a heartbeat. Read on for specifics on how to do these things.

Check for Breathing

The key to checking for breathing is to "Look, Listen, and Feel." *Look* at the person's chest for signs of movement. If you can see the chest move, the person is breathing. *Listen* for sounds of breathing by placing your ear near the person's face. *Feel* for air moving out of the person by placing your cheek close to the person's nose and mouth.

If the person is unconscious and isn't breathing, you must open and clear the person's airway. This is a four-step process.

▶ 1. Place the person on his or her back on a firm surface.

▶ 2. Put the fingers of one of your hands under the person's chin, and place the palm and fingers of your other hand on the person's forehead.

▶ 3. Lift the person's chin and press on the forehead at the same time, tilting the person's head back until his or her mouth opens. Be careful that the pressure you're applying to the chin doesn't hold the mouth closed.

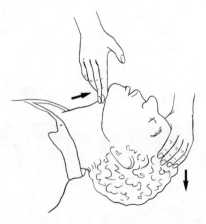

▶ 4. Look inside the person's mouth for any foreign object(s) that might be blocking the air passage. If you see a foreign object, use your index finger to remove it. Make sure the person's tongue isn't blocking his or her airway.

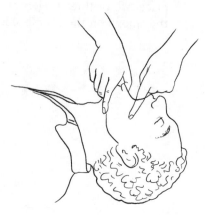

Establishing a clear airway is often enough to restore breathing. If there are still no signs of breathing, check for a heartbeat.

Check for a Heartbeat

You only need to find out if the person's heart is beating; don't try to count the number of beats per minute. You can find the pulse most easily in one of two places:

▶ 1. The side of the neck. Press two of your fingers into the person's neck, just under the sharp curve of the jawbone. Be sure to do this on the side of the person's neck closest to you to avoid putting any pressure on the person's throat.

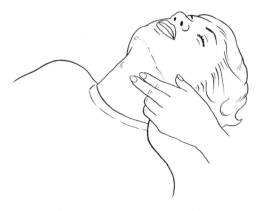

▶ 2. The wrist. Turn the person's hand so the palm is facing upward, and place two or three fingers an inch or so above the wrist joint (toward the elbow) on the thumb side of the wrist.

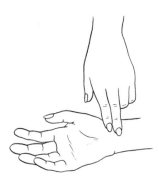

(For practice, try finding your own pulse in these two places. When checking a pulse, use your fingers, not your thumb, because there's an artery in the thumb that can give a false reading.)

If you do find a heartbeat, then keep checking for it every minute or so until help arrives. If there are no signs of breathing and no pulse, attempt CPR.

If Necessary, Attempt CPR

Cardiopulmonary resuscitation (CPR) is a two-part procedure that keeps some blood circulating in the body and is a temporary substitute for breathing. Breathing and blood flow maintain the supply of oxygen to the brain that a person needs in order to live.

> *Special Note:* Although the following instructions explain how to perform CPR, they are *not* a substitute for taking a course in CPR and practicing it under the supervision of a trained expert. The instructions are given here only as a memory refresher for those certified to perform CPR and as a possible aid if you have not had any training but must attempt to perform CPR in an emergency.
>
> *Warning:* CPR techniques are practiced on dummies, because it is extremely dangerous to perform CPR on a healthy, normal person who doesn't need it. Never practice CPR on another person!

Basic CPR is the same for adults, infants, and children, except for a few changes to account for their different sizes.

CPR for Adults

First check the person's breathing, following the directions given above. If the person isn't breathing, place the person on his or her back on a firm surface, put one of your hands on the person's chin and the other on the forehead, and tilt the person's head back until his or her mouth opens. Then do the following:

▶ 1. Check inside the person's mouth for any foreign objects or obstructions to breathing. Correct any problems you discover. Once the mouth is clear, use the fingers of your hand that is on the person's forehead to pinch his or her nostrils shut.

▶ 2. Place your mouth over the person's mouth so that your lips form a tight seal, and gently exhale into the other person's lungs for about 1 to 1.5 seconds, break away for an instant to inhale, and then do it again.

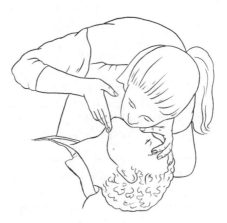

▶ 3. After two breaths into the lungs, use the hand that was placed under the person's chin to check his or her neck for a pulse. If there's a heartbeat, continue exhaling into the person's mouth until help arrives or until the person begins breathing without your assistance. If there's no heartbeat, proceed to the next step.

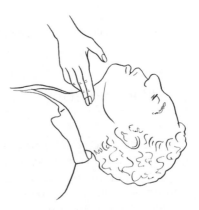

▶ 4. Kneel beside the person. With the fingers of your hand nearest the person's feet, feel his or her abdomen a few inches (centimeters) above the navel to locate the "V" notch where the two halves of the rib cage join together. Position your fingers about an inch above this "V" on the breastbone. (See diagram, top of next page.)

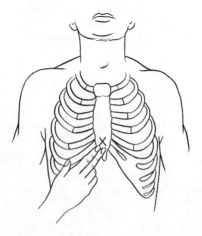

▶ 5. Place the heel of your other hand over the spot you located. You should be able to feel the bones beneath your palm.

▶ 6. Next, put your other hand on top of the hand you have in place and interlock your fingers. Use only the palms of your hands, and keep your fingers from pressing into the person's rib cage.

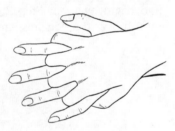

▶ 7. Straighten your arms and lock your elbows. Lean forward until your shoulders are directly above your hands on the person's chest.

▶ 8. Using the weight of your body, press down so that the person's breastbone sinks in about 1.5 to 2 inches (4 to 5 cm). Then, relax the pressure, but keep your hands in place and your arms straight. Immediately apply the pressure again—enough to let you feel the person's chest sink in and then spring back to normal. You want to press down on the breastbone hard enough to squeeze the heart, thus causing it to push blood through the arteries. Repeat this press-release cycle about 15 times in 10 to 15 seconds. It's a quick motion, a sudden pressing then a releasing, over and over again.

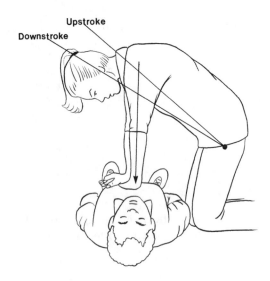

Upstroke

Downstroke

▶ 9. After doing 15 press-release cycles, stop, tilt the person's head back, and begin again at Step 2, pinching the nose closed, placing your mouth over the person's, and giving him or her two quick breaths.

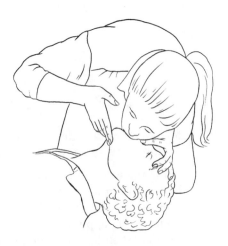

▶ 10. Continue the breathing and heart press-release cycles for a minute, then check again for a pulse. If you find signs of both a heartbeat and breathing, stop the CPR. Watch the person carefully, and if either the breathing or heartbeat stops, begin the CPR again. If the person is breathing but has no pulse, continue the chest press-release procedure. If you detect a pulse but no breathing, continue the mouth-to-mouth artificial respiration.

Even if you can't restart the person's heartbeat and breathing, continue the CPR as long as your strength holds out. Try to last until help arrives.

CPR for Infants

A baby's heart beats faster than an adult's, so you must give faster compressions. To locate the correct spot on the chest for applying pressure, put your index finger on the baby's breastbone between the two nipples: The place you want is one finger-width below that point. Use only two fingers, and press down only about an inch (2.5 cm). You want to deliver about five compressions every 3 to 4 seconds.

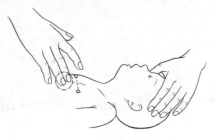

A baby's lungs are much smaller than those of an adult, so be sure to give smaller breaths. Use the same method as for adults to give one very gentle breath through the baby's mouth into the baby's lungs after every five compressions. Making a seal around the baby's mouth and nose with your open mouth may make it easier to give the breaths gently.

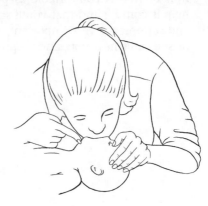

CPR for Children Up to 8 Years Old

Use the heel of only one hand to press down on the lower breastbone about 1 to 1.5 inches (2.5 to 4 cm), at a rate of about five compressions every 4 to 5 seconds. After every five compressions, give one shallow breath. For children over the age of 8, perform CPR as you would for an adult.

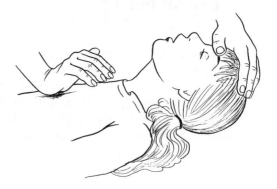

Other Things to Know about CPR

Even when CPR is given by a trained professional, it is common for the person receiving CPR to vomit as a result of air being forced into the stomach. If the person vomits, turn him or her to one side, clean out the mouth, establish an open airway as before, and resume CPR.

Once the person's heartbeat and respiration have been restored, make him or her as comfortable as possible. Offer continual reassurance that help is coming and that you'll stay right there until it arrives. Reassurance and support are very important, so talk to the person even if you think he or she can't hear you, and be positive.

CHAPTER 22

How to Choose and Work with Your Doctor

Today, high-technology diagnostic procedures and sophisticated treatments can cure diseases that in the past were incurable, including many kinds of heart disease. But these advances have not come without a sacrifice: the relationship between patient and doctor has become less personal.

How the Relationship between Patient and Doctor Has Changed

Until a few decades ago, people usually had one doctor and knew that doctor over a long period. Patients trusted that their doctors would offer the best treatment according to the doctor's judgment. Rarely did the doctor discuss alternative treatments with patients and let them decide which one they thought was best. Today, however, the medical community is larger and more business-oriented, and the patient has become a consumer of medical goods and services.

The explosion in medical knowledge has made specialization the norm, but the process of replacing one doctor with several has created a very different patient–physician relationship. More and more patients want to know their options and don't hesitate to ask questions. Moreover, informed consent—the policy that each patient must be fully informed of the consequences of a treatment before they receive it—is required for most surgical procedures.

A growing number of patients also want to participate directly in making their own health care decisions. They want to discuss the issues and options with their doctor. To do this, you must be well informed. Obtaining information isn't difficult: Reports of new medical research, revised medical theories, and refuted medical studies fill our news media. But while this unceasing flow of data can help somewhat, it often only creates confusion.

Your doctor can help resolve this confusion by talking straightforwardly with you, offering both facts and reliable reference sources. Doctors now must *guide* their patients instead of directing them. This doesn't mean that you should become your own doctor, but you now have more reason to stay abreast of medical developments.

How to Select the Right Doctor

Many people spend more time and effort finding a competent plumber than a competent doctor. Remember, though, that choosing a competent doctor can save you money and give you better health protection.

Family members, friends, and coworkers all are good sources for finding a doctor. If you know a medical professional, ask for his or her opinion. Your health insurance company may also be able to suggest names. Your local medical society and many area hospitals offer physician referral services, although they will give you only the names of those doctors who belong to the society or have privileges at the hospital. Finally, if your firm has a human resources department, someone there may be able to give you a list of reputable doctors.

Narrowing the Possibilities

Once you have a list of several recommended doctors, you can narrow the field in several ways. Since convenience is important, you may want to consider the distance between the offices of recommended doctors and your home or workplace. You may also want to consider other problems of getting to a doctor's office, including the availability of parking or public transportation.

If you're seeking a specialist, rather than a family practitioner or internist, another good idea is to look for those doctors who are board-certified in that specialty. Board certification is an added recommendation, because a doctor may specialize in a given area of medicine but not get the additional training needed to become board-certified. To find out whether a particular doctor is board-certified, call the American Board of Medical Specialties at 800–776–2378. Both the call and the service are free. All you need is the doctor's full name and the city and state in which he or she practices. You can also ask about memberships in professional societies.

After narrowing your list, you may want to arrange a get-acquainted interview. Some doctors don't charge for such a meeting, whereas others charge according to the time they spend with you.

Visiting the Office On your first visit, you should try to find out as much as you can about your new doctor. Is the staff friendly and helpful? Is the office environment pleasant?

Since you're there to learn, be sure to ask questions, and don't ignore your personal likes and dislikes. For instance, if you can't stand to wait, you may not want a doctor who's always behind schedule. Although the nature of a medical practice makes it impossible for a doctor to be on time for every appointment, you should be told if you'll be kept waiting for more than 20 minutes.

Take a little time to discuss fees. Explain that you wish to know what an office visit and typical procedures, tests, and treatments are likely to cost.

Look for a doctor with whom you're comfortable talking. Let him or her know how important you think this relationship is.

Communicating Effectively with Your Doctor You'll benefit most from a visit to your doctor if you talk as well as listen. Here are some guidelines to help you communicate better:

- Take notes. The doctor takes notes about you (which are kept in your file), and you should take notes, too. It may be hard to remember everything said during a discussion, especially if the topic is complicated. Also, taking notes may help you decide whether you have more questions.
- Be sure you understand what you're being told. Ask for clarification if you're not certain what your doctor means or if you don't understand certain words.
- Be frank and complete. Tell your doctor *all* of your problems and symptoms. Mentioning just one or two when you have three or four makes the diagnosis more difficult, and what you may regard as only minor symptoms may actually be important clues.
- Don't try to diagnose yourself. The reason you go to a doctor is to take advantage of his or her expertise.

- If possible, stay calm and don't let your emotions get the best of you until you have all the facts.
- Ask about any proposed tests or treatments. In particular, ask why the test is needed, what it will show, and if additional tests will be necessary. Find out the cost of the test and whether there's a less-expensive alternative. Inquire about the possibility of complications or risks relating to the proposed test or procedure, and whether you'll need to be hospitalized or will receive anesthesia. And last, but hardly least, ask what is most likely to happen if the test or procedure is *not* performed.
- If you're sick or don't feel well enough to receive information from your doctor or to ask questions, have someone you trust do so for you.
- If you have trouble talking with your doctor, tell him or her. If you still can't seem to communicate clearly, you should consider going to another doctor.

How to Use Medications Wisely

To become a conscientious drug consumer, you may want to ask your physician the following questions, to enable you to get the maximum benefit from the drugs you take:

- How does this drug work?
- What is its name?
- What is my exact dosage?
- Is there a certain time of day when it's best for me to take this medication?
- Is it better to take this drug before or after meals?
- May I drink alcohol while taking this drug?
- What results can I expect from this drug?
- How long must I take it before I can expect those results?
- Will this drug conflict with the other drugs I'm taking?
- How should I store the drug?
- For how long must I take it?
- How many times can my prescription be renewed?
- Are there any special instructions I need?
- Which side effects should I know about, and which can I ignore?

- Is this drug available in a less-expensive, generic form?
- What should I do if I forget to take this drug at the recommended time?
- If I don't use all of the prescription, may I save it for later?

In addition, here are some things you can do to make any medication you need to take work best, and be most cost-effective:

- Follow the storage instructions provided with your drug. If no such information is offered, ask for it.
- Follow the dosage recommendations. Don't improvise. Taking twice as much won't make you feel twice as good or work twice as fast.
- Do *not* share your prescription with someone else, even if that person has similar symptoms.
- Buy only 2 or 3 days' worth of a new drug. This will allow you to discover if you have any troubling side effects. Also, if your doctor decides to change your prescription during the first week, you won't have wasted any money.
- Ask your doctor for free samples. This is a great way to try a new drug.
- Ask about discounts when buying drugs in volume.
- Look into cost savings that might be available if you join a prescription plan and buy through the mail.
- Keep a record of the drugs you take. This is an important, valuable document and could be a lifesaver. List each drug by the name on the prescription, and note when you began taking it, the dosage, and the date of each prescription refill.

Your local library and other sources offer a number of drug reference books, many of which were written for laypersons. Learning about the drugs you're taking can often be helpful and may head off unforeseen problems.

The Value of a Good Pharmacist

Shop carefully for a pharmacist, too. A good pharmacist is an invaluable source of information about drugs. Your pharmacist keeps a list of the drugs you buy and refers to it each time you fill a prescription, to help you prevent possibly dangerous reactions between drugs or allergic reactions to them. Your pharmacist can also advise you on which over-the-counter remedies you should avoid while taking other medications. It's probably a good idea, too, to let your pharmacist know if you experience unwanted side effects from a prescribed drug. In short, your pharmacist is usually your best and most convenient source of drug information.

What You Should Know If You Have to Go to the Hospital

If your doctor recommends that you be admitted to the hospital, you should ask the following questions:

- Is there an alternative to going to the hospital?
- Is the recommended hospital the best one for this purpose? For example, you will want to make sure that the particular type of surgery or test proposed is frequently performed there.
- How long will your hospital stay last, and what are the expected costs? Is there any way to shorten your stay?

Have your doctor explain exactly what you should expect while in the hospital. If your stay in the hospital doesn't go as described, be sure to ask why while you're there.

When you're discharged from the hospital, take time to check your bill for these basics:

- Were you billed for the right kind of room (that is, private, semiprivate, or whatever)?
- Were you billed for the correct number of days?
- Were you billed correctly for the time you spent in special units, such as intensive care?
- Were you billed for only those tests you actually received?
- Were you billed for only those medications you actually received?

Hospitals go to great lengths to account properly for all charges. But occasionally they do make mistakes, so it's a good idea to check your hospital bill carefully.

Doing your part to lower medical costs by being an effective medical consumer has two advantages: First, you'll save money, and second, you'll improve the quality of health care for yourself and your community.

CHAPTER 23

The Cardiovascular System

Your heart and your circulatory system make up your *cardiovascular system*. Your heart, the main organ of your cardiovascular system, is the pump that drives life-sustaining blood to your organs, tissues, and cells. Blood from the heart is carried through *arteries* and *capillaries,* then returned to the heart through *venules* and *veins*—thus forming a closed loop. Your heart and blood vessels circulate blood throughout your body constantly. This blood delivers oxygen and nutrients to every cell, and also removes the carbon dioxide and other waste products generated by those cells.

The Heart

Your heart weighs between 7 and 15 ounces (200 and 425 grams), and it's the most dependable pump ever created. By the end of a long life, a person's heart may have beat more than 3.5 *billion* times, without maintenance or repairs—a feat that remains beyond the reach of man-made technology.

Located between your two lungs in the middle of your chest, your heart is situated with about two-thirds of it on the left side of your breastbone and about one-third on the right (see Figure 5). To hold it in place, the heart has a remarkable covering: a shock-absorbing double membrane called the *pericardium*. The outer layer of the pericardium surrounds the

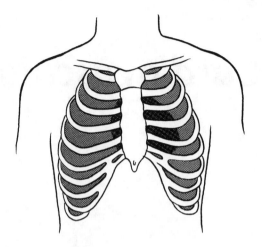

FIGURE 5   *The heart's location in the chest.*

roots of the heart's major blood vessels, and is attached by ligaments to the spinal column, the diaphragm, and other parts of the body. This outer layer is separated from the inner layer of the pericardium by a coating of fluid that acts as a lubricant; the inner layer of the pericardium is then attached to the heart muscle. This double membrane allows the heart to move during contractions yet remain firmly anchored in the body.

The central portion of the heart itself consists of four chambers (see Figure 6). The upper chambers, one on the left and another on the right, are called the *atria*. The lower chambers, again one on the left and another on the right, are called the *ventricles*. Separating the right and left atria, and the right and left ventricles, is a wall of muscle called the *septum*.

The Valves

The cardiovascular system, continuous and circular in movement, is truly a one-way street. The valves, when working properly, ensure that all traffic moves in the proper direction.

The valves accomplish this goal by opening at just the right time, then closing tight to prevent backflow. See Figure 7: After blood returning from the body fills the right atrium, it's forced from the right atrium through the *tricuspid valve* into the right ventricle. There, the right ventricle pumps the blood through the *pulmonary valve* to the lungs. Just as the right ven-

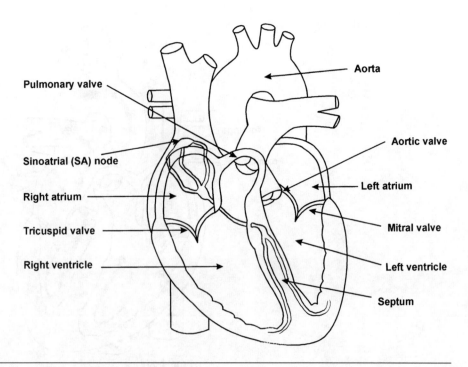

FIGURE 6   *Some important parts of the heart.*

tricle readies itself to exert this push, the tricuspid valve seals off, preventing blood from leaking backward from the right ventricle into the right atrium.

At the same time that blood from the right atrium moves into the right ventricle, the blood returning from the lungs flows into the *left* atrium and is forced through the *mitral valve* into the left ventricle. Then, just as the right ventricle is pumping blood to the lungs, the left ventricle forces blood through the *aortic valve* to the rest of the body—with the mitral valve, of course, sealing off to prevent backflow. At each juncture, the valves ensure that the blood moves in one direction only.

To enhance the flow of blood and protect heart muscle tissue from damage, the insides of each heart chamber and of the valves are lined with a smooth membrane called the *endocardium*. Behind the endocardium are the walls of the heart's four chambers. The muscle tissue that forms these walls is called the *myocardium;* it contracts when stimulated by an electrical current. Therefore, the myocardium must have a taut yet flexible strength to accomplish its job of contracting and pushing blood forward on its circulatory path.

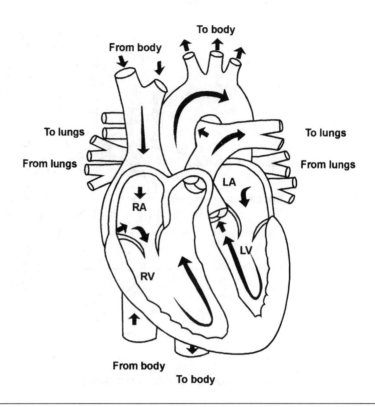

FIGURE 7   *The origins and direction of blood flow in the heart.*

The Conduction System

The heart's conduction system is similar to the ignition system of an engine. The heart contracts by means of electrical impulses generated in cells of the heart muscle, the myocardium. These specialized cells are responsible for conducting the electrical stimulus from one part of the heart to another.

This electrical stimulus originates in the *sinoatrial (SA) node*, which is located at the top of the right atrium. From there it travels through the muscle fibers of both atria to the left and right ventricles.

Because the sinoatrial node regulates the beating action of the heart, it is sometimes called the heart's natural pacemaker. At times, when the sinoatrial node fails to carry out its job, another part of the conduction system may take over ignition responsibilities, but this shift may lead to certain kinds of irregularities in the heart's rhythm (see chapter 27 for more on arrhythmias).

The Circulatory System

The circulatory system carries blood to all parts of the body—including to the heart itself. Two *coronary arteries* serve to transport blood to the heart muscle; they exit the *aorta,* the large artery that carries oxygen-rich blood throughout the body, about a half inch above the aortic valve. As these coronary arteries go around the outside of the heart muscle, they divide into smaller vessels and then into capillaries. These capillaries deliver oxygen and nutrients to the heart cells, and also remove carbon dioxide and other waste products. Then this blood returns through *coronary veins* to the right atrium, where it meets the blood returning from the rest of the body. All of it is then ready to go to the lungs for a renewed supply of oxygen that it can again deliver throughout the body.

Blood flows through your body's one-way circulatory system by means of a series of arteries, veins, and smaller blood vessels (see Figures 8 and 9). Arteries carry blood away from your heart, while veins transport it back.

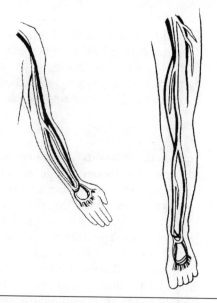

FIGURE 8   *The veins and arteries in a human arm and leg. The dark lines represent the veins, and the white lines represent the arteries.*

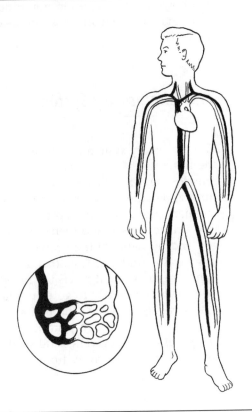

FIGURE 9   *The major arteries and veins in the human body.*
*The inset depicts capillaries in which oxygen-rich blood from the heart
(shown as white) is depleted of its oxygen by the surrounding tissue and
becomes venous (oxygen-poor) blood (shown as black), which will then
return to the heart and lungs to pick up more oxygen.*

Your body contains 20 major arteries, which trace an elaborate path
through your tissues. The arteries branch into smaller vessels called *arterioles,* and then into smaller and smaller vessels, known as *capillaries.*

Capillaries are the true deliverer of the goods—oxygen and nutrients—
to the cells. Many of these capillaries are thinner than a hair; in fact, the
walls of most capillaries are just one cell thick, and many capillaries are so
tiny that only one blood cell at a time can move through them.

Once capillaries complete their task of delivering oxygen and nutrients and picking up carbon dioxide and other waste products, the route
back to the heart is through ever-widening vessels called *venules* that even-

tually join to form veins. Because the blood pressure in the veins is signifi-cantly lower than that in the arteries, the walls of veins don't need to be as thick as the walls of arteries. But this lower pressure also means that a series of valves is needed inside the largest veins. These valves ensure that blood pushed upward against the force of gravity will continue to the heart instead of flowing backward and pooling in the legs or feet. Gener-ally, the paths of arteries and veins run quite close together.

Your heart and circulatory system are adept at making adjustments based on your level of activity. When you increase your level of physical activity, your heart begins to work harder to meet your body's need for oxygen in its cells. The heart beats faster and with more force, the two coronary arteries expand, and blood is moved more quickly to all organs. To keep up with very vigorous exercise, your heart can increase its flow of blood through the arteries up to five or six times its normal rate.

The arteries and arterioles also help control your blood pressure by en-larging or contracting as needed to increase or decrease blood flow. The walls of the medium-sized and larger blood vessels are made up of a layer of smooth muscle tissue lined with a layer of smooth cells, the *endothe-lium*. This combination forms a smooth pipeline within a pipeline, which helps protect the walls of the vessels and facilitate the flow of blood.

Blood

While the circulatory system is the route by which cells receive life-sus-taining nutrition, the blood is the actual *carrier* of that nutrition. Blood is a fluid containing a great variety of cells within *plasma*, a yellowish liquid that's 90 percent water. But in addition to the water, plasma contains vari-ous salts, sugar (glucose), and other substances. And, most important, plasma contains proteins that carry vital nutrients to all body cells and bolster the functioning of the immune system.

Three types of blood cells circulate with the plasma: *platelets, red blood cells,* and *white blood cells.* The platelets help blood to clot, which stops it from flowing out of the body when a vein or artery is broken. Red blood cells—the most numerous of the three types, with about 35 trillion in a healthy adult—are the oxygen-carriers. The body creates these cells at a rate of about 2.4 million a second, and they each have a life span of about 120 days. White blood cells ward off infection. These cells, which come in a variety of shapes and sizes, are vital to the immune system. When the body is fighting off infection, it makes them in ever-increasing numbers. Still, compared to red blood cells, their quantity is low: Most healthy adults have about 700 times as many red blood cells as white ones.

The Cardiovascular System at Work

You've just read how various parts of the cardiovascular system operate; now here's a look at the whole system in action.

Although your heart's entire double-pump sequence takes only about a second, a lot happens in that short time. See Figure 10. As blood flows into and collects in the right and left atria, the sinoatrial node sends out an electrical impulse. This impulse causes the atria to contract, sending blood through the open tricuspid and mitral valves into the right and left ventricles, respectively. This part of the two-part pumping sequence is called the *diastolic phase;* it takes up more than half the time of the full cycle.

At the end of the diastolic phase, the right and left ventricles are full of blood from the right and left atria. The electrical impulse from the sinus node spreads along its cellular pathway to the ventricles, causing them to contract—which begins the shorter *systolic phase.* As pressure inside the contracting ventricles builds, the tricuspid and mitral valves shut tight, preventing blood from flowing backward into the atria. At the same time, the pulmonary valve in the right ventricle and the aortic valve in the left

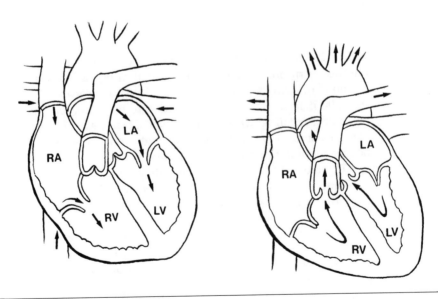

FIGURE 10   *The direction of blood flow and the opening and closing of heart valves during the diastolic (shown on the left) and systolic (shown on the right) phases of a heartbeat.*

ventricle are pushed open. From the right ventricle, blood flows to the lungs to pick up oxygen. From the left ventricle, blood flows to the heart and other parts of the body carrying oxygen-rich blood.

When they have finished contracting, the ventricles relax. The blood that has now moved out of the ventricles into the pulmonary artery and the aorta exerts pressure backward on the ventricular valves, forcing them to close. The atrial valves, no longer forced shut by blood pressure in the ventricles, open up, and the cycle begins again. This series of smoothly synchronized contractions is repeated continuously—more times per minute when you're exerting yourself, and fewer times per minute when you're at rest.

The amount of blood the heart pumps depends on two factors: (1) the number of times it beats per minute, and (2) the volume of blood that the ventricles eject each time they contract, which is known as the *stroke volume*. The ventricles normally squeeze out about half the blood they contain with each contraction—about 3 ounces (90 ml) from each ventricle. At a rate of 70 beats per minute (which is normal for a resting adult), the ventricles are moving 210 ounces (6.2 liters) of blood through the circulatory system every minute, or about 100 gallons (379 liters) every hour!

On its one-way journey through the circulatory system, all blood travels to the lungs for oxygen before setting off throughout the rest of the body. In the lungs, the blood exchanges carbon dioxide for oxygen. As this trade takes place, the color of the blood changes from a bluish red to a brilliant scarlet. Then the oxygen-rich blood travels to the left atrium and from there on to the left ventricle.

The left ventricle, the largest and strongest chamber in the heart, serves as the main pumping station for the entire body. Its chamber wall is often a half inch thick, with enough contraction power in its muscle to push blood through the aortic valve and into the main arterial system. Its pumping action *must* be forceful: It has to overcome the resistance of gravity and maintain the body's circulation.

As you've just read, each heartbeat consists of a double-pump sequence: First the atria squeeze blood into the ventricles, then the ventricles pump blood out of the heart. In addition, the heart can also be thought of as a double pump in a different way: One stroke sends oxygen-depleted blood to the lungs, and a second, simultaneous stroke sends the oxygen-enriched blood from the lungs through the body. Since your body's cells need oxygenated blood constantly, your heart can never rest. No wonder it's called the hardest working muscle in your body.

Your heart doesn't, however, act as a fully independent agent. Other parts of the body control and interact with it in vital ways. Your brain and other nerve centers are constantly tracking the conditions in your physical world, such as climate and your level of physical activity. They then use this information to adjust your cardiovascular system to changing circumstances. When you exercise, for example, your brain sends a series of chemical commands to your cardiovascular system. These include instructions for your blood to flow faster to your lungs, your arteries to expand, and your heart and breathing rates to increase. The kidneys also directly affect the heart by signaling how much fluid to retain. *Renin*, a substance produced by the kidneys, increases the retention of water and sodium—and, therefore, also increases blood pressure.

Don't Ignore a Heart Problem

During the hours and days that make up their lives, most healthy people give little or no thought to the constant and regular pumping action of their hearts. The quiet beat and the modest amount of movement in their chests don't attract their conscious attention. Yet the distinctive sounds produced by vibrations in the heart structure, the noise of the valves in operation, and the turbulence created by the circulating blood are all very revealing to a physician listening with a stethoscope. To a trained ear, these sounds tell a great deal.

The human heart is a muscle that's capable of remaining strong and reliable for 100 years or longer. Yet it may also malfunction. The cardiovascular system is a set of components that must function in perfect harmony. When heart function or blood circulation is interrupted or disturbed for even short periods of time, life is at risk. For these reasons, any breakdown in the cardiovascular system calls for your *immediate* attention. And in most cases, the care you get will extend your life.

CHAPTER 24

The Symptoms of Heart Disease

The earlier you can spot a heart problem and get medical attention, the sooner you can begin getting the treatment you need. Any signs of heart disease should send you to your doctor without delay—so it's important to know what they are. But you also need to know that it's possible to have some forms of heart disease without noticing any symptoms.

Each of the symptoms of heart disease may stem from a problem other than your heart. Yet you need to pay attention to your body's signals and act if you experience one or more of these warning signs: shortness of breath, fatigue, fainting, palpitations, swelling of tissue, skin discoloration, and chest pain.

Shortness of Breath

The single most common symptom of heart disease is shortness of breath. But the kind of shortness of breath that's related to heart disease is *not* the kind you experience after exercising vigorously, having sex, or walking up a flight of stairs. After all, it's normal to feel winded after activities requiring physical exertion.

The type of breathlessness that may signal heart disease is when you feel short of breath after doing routine things—such as walking at your usual pace or even sitting quietly. Sometimes this type of shortness of breath seems to come on suddenly, without any special reason. If you notice shortness of breath that you can't associate with any physical exertion, pay attention. It's a sign that something is wrong. Although the cause may not be heart-related, you should see your physician as soon as possible.

Fatigue

Fatigue is another common sign of heart disease, although there can also be many other reasons for it, both physical and psychological. Depression, for instance, can often make a person feel generally tired all the time. And fatigue is often associated with diabetes, some lung diseases, and hypothyroidism. Several medications, including some used to treat high blood pressure, can also contribute to fatigue.

Heart-related fatigue comes from a weakening of the heart muscle such that the heart can't pump enough blood to nourish the cells in the body. Usually, a person experiencing heart-related fatigue feels a normal amount of energy upon waking in the morning, but feels more and more tired as the day wears on. By late in the day, the person may feel completely exhausted, may lose all appetite for food, and may feel great weakness or heaviness in the legs.

Don't ignore fatigue. Although it could be caused by not eating or sleeping properly, or by a high level of stress, it can also be a warning sign of a heart problem. Your physician can determine whether or not it is heart-related and can recommend appropriate treatment for you.

Fainting

Fainting, which is the sudden loss of consciousness, can be triggered by stress from a number of sources, both physical and emotional. Fright, extreme shock, or pain can all make a person faint. But both fainting and a feeling that you are about to faint (light-headedness, sometimes referred to as dizziness) can also be a sign of heart disease. In either case, the heart fails to deliver sufficient oxygen-rich blood to the brain. If the brain doesn't receive oxygen for a period of about 10 seconds, fainting results.

Abnormalities of the heart, circulatory system, and brain can cause fainting. The most common cause of heart-related fainting is an irregular heartbeat, called *arrhythmia*. The heart either beats too slowly to deliver enough blood to the brain, or beats so fast that the heart's pumping action is interrupted, again causing too little blood to be delivered to the brain. Fainting can also be caused by blocked arteries, especially those in the neck that carry blood to the brain.

You should consider any fainting spell serious enough to warrant a doctor's attention—especially if you can tell that it's related to an irregularity or change in your heart rate.

Palpitations

Like most people, you've probably experienced a skipped or missed heartbeat at one time or another. What has really happened is that your heart has experienced an *early extra* beat. That is, your heart has displayed a minor irregularity by beating prematurely and then immediately beating more strongly—a sort of catch-up beat. It is the strength of this catch-up beat that makes you feel as if you've skipped a beat. This is a common type of heart palpitation: Unless you experience it frequently, it shouldn't give you reason to worry.

When palpitations are severe, they would likely give you a fluttering sensation or a sudden thudding as if your heart were trying to roll over. Certainly any sudden awareness of the force or irregularity of your own heartbeat can be disturbing as well as physically uncomfortable.

Various substances and events can cause your heart to palpitate. For example, caffeine, smoking, overeating, hard exercise, emotional stress, and some medications can alter your heartbeat. Because so many different things could be the cause, it's often difficult for you to know if your palpitations are serious. But any extremely rapid series of heartbeats that lasts for more than 2 or 3 minutes and that you cannot relate to strenuous physical activity is good reason to contact your doctor. And if you notice that palpitations are accompanied by chest pain, shortness of breath, or an overall feeling of weakness, you should seek help immediately.

Swelling of Tissue

The swelling of tissue, called *edema*, is frequently a sign of heart disease. It may occur around the eyes or on the chest, abdomen, legs, or ankles. Exactly where it occurs could be a sign of what kind of heart problem there is.

Swelling in the abdomen or legs usually indicates that the muscle on the right side of the heart may be weakened. This weakness means that the right ventricle is pumping a lesser volume of blood to the lungs—and that more blood is therefore building up in the veins in the body that lead back to the right atrium. As a result, the abdomen and legs swell. Ankles that become puffy after standing for a short time can also be related to this right-sided heart failure. The most common cause of right-sided heart failure is left-sided heart failure.

Failure of only the heart's left side may cause swelling of tissue. Usually, however, weakness there tends to cause shortness of breath as pressure builds in the veins branching out from the pulmonary veins and in the lungs themselves.

Of course, not all swelling is caused by heart disease. Often women experience swelling in their ankles and feet during the final portion of their pregnancies. And travelers who sit for long periods in cars, planes, and trains, or anyone whose movement is restricted, may experience some swelling as well.

With these exceptions, however, tissue swelling is abnormal. It's a sign of serious disease, whether heart disease, kidney disorder, liver disease, certain forms of cancer, or diseases affecting the lymphatic system. So if you have any type of chest, abdominal, leg, or ankle swelling, or if you're consistently puffy around the eyes, you should check with your physician.

Skin Discoloration

When the circulatory system can't deliver enough oxygen-rich blood to body cells, the skin, lips, and fingernails turn blue. Called *cyanosis* (cyan = blue), this discoloration usually indicates heart disease or a damaged heart.

A similar discoloration can also be caused by exposure to the cold. In that instance, the cold outdoor temperature signals the body to reroute the flow of blood by constricting the capillaries in the skin. There's a big difference between heart-related discoloration and this kind, however: The cold-related kind disappears as the body warms up again.

Anyone who has a persistent bluish coloring to the skin that's not related to being out in cold weather should visit a doctor right away.

Chest Pain

The most obvious symptom of heart disease is chest pain. If you experience it, you should be examined by a doctor without delay—even though, again, heart disease is not the only possible cause of it.

Angina

One type of chest pain is called *angina pectoris* (or just *angina,* for short). The name *angina pectoris* comes from Latin and means "strangling in the chest." People who experience it often describe it as a squeezing, suffocating, or pressure sensation. Angina occurs when a narrowed coronary artery (often blocked by plaque) can no longer deliver enough blood to a portion of the heart. Typically, this happens at a time when the heart has a greater-than-usual need for blood, especially during exercise.

The pain of angina is different from the pain that accompanies a heart attack, but angina may precede a heart attack. The pain of angina tends to start in the center of the chest, but it may radiate to the arms, neck, or jaw. Some people feel a numbness or loss of sensation in their arms, shoulders, or wrists. Most episodes last from 1 to 15 minutes. If the pain lasts longer than that, the person may be having a heart attack. The pain of angina usually occurs in response to physical exertion and emotional stress; it goes away with rest.

More than 85 percent of all cases of angina are directly related to atherosclerotic coronary artery disease. However, a few may result from spasms in an artery's muscular wall, disease of a heart valve, or abnormalities of the left ventricle.

In a way, those who experience an attack of angina are fortunate. They have received a warning about a heart problem. Because the inadequate supply of blood to their heart muscle (called *ischemia*) has caused physical pain, they have an opportunity to act. Certain other cases of inadequate supply of blood to the heart muscle do not cause pain; these cases are called *silent ischemia.*

Heart Attack

Most heart attacks, or *myocardial infarctions,* result from the complete blockage of a coronary artery. Such a blockage shuts off the blood flow, preventing oxygen and nutrients from reaching a section of the heart. Prompt medical treatment can minimize damage to the heart, but once tissue damage has occurred in a section of heart muscle, that destruction is generally permanent.

In most cases, a physician can diagnose that a patient has had a myocardial infarction by giving the patient a physical exam, taking his or her medical history, analyzing blood samples, and performing an electrocardiogram, which is an electronic assessment of heart muscle condition and electrical activity.

The classic heart attack begins with a sudden, powerful chest pain that patients describe as a crushing sensation or the feeling of being crushed by an incredibly heavy weight. Like the pain of angina, the pain of a heart attack may move to the arms, neck, or jaw.

Not everyone experiences exactly those classic symptoms, however. For some, the experience of a heart attack starts as a burning sensation very similar to indigestion or heartburn. For them, the pain may be limited to a fairly small area of the chest.

If you feel crushing chest pain that lasts 5 minutes or any chest pain that lasts 20 minutes or longer, don't try to decide exactly what's causing it. Instead, go immediately to your nearest emergency room for evaluation by a physician. If you're experiencing a heart attack, the important goal is to survive and salvage as much heart muscle as possible. *So don't delay.*

Combination of Symptoms

If you experience even one of the symptoms of heart disease described above, you should see your physician. Don't decide that you don't have "enough" symptoms.

Moreover, a combination of symptoms, such as chest pain along with palpitations of the heart and dizziness, calls for more immediate action. You need medical evaluation, and you may need swift treatment. Dialing 911 or having someone drive you straight to a hospital emergency room would not be an overreaction.

Remember, if you have a serious heart problem, prompt treatment may save your life. Therefore, you need to be familiar with all the symptoms of heart disease, spot them when they occur, and act immediately to get help.

CHAPTER 25

Congenital Heart Disease

Congenital heart problems are those present at birth. They include defects in the valves and chambers and also circulatory problems. About eight of every 1,000 infants are born with one or more heart or circulatory problems, and about half these cases are serious enough to require treatment.

The good news is that congenital defects are being detected earlier than ever—sometimes in the womb—and are being treated with refined medical and surgical methods, including less invasive methods than those used in the past.

Causes of Congenital Heart Disease

We can very rarely identify the exact cause of a congenital heart defect. Although genetic factors seem to play a part, families should be aware that medical researchers cannot predict most cases. Therefore, there's no point in trying to assess genetic "blame" or determine which side of the family "caused" the problem.

In addition to genetic factors, certain environmental and behavioral factors have been identified as interfering with the development of the fetus's heart during the first 10 weeks of gestation. Some conditions that alert a physician to the possibility of congenital heart disease in an infant include:

- Congenital heart disease in the mother or father.
- Congenital heart disease in a previous child or other relative.
- Diabetes in the mother.
- Rubella (German measles), toxoplasmosis (a protozoal infection transmitted via cat feces), or HIV infection in the mother.
- The mother's excessive use of alcohol.
- The mother's use of cocaine or other drugs.
- The mother's exposure during pregnancy to certain anticonvulsant and dermatologic medications.

Some of these conditions are far more preventable than others. The goal of medical researchers who identify these links is to encourage people to take all the reasonable preventive steps they can in preparing for their baby.

Even though there seem to be both genetic and environmental links to congenital heart disease, a pregnant woman's exposure to one or more of these environmental threats doesn't necessarily mean that her baby will be born with a heart defect. For example, not every mother who contracts rubella during pregnancy delivers a baby with a defective heart. Likewise, unless a specific chromosomal defect has been identified, the fact that an earlier child or close family member had a congenital heart defect does not guarantee that a baby will have a similar problem.

The Fetal Heart

During development inside the uterus, the growing fetus is fully dependent on the mother's circulatory system and the placenta for nourishment. The fetus is also dependent on the placenta as its source of oxygen and its means of removing carbon dioxide.

The fetus doesn't use its own lungs until birth, so its circulatory pathway is different from that of a newborn infant: Before birth, the heart doesn't have to pump blood to the lungs to pick up oxygen. So instead of having a separate left pulmonary artery and aorta, in the fetal heart, these two blood vessels are connected via a blood vessel called the *ductus arteriosus*. In addition, there is an opening between the right and left atria in the fetal heart, called the *foramen ovale*, which allows blood to circulate more directly from the *right* atrium to the *left* atrium during fetal development.

The ductus arteriosus and the opening between the two atria exist as parts of the circulatory system before birth, but that system changes after birth.

These temporary routes naturally close up shortly after birth, when the baby's lungs and cardiovascular system take over. And because the fetal heart has a circulatory system different from the one the baby uses after birth, some heart defects become apparent days or weeks after birth that weren't spotted earlier.

Types of Congenital Heart Disease

The most common congenital heart defects are:

- Abnormalities that impede the flow of blood through the vessels.
- Heart valves that are malformed, missing, or blocking blood flow.
- Problems with the structure of the heart that allow blood to flow from one side to the other outside the normal circulatory path.
- Problems with the connections between the main arteries or veins and the heart.

The outlook for most children born with heart problems is optimistic. Although in some cases physicians may recommend that the children limit their physical activity, young patients can often expect to live normal lives.

More than one congenital problem may be present at the same time, but we'll discuss each of 12 specific diagnoses separately in the next few pages. We've included an illustration of a normal heart here (see Figure 11) for comparison with the illustrations of the various defects.

Ventricular and Atrial Septal Defects

A *septal defect* is a hole in the septum, the muscle wall separating the right from the left atrium and the right from the left ventricle. When a child is born with a hole in the septum, blood leaks back from the left side of the heart, where the pressure is higher, to the right. If the leakage is minor, it may create only minor problems, but if it's significant, it can make for inefficient blood flow throughout the body and lead to enlargement of a heart chamber. When such a leakage occurs, the heart may be overworked, and a child will have difficulty breathing and growing normally.

Septal defects are named for the location of the hole: a ventricular septal defect or an atrial septal defect.

A *ventricular septal defect* is a hole in the septum between the right and left ventricles (see Figure 12). In normal circulation, of course, blood

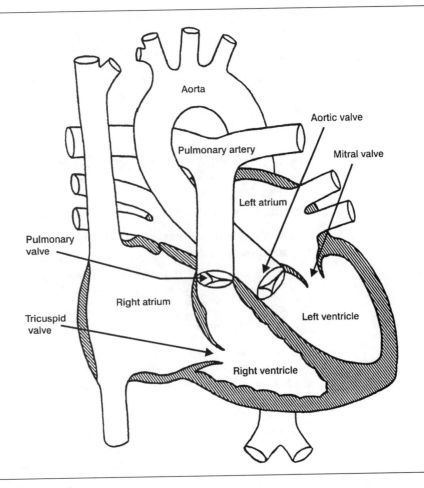

FIGURE 11

A normal heart.
Adapted from Mullins DE, Mayer DC. Congenital heart disease: A dia-
grammatic atlas. *© 1988 Wiley-Liss, Inc. By permission of Wiley-Liss, Inc.,*
a division of John Wiley & Sons, Inc.

moves from the right ventricle to the lungs to pick up oxygen before moving on to the left atrium and left ventricle, from where it's then pumped
out through the aorta to all body organs. With a ventricular septal defect,
some of the oxygen-rich blood in the left ventricle leaks back to the right
ventricle and is unnecessarily recirculated to the lungs.

The result, in addition to extra blood being sent to the lungs, is a reduced amount of blood sent throughout the body. In response, the left
ventricle works harder than ever to maintain adequate circulation. Eventually, the heart may become enlarged, which can bring about even poorer

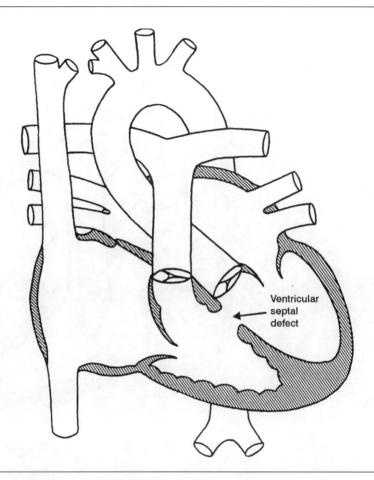

Ventricular
septal
defect

FIGURE 12

The ventricular septal defect is a hole in the wall (septum) between the two ventricles.

Adapted from Mullins DE, Mayer DC. Congenital heart disease: A diagrammatic atlas. © 1988 Wiley-Liss, Inc. By permission of Wiley-Liss, Inc., a division of John Wiley & Sons, Inc.

heart function and further reduce the amount of blood circulated throughout the body. Symptoms of ventricular septal defects, including respiratory distress, heart failure, and failure to grow, may not become evident for weeks after birth. Surgical repair of the hole will probably be recommended unless spontaneous closure occurs.

Fortunately, many ventricular septal defects naturally close—either partially or completely—during the first 7 years of life. And some cases of partial closure don't require surgery unless the remaining hole causes heart enlargement.

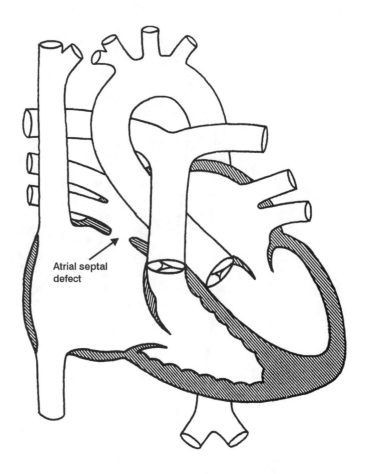

Atrial septal
defect

FIGURE 13   *In the ostium secundum atrial septal defect, the normal hole present in the wall (septum) between the two atria fails to close after birth.*
Adapted from Mullins DE, Mayer DC. Congenital heart disease: A diagrammatic atlas. *© 1988 Wiley-Liss, Inc. By permission of Wiley-Liss, Inc., a division of John Wiley & Sons, Inc.*

An *atrial septal defect* most frequently involves the failure of the normal hole present between the fetus's two atria to close (see Figure 13). In this defect, called an *ostium secundum defect*, the oval-shaped hole in the fetus's atrial septum fails to close naturally soon after birth.

About one-fourth of atrial septal defects close by themselves before the child is 2 years old. After that time, natural closure is rare, so serious cases (those in which the right side of the heart is enlarged) typically require surgery. Traditional surgery usually involves repairing the hole with a fabric patch graft. Recent advances have also been made in less invasive repair methods: Through a catheterization procedure, a small umbrella-like device can be implanted to cover the hole.

Often, the symptoms of atrial septal defects don't appear during childhood. Instead, the effects are quite gradual. A child with the defect may be unusually slender, but not until adulthood does the gradual enlargement of the right atrium take its toll. Then, the person may experience arrhythmias, especially *atrial fibrillation* or heart failure, a condition in which the heart can't pump enough blood to supply the body's needs. Heart failure can cause congestion of blood and fluid in the body tissues, such as the lungs, liver, abdomen, and legs.

Common Atrioventricular Canal Defect

Commonly known as a *complete atrioventricular canal,* this septal defect is a complex problem—and about half the babies with it also have Down syndrome. In all forms, it involves a defect right at the part of the septum where the atria and ventricles meet—the "four-corners" spot (see Figure 14).

At this spot, the tricuspid valve normally directs blood from the right atrium to the right ventricle, while the mitral valve allows blood to move from the left atrium to the left ventricle. But if the canal defect is complete, just one large hole and one valve are there instead, and the valve may not close all the way, allowing free communication of blood among all four chambers.

Children with a complete canal defect develop heart failure and lung problems. Their hearts work overtime, producing heart enlargement, emaciation, and at times blue discoloration in their lips and fingernails. Nearly always, surgery is needed in the first few months after birth to correct a complete canal defect.

Patent Ductus Arteriosus

Patent ductus arteriosus (PDA) is a defect in which the temporary blood vessel connecting the left pulmonary artery to the aorta in the fetus fails to close in the newborn (see Figure 15). As discussed earlier, fetal circulation bypasses the lungs and gets its oxygen from the placenta. But at birth, the newborn's lungs take over, the body stops producing the chemicals that have kept the ductus arteriosus open, and it naturally closes.

If it fails to close completely, the baby has the defect PDA. While the problem is relatively uncommon, it is sometimes associated with mothers who have had rubella (German measles) during pregnancy and with infants born prematurely. The result of this defect is that too much blood travels to the lungs. The severity of the problem depends on how large the opening remains and how prematurely the baby was born.

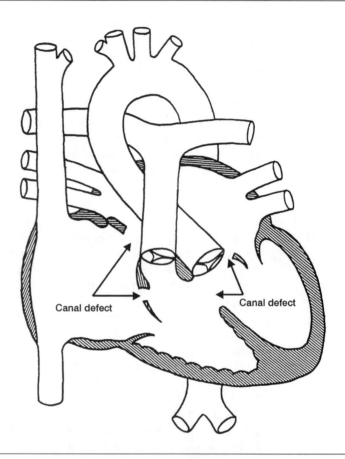

Canal defect

Canal defect

FIGURE 14

In the canal defect, a large hole exists between both the atria and both the ventricles, and the tricuspid and mitral valves are deformed.
Adapted from Mullins DE, Mayer DC. Congenital heart disease: A diagrammatic atlas. *© 1988 Wiley-Liss, Inc. By permission of Wiley-Liss, Inc., a division of John Wiley & Sons, Inc.*

Mild cases of PDA may be noticed only by a heart murmur that presents no problems, but severe cases involve a great excess of blood being sent to the lungs, which may increase the pulmonary artery pressure and fluid buildup, making the child short of breath and excessively tired. Sometimes, PDA is hard to diagnose in premature babies because they may need to be on a ventilator while their lungs mature; the ventilator relieves any fluid buildup in the lungs, and may mask the underlying problem, which is PDA.

Correction of PDA in premature infants sometimes entails treatment with medications that stimulate the ductus to close. At other times, sur-

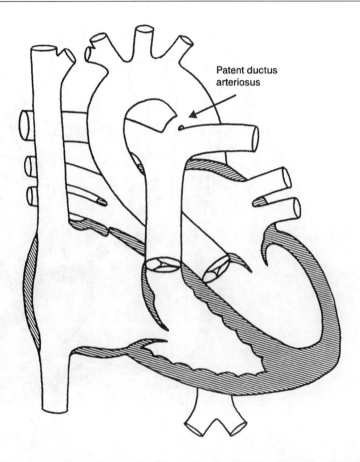

Patent ductus arteriosus

FIGURE 15

In patent ductus arteriosus, the blood vessel connecting the left pulmo-nary artery and the aorta, which is supposed to close after birth, instead remains open.
Adapted from Mullins DE, Mayer DC. Congenital heart disease: A dia-grammatic atlas. *© 1988 Wiley-Liss, Inc. By permission of Wiley-Liss, Inc., a division of John Wiley & Sons, Inc.*

gery is used to tie off the ductus. Another surgical solution involves using a catheter to insert a tiny umbrella-like device that blocks the hole.

It's important that PDA be corrected because its presence can lead to congestive heart failure or *cor pulmonale* (a disease of the right side of the heart) in later life; PDA also increases the risk of *endocarditis*, a life-threatening bacterial infection of the lining that covers the heart chambers, valves, and main arteries.

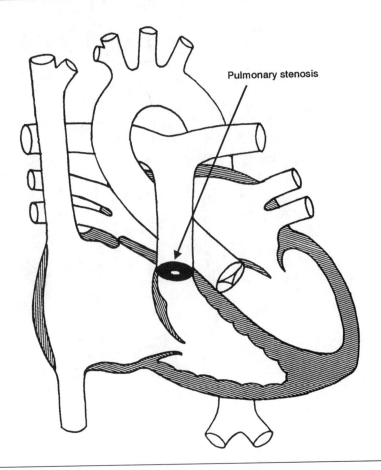

Pulmonary stenosis

FIGURE 16   *In pulmonary stenosis, the pulmonary valve is too narrow and thus inter-feres with the flow of blood.*
Adapted from Mullins DE, Mayer DC. Congenital heart disease: A dia-grammatic atlas. *© 1988 Wiley-Liss, Inc. By permission of Wiley-Liss, Inc., a division of John Wiley & Sons, Inc.*

Aortic or Pulmonary Valve Stenosis

Valve stenosis, a narrowing, may affect the pulmonary or aortic valves. *Pul-monary stenosis* is a constriction of the valve that lets blood flow from the right ventricle to the lungs (see Figure 16). When it occurs, the right ven-tricle has to work harder and so tends to become enlarged. An infant with a severe case of pulmonary stenosis may also appear bluish because not enough oxygen-rich blood is reaching all parts of the body. In this case, the child would need immediate surgery or *balloon valvuloplasty* (described below).

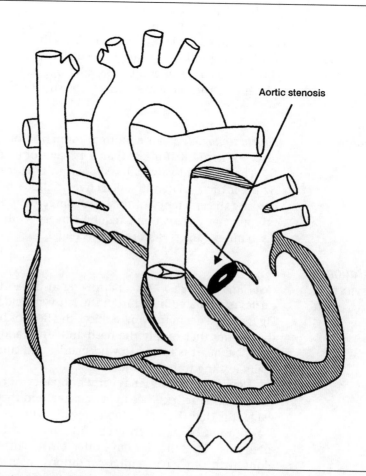

Aortic stenosis

FIGURE 17

In aortic stenosis, the aortic valve is too narrow and thus interferes with the flow of blood.

Adapted from Mullins DE, Mayer DC. Congenital heart disease: A dia-grammatic atlas. © 1988 Wiley-Liss, Inc. By permission of Wiley-Liss, Inc., a division of John Wiley & Sons, Inc.

Aortic stenosis is a constriction of the valve that lets blood flow from the left ventricle to all parts of the body (see Figure 17). When the left ventricle can't force enough blood through the aortic valve, the ventricle increases its pumping action, which causes it to enlarge. This condition may ultimately lead to heart failure.

Mild cases of stenosis require careful monitoring but not necessarily treatment. Surgery is the traditional remedy for narrowed valves, but a catheterization procedure called balloon valvuloplasty has become widely used, especially to treat pulmonary stenosis. In balloon valvuloplasty, a "balloon" is guided into the heart on the tip of a catheter. When it has been positioned precisely at the constricted valve, the balloon is then inflated to force a wider opening of the valve.

Lifelong follow-up care is needed after balloon valvuloplasty or valve surgery, because sometimes the valve degenerates or the stenosis recurs, in which case the valve may need to be surgically replaced.

Ebstein's Anomaly

Ebstein's anomaly is an abnormal formation of the tricuspid valve. A rare defect, it accounts for less than 1 percent of all congenital heart defects.

The tricuspid valve allows blood to flow from the right atrium to the right ventricle. When it is defective, it allows blood to flow backward, decreasing the efficiency of the heart. Surgery on the valve is usually successful, but many cases don't require surgery. Only when symptoms become disabling is surgery seriously considered.

Coarctation of the Aorta

Coarctation of the aorta is a narrowing in the aorta, which is the artery that carries oxygenated blood from the left ventricle to the rest of the body (see Figure 18). This narrowing reduces the flow of blood, increases pressure in the arteries that supply the head and arms, and impairs circulation to the legs. The heart is forced to work harder and thus becomes enlarged, eventually leading to heart failure.

Detecting this defect as early in infancy or childhood as possible is important because it causes hypertension, and the later it's treated, the more likely it is that the high blood pressure will persist.

In a newborn, a narrowed aorta may not be noticed until the ductus arteriosus closes in the days after birth. This defect sometimes appears along with other congenital conditions, such as septal defects and valve problems.

Traditional surgery may be used to take out the narrowed segment of artery and replace it with tube graft made of fabric, a fabric patch, or a flap of tissue from a blood vessel close to the site of the narrowing. Repair done early in life is successful in two-thirds of cases. Or balloon angioplasty may be used: This is a procedure in which a balloon-tipped catheter is threaded to the area and the balloon inflated to widen the passage.

Tetralogy of Fallot

Tetralogy of Fallot is a combination of four heart defects; it accounts for about 10 percent of all congenital heart disease in the United States. The four defects that make up the tetralogy of Fallot are:

▶ 1. A hole between the ventricles (a ventricular septal defect), which allows oxygen-poor blood to mix with oxygen-rich blood.

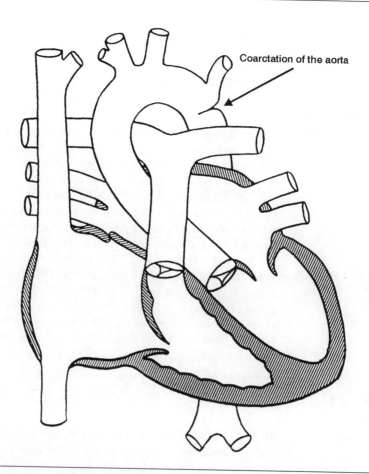

Coarctation of the aorta

FIGURE 18

In coarctation of the aorta, the aorta is narrowed, which interferes with the flow of oxygenated blood from the left ventricle to the rest of the body.
Adapted from Mullins DE, Mayer DC. Congenital heart disease: A diagrammatic atlas. © 1988 Wiley-Liss, Inc. By permission of Wiley-Liss, Inc., a division of John Wiley & Sons, Inc.

▶ 2. A narrowed outlet to the pulmonary artery, often in conjunction with an abnormal pulmonary valve, which partially blocks blood flow from the right ventricle to the lungs.

▶ 3. An aorta that overrides or straddles the wall (septum) between the ventricles, allowing oxygen-poor blood to flow through the ventricular septal defect and into the aorta.

▶ 4. Thickened and enlarged heart muscle tissue in the right ventricle.

The hole between the ventricles and the narrowed pulmonary outlet seriously hinder the flow of blood to the lungs; these defects also keep the level of oxygen in the blood too low, causing *cyanosis,* a blue tint to the skin. To correct this combination of defects, open-heart surgery is usually performed between infancy and age 12. Research has found that the sooner the surgery is done, the better the heart works later in life.

Transposition of the Great Arteries

In *transposition of the great arteries,* the normal position of the two arteries that emerge from the heart is reversed: The aorta comes out of the right ventricle (rather than the left), while the pulmonary artery emerges from the left ventricle (see Figure 19).

The biggest problem resulting from this reversal is that oxygen-rich blood recirculates to the lungs, while oxygen-poor blood gets carried to the rest of the body. A bluish skin color, most noticeable on the lips and the fingernails, is a major sign of this condition.

If a baby is also born with another defect that lets some oxygen-rich blood circulate, he or she can survive. Otherwise, an emergency catheterization procedure known as *balloon septostomy,* in which a balloon-tipped catheter is used to create a septal defect, may allow temporary relief. Or the ductus arteriosus may be kept open through drug treatment. But both of these solutions are temporary: They merely allow the body to get some oxygenated blood until surgery can be performed to correct the transposition.

Persistent Truncus Arteriosus

In this rare condition, the coronary arteries and one or two pulmonary arteries branch out of a great artery at the base of the heart. *Persistent truncus arteriosus* is a form of *cyanotic heart disease,* because blood oxygen is low, and the skin therefore has a bluish color. Babies born with this condition have difficulty breathing and feeding, and only half of them live longer than 1 month without surgery. Moreover, repeated surgeries may be needed as the child grows.

Atresia

Atresia is the absence of an opening; it most commonly affects the tricuspid and pulmonary valves.

In *tricuspid atresia,* the valve between the right atrium and right ventricle is missing. It usually occurs along with an atrial septal defect—which lets blood leave the right atrium. But that oxygen-poor blood mixes with the oxygen-rich blood in the left atrium and is sent throughout the body, causing the skin to look blue. Surgery is needed to make the blood flow in a normal path.

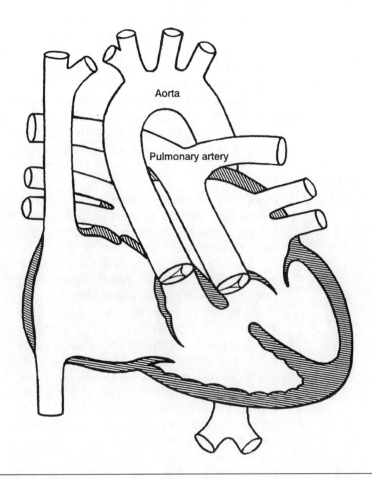

Aorta

Pulmonary artery

FIGURE 19   *In transposition of the great arteries, the normal position of the two arteries that emerge from the heart is reversed.*
Adapted from Mullins DE, Mayer DC. Congenital heart disease: A diagrammatic atlas. © 1988 Wiley-Liss, Inc. By permission of Wiley-Liss, Inc., a division of John Wiley & Sons, Inc.

In *pulmonary atresia,* the pulmonary valve (the one that allows blood to flow from the right ventricle to the lungs) has not formed or is closed. As a result, the oxygen content of the blood reaching the rest of the body will be drastically lowered. As a temporary remedy to this serious condition, physicians may give an infant drugs to keep the ductus arteriosus open for a time, thus increasing the supply of oxygenated blood until surgery can be performed to open the pulmonary valve.

Total Anomalous Pulmonary Venous Connection

Total anomalous pulmonary venous connection is a rare condition in which oxygen-rich blood returning from the lungs flows into the right atrium or right-sided systemic veins instead of into the left atrium. This oxygen-rich blood mixes with oxygen-depleted blood and flows through an atrial septal defect into the left atrium, then into the left ventricle, from where it is pumped to the body.

Because not enough oxygen is reaching all body cells, the baby's skin looks bluish. In cases where the blood flow is obstructed, babies need emergency surgery soon after birth to repair the septal defect and redirect blood flow from the lungs to the left atrium.

Hypoplastic Left Heart Syndrome

Hypoplastic left heart syndrome is rare, but it's the most serious of all congenital heart defects. Even with surgery, only about half of affected infants survive. However, heart transplantation offers one more promising treatment possibility.

An infant with hypoplastic left heart syndrome has an underdeveloped left ventricle, the heart chamber responsible for pumping blood through the aorta to the entire body. In some cases, atresia of the mitral or aortic valves, or both, may occur, isolating the left ventricle completely. The patient is kept alive only by the pumping action of the right ventricle, which sends blood through the ductus arteriosus into the aorta.

In the days following birth, the baby may seem normal, because the ductus arteriosus hasn't yet closed. But when that ductus closes, the right ventricle is cut off from its outlet to the aorta. The outward sign of this deprivation is cyanosis, the bluish color of the skin. The infant soon goes into shock and multiorgan failure, so emergency surgery or a heart transplant must be performed.

High Blood Pressure and Cholesterol

Although *hypertension,* or high blood pressure, is not considered a congenital heart disease, it sometimes has a hereditary link. For that reason, children born in families with a history of high blood pressure need to have their blood pressure monitored with special care.

Fewer than 3 percent of children in the United States have high blood pressure. But high blood pressure is serious when it is present during childhood and remains undetected for years. Therefore, it's wise to make sure that measuring a child's blood pressure is a part of his or her annual checkup. (Table 12 in chapter 8 lists normal and high blood pressure values for children at different ages.)

Very high levels of LDL ("bad") cholesterol also sometimes run in families: One inherited condition that affects 1 to 2 percent of children is *familial hypercholesterolemia*. Very high levels of LDL cholesterol may contribute to *atherosclerosis*, which is the buildup of plaque in the arteries. Therefore, children with familial hypercholesterolemia need to have their cholesterol levels tested before they're 5 years old, and regularly thereafter. Treatment for high cholesterol may involve the child's getting more exercise and eating foods with low levels of fat and cholesterol. Medication to lower cholesterol levels may be prescribed for children whose LDL cholesterol after 1 year of diet therapy remains greater than 190 mg/dL (5.0 mmol/L), or for children over 10 who have additional risk factors for heart disease and whose LDL cholesterol remains greater than 160 mg/dL (4.1 mmol/L).

The Outlook for Congenital Heart Disease

Rarely can families predict or prevent congenital heart defects. Of course, every pregnant woman needs to take all appropriate preventive measures to ensure the health of her baby—including avoiding excess alcohol, exposure to rubella, environmental toxins, and drugs.

Unfortunately, a small percentage of babies will be born with congenital defects—in spite of their parents' good health and healthy behaviors. The good news is that many defects that would have been fatal just decades ago are now being treated successfully.

Strides are also being made in diagnosing heart defects while the fetus is still in the womb. In the future, some forms of treatment may be available to correct some defects before the baby is even born.

CHAPTER 26

Diseases of the Heart Muscle

Cardiomyopathy is the medical term for diseases of the heart muscle (*cardio* = heart, *myo* = muscle, and *pathy* = disease). Heart muscle disease damages the muscle tone of the heart, dangerously reducing its ability to pump blood effectively.

Heart muscle diseases constitute one of the four most common causes of heart failure in the United States. However, when compared with other cardiovascular diseases, the number of cases each year is relatively low. They account for approximately 50,000 of the 400,000 new cases of heart disease each year, and for only about 1 percent of all deaths in the United States due to heart disease.

Still, cardiomyopathy is a significant threat, one that's all the more disturbing because it can go unrecognized and untreated. It is also different from other heart problems in that it frequently affects younger people, and often results in quick death.

Dilated Cardiomyopathy

The most common form of heart muscle disease is called *dilated cardiomyopathy*. This form of the disease, also called *congestive cardiomyopathy*, damages the muscle tissues that make up the pumping chambers of the heart.

Dilated cardiomyopathy usually affects all the chambers of the heart, weakening their walls. When these walls become weak enough, the heart can no longer perform its pumping action with normal force. Other parts of the body do their best to compensate for this deficiency in pumping power by increasing the quantity of fluid they retain—and by producing a greater volume of blood than usual. The heart chambers then dilate (expand) to accommodate the greater blood volume.

In the short run, bodily functions remain near normal. More blood is moved with less pressure, and circulation is maintained. Stretching the heart muscle tissue by increasing the chambers' volume also restores some of the heart's pumping strength because the more a muscle is stretched—up to its elastic limit—the more forcefully it will contract.

Over the long term, however, the effects of these changes are not positive. Other body mechanisms act to make the heart pump faster than normal. The added fluid, combined with the less efficient heart action and less adequate circulation, causes fluid to accumulate in the lungs, abdomen, and legs. This fluid accumulation produces two common symptoms, breathing difficulties and swelling, both of which indicate heart failure.

Thus the body's own efforts to compensate for the impaired heart create a self-defeating cycle: The muscle-damaged heart chambers enlarge, the volume of blood in the body increases, more fluid is retained, and muscle fibers are stretched even more. All this causes the heart to work harder and faster than ever. Finally, when the heart muscle is stretched to its limit and the heart can no longer pump enough blood to the rest of the body, the heart fails.

What Causes It

No exact cause can be determined for roughly 80 percent of all cases of dilated cardiomyopathy. Therefore, these cases are called *idiopathic*—meaning "of unknown origin."

Although cardiology specialists aren't sure, many suspect that a great number of cases of idiopathic dilated cardiomyopathy may be caused by a viral infection. Unfortunately, viruses are very difficult to detect in laboratory samples from a person who is ill: Because such a viral infection might have occurred months or even years before the person showed any sign of a weakened heart muscle, this cause is difficult to pinpoint with certainty.

Other cases of dilated cardiomyopathy can be traced to separate roots: alcohol or some other toxic substance, poor nutrition, inflammation caused by infection, complications during pregnancy or childbirth, and heredity.

Alcohol and Other Toxic Substances

Among men in the United States, excessive consumption of alcohol is thought to cause some cases of dilated cardiomyopathy. Researchers have found that after years of heavy drinking, a person's heart muscle can be weakened by alcohol's toxic effect on muscle cells. (Alcohol can also attack cells in the liver, but typically it damages *either* the liver or the heart muscle, not both at the same time!)

Also, because heavy drinkers may substitute alcohol for food, alcoholism may play another, less direct role in the development of dilated cardiomyopathy: Nutritional deficiencies are also related to the disease.

Other toxic substances, including some chemicals and pesticides, have also been shown to weaken the heart muscle.

Poor Nutrition

People who suffer from severe deficiencies in essential vitamins and minerals—especially thiamine (also known as vitamin B-1)—may develop dilated cardiomyopathy. However, such deficiencies are found far more commonly in underdeveloped nations of the world than they are in the United States.

Inflammation

In a condition called *myocarditis*, the heart muscle becomes inflamed as a result of infection by a virus or, less often, by bacteria. Not all inflammations of the heart muscle lead to dilated cardiomyopathy, but often it's an underlying cause.

Myocarditis is a relatively rare problem. Sometimes a person may feel no symptoms at all; in other cases, he or she will feel acute chest pains with the overall weakness one feels with a bad cold or the flu. While mild cases of myocarditis may go completely undiagnosed, severe cases are frequently not diagnosed until the symptoms of heart failure appear. Usually, the mild cases disappear and cause no lasting damage. Even a severe case occasionally goes away spontaneously, but intense bouts of inflammation usually cause progressive and irreversible damage to the heart muscle.

Pregnancy and Childbirth

In rare cases, a woman may develop heart muscle disease late in pregnancy or during the first few months after she has given birth to a child. The term *peripartum* (*peri* = around the time of, *partum* = birth) is therefore applied to this type of dilated cardiomyopathy.

Without having a viral or bacterial infection, the woman with *peripartum dilated cardiomyopathy* experiences an inflammation of her heart muscle. Why this happens hasn't been determined. However, if the woman recovers from the disease and becomes pregnant again, she is again at high risk for developing the condition. Researchers haven't been able to discover why this heart muscle disease occurs in some women, although they have noted that the incidence of peripartum dilated cardiomyopathy is higher in black women than in other women in the United States.

Heredity

Research studies haven't identified an abnormal gene related to the development of dilated cardiomyopathy. However, because at times several members of a family are affected by the disease, some experts suspect that there may be a genetic link. They also point to instances in which dilated cardiomyopathy occurs within families that also experience a genetic neurologic disorder, such as muscular dystrophy. Further research may one day lead to pinpointing a genetic factor more precisely.

How It's Diagnosed

As mentioned earlier, sometimes an inflammation of the heart muscle causes no immediately noticeable symptoms. At other times, the person affected may feel symptoms most often associated with the common cold or flu: chills, fever, overall aches, and weariness.

When the heart becomes very enlarged, a person eventually *does* feel definite symptoms. These include chest pains, extreme tiredness, shortness of breath, and swelling of the legs and ankles. All these, as well as fluid retention in the lungs (which wouldn't be felt), are signs of the early stage of heart failure.

Examination and testing by a cardiologist generally would provide a precise diagnosis. A chest X ray could show that the heart is enlarged and that there is an accumulation of fluid in the lungs—the two main indicators of dilated cardiomyopathy. Upon recommendation of the physician, one or more of the following follow-up tests could then provide full details of the state of the disease.

■ An *electrocardiogram,* which is a record of the changes in electrical potential occurring in the heart muscle during the heartbeat, may be ordered to show the extent of damage to the heart walls.

■ *Echocardiography* may show a picture of the heart's activity through the use of sound waves. Specifically, echocardiography details the dimensions of the heart and the degree of damage.

- *Angiography,* a cardiac catheterization procedure, may give cardiologists a detailed view of how well the heart's arteries and chambers are functioning.

- A *biopsy* of tissue from the wall of the heart may also aid in determining how seriously the heart has been damaged and what may have initially caused the damage.

Treatment for Dilated Cardiomyopathy

Before a specific course of treatment is decided on, physicians will try to identify what has caused the dilated cardiomyopathy. In most cases, however, the cause cannot be determined. But when a nutritional deficiency, excess alcohol, infection, or exposure to a toxin can be identified as the cause, the patient and physician can take immediate action. In some cases, correcting the deficiency or eliminating the toxin can actually reverse the damage that's been done to the heart. For example, in some cases of alcohol-caused dilated cardiomyopathy, total abstinence allows the body to repair itself.

Whether an underlying cause can be identified or not, treatment for the condition is focused on relieving symptoms—as well as relieving the extra load the heart is bearing. Drugs can help with both managing symptoms and improving heart action. Among the various medications that a physician may prescribe are ones intended to reduce salts and the excess fluids that the body is retaining, improve the heart's contracting, and lower blood pressure so blood can flow more effectively throughout the body.

Patients may also be asked to modify their lifestyles. In certain instances, they may need to lose weight, stop smoking, or begin a moderate exercise program. All these ways of improving overall fitness help to ease the demands on the heart and improve the chances that the prescribed medications will work effectively.

For some patients, the amount of damage to the heart muscle is so great that medications aren't effective—nor are additional medical options for repairing the damage promising. In those cases, physicians may recommend that a heart transplant be considered.

Hypertrophic Cardiomyopathy

Hypertrophic cardiomyopathy is sometimes called "athletic" heart muscle disease because fainting on the part of a young athlete during strenuous exercise is often the first and most dramatic symptom of the disease.

Hypertrophic cardiomyopathy is characterized by a thickening of the walls of the heart's chambers as a result of abnormal muscle tissue growth. Some thickening of these walls is typical for healthy athletes, but when the disease strikes, this thickening is extreme. The septum, which separates the left and right sides of the heart, intrudes into the left ventricle. Muscles in both ventricles often become enlarged, and these thickened muscle walls may partially block the flow of blood through the aortic valve or prevent the heart from stretching properly and filling with blood.

Although the sudden deaths of athletes from heart muscle disease make the headlines, such incidents are in fact rare. According to the *American Journal of Diseases of Children,* each year there are only one or two such deaths per 200,000 athletes aged 30 and younger.

Sometimes no symptoms of hypertrophic cardiomyopathy precede sudden collapse and death. That's why hypertrophic cardiomyopathy is usually suspected when an apparently healthy athlete dies while exercising vigorously.

When symptoms do occur, the most common ones are shortness of breath, chest pain, fatigue, and fainting. The amateur athlete should pay attention to any of these warning signs rather than ignoring them. In fact, anyone who exercises regularly and feels athletically fit should pay attention to unusual shortness of breath or unnatural tiredness—rather than push on in the face of such signals.

Athletic 25-year-olds who die of hypertrophic cardiomyopathy usually die undiagnosed, because most young adults assume that they don't need the thorough physical exam that a 50-year-old might get before beginning a new exercise program. But anyone—young or old—who wants to participate in strenuous athletic competition should have an exam that includes a chest X ray.

The American Academy of Pediatrics has issued specific guidelines for children's participation in competitive sports, and the American College of Cardiology has issued guidelines for determining the eligibility to compete for athletes of all ages who have cardiovascular abnormalities. The publications containing these guidelines are listed under "Chapters 23 to 34" in the references section at the back of this handbook.

What Causes It   A hereditary link has been established for this form of cardiomyopathy. In about half the cases, the person has inherited an abnormal gene from a parent, while in the rest of cases, a gene that's normal at birth later undergoes mutation.

Fortunately, a genetic test has recently been developed to identify those at risk for hypertrophic cardiomyopathy. Using the results of this test, doctors can warn children at risk to avoid extra exertion and refrain from participating in competitive sports.

Causes other than hereditary ones may also lead to hypertrophic cardiomyopathy. A buildup of heart muscle can sometimes be traced to hypertension (high blood pressure) and heart valve disease.

How It's Diagnosed

When a chest X ray reveals that a person has an enlarged heart, further investigation is pursued before a diagnosis of the condition is made. A cardiologist may use *echocardiography*, a noninvasive method that uses sound waves to create a picture of the heart's activity. When necessary, the physician will also perform a *diagnostic angiography procedure,* a more invasive means of viewing heart activity.

Not everyone with hypertrophic cardiomyopathy experiences symptoms, but when they do, the symptoms are usually shortness of breath, chest pain, fatigue, or fainting during strenuous exercise.

Treatment for Hypertrophic Cardiomyopathy

Often the treatments for this condition address the symptoms rather than the disease itself. Among those treatments are lifestyle modifications, medications, and surgery.

The patient and physician would need to discuss what restrictions on physical exertion and what changes in daily habits would best promote future heart health. Along with these changes, drugs would likely be prescribed to relieve symptoms and ease the load on the heart, helping it pump more easily. For example, beta-blockers could reduce the force of the heart's contractions, or calcium channel blockers could make the muscle-stiffened heart chambers more flexible. Drugs to combat arrhythmias (particularly the drug disopyramide) may also be helpful.

Surgical removal of the excess tissue interfering with blood circulation is an option if medications fail to bring relief. More recent treatment sometimes includes implanting a pacemaker (or, in certain cases, a defibrillator) to control the heart rate. If these options fail to control the condition, or if the person's condition deteriorates to heart failure, a heart transplant would then need to be considered.

Restrictive Cardiomyopathy

Restrictive cardiomyopathy gets its name from the fact that the condition restricts the proper stretching and filling of the heart with blood. In this rare disorder, muscles of the heart grow inflexible, so while the rhythm and pumping action of the heart may be healthy, the stiff walls of the heart chambers prevent them from filling normally. As a result, blood flow is reduced—and some blood that would normally enter the heart is backed up in the circulatory system. Eventually, the heart fails.

What Causes It

One known cause of restrictive cardiomyopathy is *amyloidosis*, a condition sometimes associated with cancers of the blood. Proteins from certain blood cells get deposited in heart tissue, making the tissue stiff and thickened. In other rare cases, diseases can create deposits that can make the heart walls thick and stiff.

*How It's
Diagnosed*

Physicians want to be sure to diagnose restrictive cardiomyopathy accurately, because it can be mistaken for a more treatable heart disease. When the pericardium, which is the membrane surrounding the heart, becomes inflamed and thickened, the condition is called *constrictive pericarditis*— and surgery can frequently correct it. Restrictive cardiomyopathy, on the other hand, *cannot* be corrected surgically; instead, attention must focus on controlling its symptoms.

One tool that's important in the diagnosis of restrictive cardiomyopathy is *echocardiography*, which uses sound waves to provide an image of the heart's activity. Additional diagnostic tools include the imaging techniques of *computed tomography (CT) scanning* and *magnetic resonance imaging (MRI)*. A biopsy of tissue from the wall of the heart may also help determine an accurate diagnosis.

*Treatment for
Restrictive
Cardiomyopathy*

Restrictive cardiomyopathy cannot be reversed, and medical experts currently have no means of repairing damaged heart muscle. Therefore, treatment is confined to controlling its symptoms: Drugs are used to lessen the workload placed on the heart and to regulate heart rhythm. When the condition is severe, a heart transplant may become necessary.

Ischemic Cardiomyopathy

Ischemia describes a lack of oxygen in a part of the body; it's caused by a constriction or blockage in a blood vessel, which cuts off the supply of blood to that part of the body. In *myocardial ischemia,* or ischemia of the heart muscle, constriction or blockage of the coronary arteries reduces the supply of oxygen to the heart muscle itself. The heart muscle can be damaged in this way by one or more heart attacks.

Ischemic cardiomyopathy, therefore, is the loss or weakening of heart muscle tissue that results from coronary artery disease and subsequent heart attacks.

The damage that occurs to the heart muscle from a lack of oxygen is similar to other forms of heart muscle disease. And the result is the same: The heart is prevented from functioning. Therefore, treatment for ischemic cardiomyopathy is similar to that for other forms of cardiomyopathy—with special attention given to correcting the reversible aspects of coronary artery disease.

How You Can Protect Yourself against Cardiomyopathy

Although cardiomyopathy is among the less frequent forms of heart disease, it's still important to be aware of the role heredity plays in this disease and to be familiar with its symptoms.

Because heredity is a factor in some cases of cardiomyopathy, you need to investigate your family's medical history to learn if you are at special risk. And regardless of your genetic predisposition to some form of cardiomyopathy, you need to know that if you experience unexplained shortness of breath, fainting, or chest pains, *you need to see your doctor.* In addition, because excess alcohol, inadequate nutrition, and exposure to toxins can all cause cardiomyopathy, you need to reduce your risks by practicing the habits of a heart-healthy life.

CHAPTER 27

Arrhythmias

Any abnormality in the rate or regularity of the heart's natural rhythm is called an *arrhythmia*. Arrhythmias range in severity from the single extra beat, which almost everyone has experienced, to an uncontrolled flurry of contractions that may lead to cardiac arrest. In fact, arrhythmias are the main cause of sudden cardiac death in the United States, accounting for over 400,000 deaths annually.

Many arrhythmias are minor and may simply be caused by alcohol, caffeine, fatigue, or stress. However, if you experience noticeable irregularity in your heartbeat, you need to see your physician. Certain arrhythmias can be controlled with medications, while others require surgery or the implantation of a rhythm-regulating device to stop the arrhythmia.

Your Heart's Electrical System

Your heart is like a pump, with each squeeze activated by an electrical impulse. This impulse originates in the heart's "natural pacemaker"—the sinoatrial (SA) node, which is located at the top of the right atrium.

Without an electrical charge from the SA node, the heart cannot contract normally. So both the timing of the charge and the route it takes are crucial for the proper functioning of your entire cardiovascular system.

Here's how the system works: The SA node sets off its electrical impulse about 60 to 100 times a minute when you're sitting quietly. Each impulse first travels through the atria, making the muscle there contract and push blood into the ventricles. The impulse then reaches the atrioventricular (AV) node in the septum, the muscle wall between the ventricles. There the impulse is delayed briefly until atrial contraction is complete, at which time it's sent on to the ventricles through a network called the *His-Purkinje system*. The impulse causes the ventricles to contract, and the result is a steady pushing of the blood out to the lungs and the rest of the body.

The rhythmic pace of your heart increases, of course, whenever you begin exerting yourself physically or when your emotional level is raised. It decreases during sleep. These changes come as a result of messages sent by your brain, hormones, and autonomic nervous system. Probably the best-known example is adrenaline: Danger or sudden fear can send this hormone through your bloodstream, triggering a near-instant increase in your heart rate.

When it functions well, the electrical process that controls your heart rate is wonderfully consistent and reliable. But it can go awry, either in its speed or in the route the electrical stimulus takes.

Speed irregularities are usually categorized as too slow—*bradycardia*—or too fast—*tachycardia*.

Bradycardia

An abnormally slow heart rate, *bradycardia* involves a heart rate of less than 60 beats per minute.

One form of bradycardia generally presents no problem at all: *Sinus bradycardia* is a heart rate of less than 60 beats per minute with a regular rhythm. This form may be found in young, physically fit people, and it may not interfere with their normal activities.

But bradycardia becomes serious when it results in too little oxygen reaching body cells. When this happens, a person may experience shortness of breath or fainting.

The cause of the overly slow rhythm usually stems from one of two sources: The central nervous system may fail to signal that the body needs more heart-pumping action to get the oxygen it needs, or the SA node may be damaged. This damage might be related to aging or heart disease, or it might be caused by certain medications—including some used to control arrhythmias and hypertension.

Tachycardia

Tachycardias, abnormally fast heart rates, take many forms. But all involve heart rates greater than 100 beats per minute. One common means of categorizing tachycardias is by where the fast rate originates: If it originates *above* the ventricles, it's called *supraventricular tachycardia*, while if it originates *in* the ventricles, it's called *ventricular tachycardia.*

Supraventricular Tachycardia

Supraventricular tachycardia is any very rapid rhythm (or heartbeat) that originates above the ventricle. *Atrial tachycardia* is characterized by a rapid, regular heart rate greater than 150 beats per minute arising from an area in the atrium other than the SA node. Atrial tachycardias include *atrial fibrillation*, a rapid, irregular rhythm that involves an ineffective twitching or contraction of the individual muscle fibers; *Wolff-Parkinson-White (WPW) syndrome*, a group of abnormalities caused by extra muscle pathways between the atria and the ventricles; and *atrial flutter*, a rapid electrical impulse radiating in regular succession down toward the ventricles.

Ventricular Tachycardia

Ventricular tachycardia is a condition in which the SA node no longer influences the contraction of the ventricles. Instead, some other area along the lower electrical pathway takes over the signaling work. Since the new signal doesn't proceed through the heart muscle along the regular route, the heart muscle fails to contract normally. The heartbeat quickens, with the person feeling as if the heart is "skipping beats."

The most serious arrhythmia is *ventricular fibrillation (VF)*, a condition similar to ventricular tachycardia. VF involves an uncontrolled fast beating. Instead of the one misplaced ventricular impulse, a person may have *several* impulses that originate simultaneously from different locations—all signaling the heart to beat. The result is a much faster heartbeat that sometimes reaches 300 beats per minute! Yet because very little blood is actually being pumped from the heart to the brain and body, the person loses consciousness. Medical attention is needed immediately. If cardiopulmonary resuscitation (CPR) can be started, or electrical energy used to "shock" the heart back to a normal rhythm, damage to the heart may be reduced.

In addition, healthy people may commonly experience single, unrelated ventricular impulses called *premature ventricular contractions*. In the absence of other heart disease, these palpitations are generally harmless.

Heart Block

Heart block takes place when the SA node sends its electrical signal properly but that signal isn't conducted through the atrioventricular (AV) node or lower electrical pathways as it should be. The condition is most often caused by aging or by the inflammation or scarring that sometimes results from coronary artery disease. There are several types of heart block, and they're named after the site where the blockage occurs.

Instances of heart block are also categorized by their degree of severity. In *first-degree heart block,* conduction through the AV node is too slow. In *second-degree heart block,* impulses travel through the atria but are delayed in the AV node and therefore fail to stimulate the ventricles at the right moment. Finally, in *third-degree heart block,* no impulses reach the ventricles from impulse-generating sites above them. To compensate, the ventricles use their own "backup" pacemaker. Sometimes, however, because a gap in time is likely to occur between the last conducted impulse from the atria and one from the backup unit, the person may faint. This disorder is known as a *Stokes-Adams attack.* Third-degree heart block is very serious and can lead to heart failure, fainting, or death.

Diagnosing Arrhythmias

People with suspected arrhythmias need to receive a thorough cardiac examination, which may include a combination of simple and very sophisticated testing procedures, such as electrocardiograms, monitoring devices, tilt-table evaluations, and electrophysiology studies.

A standard electrocardiogram (ECG) may be used to show the heart's rhythm patterns. Sometimes a computer is used to analyze the standard ECG readings to identify electrical signals that may predict arrhythmic events. This analysis is known as a *signal-averaged ECG.*

Alternatively, *esophageal electrocardiography* may be performed. In this exam, an electrode is inserted into the esophagus through the mouth or nose of a patient. Some difficult arrhythmias may be better detected in this way, because the esophagus lies just behind the atria near the natural-pacemaker site.

Another means of evaluating rhythm disturbances is to have an individual wear an arrhythmia monitoring device for a period of 24 hours or more. This process is known as *Holter monitoring.* The person's heart rate and rhythm can be monitored continuously, or the wearer can push a "record" button on the monitor when he or she feels symptoms. At the end of the designated period, a physician can examine the printout of the monitoring to determine the nature of the arrhythmia.

A tilt-table evaluation is a noninvasive way for physicians to evaluate the heart's rhythm in cases of fainting. The patient is monitored for heart rate and blood pressure while lying flat, and continues to be monitored as the table is tilted (head up) to 65 degrees. The changing angle exerts stress on the part of the nervous system responsible for maintaining heart rate and blood pressure, so the technique lets physicians observe exactly how the heart responds under carefully supervised conditions of changing stress. This test can reveal the presence of bradycardia.

Electrophysiology (EP) studies are typically performed in a cardiac catheterization laboratory. The EP study involves having a small wire inserted through a vein in the leg and then guided to the heart. Electrical impulses are then sent through this wire to reveal the nature and location of the rhythm disturbance. An EP study shows how the heart reacts to the controlled electrical stimulus that a physician administers. During the study, medications may also be given to test how the heart responds to specific antiarrhythmic drugs.

Treating Arrhythmias

A number of treatment options are available for arrhythmias, but of course the appropriate treatment depends on each person's symptoms, physical condition, medical history, and exact diagnosis. Among the most frequent options are drug therapy, implantable devices, ablation procedures, and surgery.

Drug therapy is often the first approach taken to treating an arrhythmia. A wide variety of antiarrhythmic medications have proven quite effective, including digitalis, beta-blockers, calcium channel blockers, and a variety of more potent drugs. Single medications or combinations of them may be prescribed.

In addition, different kinds of implantable pacemakers and defibrillators are available, and each device is specifically set to regulate the heartbeat of the individual in whom it's implanted.

A *pacemaker* may be chosen to regulate heart rhythm in some cases of slow heart rate, blockage in the conduction system, or a combination of fast and slow heart rates. About the size of a small matchbox, the pacemaker is surgically implanted near the collarbone. Its batteries supply the electrical energy to replace the heart's natural stimulation. A pacemaker may pace the atria, ventricles, or both; it may inhibit extra impulses, trigger impulses, or do both—depending on what's needed at the moment. When set to an appropriate rate for the individual, the pacemaker can sense the heart's rhythm and deliver a stimulus when necessary. Pacemakers can also be adjusted to the physical demands and lifestyle of the individual.

The *implantable cardioverter-defibrillator (ICD)* is a new option for treating serious ventricular arrhythmias. In *acute ventricular arrhythmias,* the ventricles contract so rapidly that the heart may stop pumping completely, leading to cardiac arrest. However, about 20 percent of those who have an acute ventricular arrhythmia survive, and they are prime candidates for an implantable defibrillator. This device quickly detects an episode of acute arrhythmia, such as fibrillation, and responds with a shock that restores normal rhythm, or delivers a set of specific overriding impulses. Implantation of an ICD usually requires open-chest surgery, but systems are now being tested that can be implanted, like pacemakers, beneath the skin.

Another treatment option is *radio-frequency ablation,* which is performed in the catheterization laboratory. After the patient is sedated, a catheter is inserted into a vein and maneuvered into the heart. The end of the catheter is equipped with a device that permits mapping of the electrical pathways of the heart. Once the cardiologist sees the complete map, he or she can use high-frequency radio waves to ablate—meaning, eliminate—the additional pathway or pathways causing the arrhythmia.

Surgery is sometimes considered the treatment of last resort for arrhythmias, but it may be appropriate for very serious cases and for younger individuals who can better handle the stress of surgery. *Surgical ablation* is similar in principle to radio-frequency ablation. Using advanced computerized mapping techniques and *cryoablation*—the elimination of tissue with a cold probe—surgeons can destroy the "misfiring" cells.

Maze surgery may be suitable for a patient with atrial fibrillation who hasn't responded to drugs or to electrical shock (cardioversion therapy). Through a recently developed surgical procedure, surgeons create a "maze" of carefully planned sutures that permit electrical impulses to travel effectively.

Living with an Arrhythmia

Arrhythmias are serious, so if you experience episodes of irregular heart rhythm, you need to be evaluated by a physician. However, you can also take certain steps to prevent arrhythmias from occurring.

Some steps relate to the emotional side of your life: managing your level of stress and controlling your anxiety. Others involve daily habits: Caffeine, alcohol, and cigarettes are all known to contribute to arrhythmias (although there is some debate about how much caffeine you'd have to consume before you'd experience any effect; the current thinking is that one or two cups of coffee or tea a day won't disturb heart rhythm).

In addition, many people find that they can stop a sudden, rapid heartbeat (supraventricular tachycardia) with an exercise that slows the heart rate. To try this, sit erect with your feet flat on the floor. Then, with both hands, press on your stomach just below your rib cage. Press firmly inward, then, using the strength of your abdominal muscles, resist the pressure of your hands and try to push them outward. Hold this pressure for 10 to 15 seconds, then relax. After a half-minute break, do the exercise again.

Other techniques for stopping a rapid heart rate include holding your breath, rubbing your neck, splashing your face with cold water, and coughing. You might discuss these techniques with your doctor to see if they're appropriate for your condition.

Everyone at some time or another has felt a minor fluttering or an unpleasant pounding in the chest. Sometimes the experience is more upsetting than actually dangerous. But remember, arrhythmias are serious—and at times fatal. Therefore, don't try to diagnose the seriousness of your own heart irregularity. Instead, see your physician for examination and any testing that may be appropriate.

CHAPTER 28

Diseases of the Heart Valves

The proper functioning of your four heart valves is crucial to the efficient operation of your whole cardiovascular system.

These valves—the *tricuspid, pulmonary, mitral,* and *aortic*—control how blood travels on its one-way path. Figure 20 shows the structure of the mitral valve (on the right) and the aortic valve (on the left). For everything to work well, they must open at just the right moment, let blood flow through, then close securely so that no blood moves backward along the path.

How the Valves Work

The valves regulate the flow of blood through the heart. From the right atrium, blood is sent through the *tricuspid valve* to the right ventricle, and from there through the *pulmonary valve* to the lungs to pick up oxygen. After the blood travels back from the lungs to the left atrium, it's sent through the *mitral valve* to the left ventricle, and from there pumped to all body organs through the *aortic valve*. (See Figures 6 and 7 in chapter 23.)

The valves are actually thin flaps of tissue, also called *leaflets* or *cusps,* that open and close as the pressure behind and in front of them changes. For example, when the right atrium contracts, blood that has returned there from the rest of the body is sent through the open tricuspid valve to

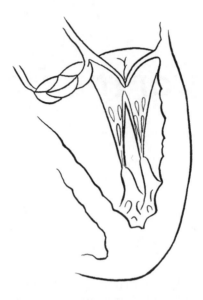

FIGURE 20   *The mitral valve (right) and aortic valve (left) within the left ventricle.*

the right ventricle. At the time of atrial contraction, the pressure in the right atrium is high, and that pressure helps keep the tricuspid valve open, but by the end of the atrial contraction, pressure from the atrial side of that valve has decreased, while pressure from the ventricular side of that valve has increased, and the valve naturally closes.

How Valve Disease Develops

Because the main functions of heart valves are to open and close, it's probably no surprise that the two major problems associated with valves are the failure to open properly and the failure to close properly.

Stenosis, the narrowing of a heart valve, is the biggest problem related to a valve's opening properly. If the leaflets that make up a valve stiffen, become thickened or narrowed, or fuse together, the valve cannot open fully. Therefore, less blood can flow through the valve, and the heart has to work harder to maintain circulation.

The valve's failure to close—called *regurgitation, insufficiency,* or *incompetence*—means that blood flows backward through the valve. In severe cases, most of the pumped blood flows back through the valve, leaving only a little blood to travel forward in the cardiovascular system. As with valvular stenosis, the heart tries to make up for this problem by working harder, but gradually this makes the heart enlarge and become less and less effective in moving blood through the system.

More valve problems are evident on the left side of the heart than on the right, because the left chambers have a harder job to do than those on the right. While the right chambers deliver blood to the nearby lungs, the left chambers must pump it through the whole arterial system. For this reason, valve disease in the mitral and aortic valves most frequently produces symptoms and requires treatment.

Some valve problems cause no real disturbance in people's lives. In other cases, valve disease takes its toll over many years, gradually causing the heart to enlarge and its muscle walls to weaken. Eventually—sometimes after 20 or 30 years—the person feels symptoms, but by then the symptoms likely indicate a very serious condition. Congestive heart failure may occur: The heart can't pump enough blood, and fluid is retained in the lungs, causing shortness of breath, and in the legs and ankles, causing swelling. In addition to congestive heart failure, valve disease can lead to heart muscle disease, arrhythmias, and blood clots.

Types of Valve Disease

Diseases of the heart valves are often classified according to which valve or valves are involved and how much disruption in blood flow is created by the problem.

Defects in the tricuspid and pulmonary valves are relatively rare. While the tricuspid valve is subject to both narrowing and backflow problems, these difficulties are usually related to other kinds of heart problems—and account for only about 5 percent of valve defects. Pulmonary valve problems are also rare, although some infants are born with narrowed pulmonary valves and need surgery immediately. However, the most frequent and serious valve problems involve the mitral and aortic valves. These are described below.

▶ **1.** *Mitral valve prolapse (MVP)* is a defect in the closing of the mitral valve, the one that regulates the flow of blood from the left atrium to the left ventricle. It's the most common type of valve disorder, and is often called the *click-murmur syndrome* in imitation of the distinct heart sound that is caused by the incomplete closure of this two-leaflet valve.

Mitral valve prolapse tends to affect more women than men, and it does run in families. An estimated 5 to 10 percent of the U.S. population have some degree of MVP, but most people have mild cases with no symptoms. When MVP does cause symptoms, they include shortness of breath, chest pain, great fatigue, and palpitations.

Infrequently, mitral valve prolapse leads to mitral regurgitation, in which case patients might need to limit their strenuous exercise. The condition can also lead to an overly rapid heartbeat (tachycardia, a rhythm disorder discussed in chapter 27).

▶ **2.** *Mitral stenosis* is a narrowing of the mitral valve. A very few infants are born with it, but adults who develop it usually had rheumatic fever earlier in life. Now that antibiotics are used to combat infections leading to rheumatic fever, there are far fewer cases of mitral stenosis in industrialized countries.

Adult cases of the disease are often identified 10 to 20 years after they have begun; these cases tend to become progressively more serious. The narrowed valve creates a traffic backup: Blood doesn't flow efficiently to the left ventricle; instead, pressure remains in the left atrium, causing congestion in the lungs. So the major symptom a person may feel is shortness of breath. Mitral stenosis may lead to heart failure, but treatment—either with diuretics or surgery—is highly effective in relieving the problem.

▶ **3.** *Mitral regurgitation* is a backward flow of blood through the mitral valve. It is rarely present at birth, but may be caused by rheumatic fever, heart attack, or a defect in the muscles that help control the valve's closure.

Like mitral stenosis, mitral regurgitation may take years to reveal itself. But if leakage back from the left ventricle to the left atrium goes on long enough, it may cause pressure to build in the lungs, and the person may experience shortness of breath. Medications would probably then be prescribed to relieve that breathlessness.

In most cases, symptoms come on gradually. Sometimes, however, such as after a heart attack, the effects of mitral regurgitation will be severe and the person may need emergency treatment.

▶ **4.** *Aortic stenosis* is a narrowing of the aortic valve, the one that regulates the flow of blood from the left ventricle into the aorta—and on to the rest of the body. Again, congenital defects and rheumatic fever account for most cases in people under 50. In the elderly, calcium deposits and *fibrosis,* which is the growth of fibrous tissue, on the valve also lead to aortic stenosis.

Whatever the cause, the result is that the valve leaflets become coated with deposits that distort their shape and reduce blood flow through the valve. To compensate, the left ventricle pumps harder in an attempt to expel enough blood for the body. But the extra exertion tends to weaken the heart muscle over time.

While a person with aortic stenosis may feel no symptoms for years, he or she may eventually feel chest pain or experience shortness of breath or fainting, especially during exercise. After being diagnosed with aortic stenosis, patients are advised not to exercise strenuously.

▶ 5. *Aortic regurgitation* is a condition in which blood flows backward from a widened aortic valve into the left ventricle. In its less common but most serious form, it is known to be caused by an infection that leaves holes in the leaflets of the valve.

As is common with valve defects, symptoms of aortic regurgitation may not appear for years. When they do appear, these symptoms are the result of the left ventricle's working harder to make up for the backward flow of blood: The ventricle eventually enlarges, and fluid backs up. So the person feels short of breath and has chest pain and swelling in the ankles. Severe cases lead to heart failure and require emergency surgery for valve replacement.

Major Causes of Valve Disease

Before antibiotics became widely used, rheumatic fever was the single biggest cause of a person's later developing valve disease. The inflammatory condition could attack body tissue, including the heart, leaving scars on the heart muscle and the valves. Because rheumatic fever typically starts with strep throat, it continues to be important today to prevent rheumatic fever through early diagnosis of strep throat and appropriate treatment with antibiotics.

In the elderly, a childhood bout of rheumatic fever—which usually strikes those between 5 and 15 years old—is implicated as the major cause of valve disease. Today, in younger people who experience valve disease, the source is probably one of these four other possibilities:

▶ 1. *Myxomatous degeneration* is a weakening of valve tissue caused by unexplained metabolic changes. This loss of elasticity of the valves happens most often in the elderly and most often in the mitral valve. The condition may sometimes be diagnosed without leading to further heart problems.

▶ 2. *Calcific degeneration* may affect the elderly with a buildup of calcium deposits on the aortic or mitral valve. On the aortic valve, this buildup tends to cause narrowing, while on the mitral valve, it causes regurgitation.

▶ 3. One common *congenital defect* (present at birth) is an irregularly shaped aortic valve, while a less common congenital problem is a narrowed mitral valve.

▶ 4. *Infective endocarditis* is an infection in the lining of the heart walls and valves—the endocardium. It tends to affect men more often than women, and it's usually a problem associated with people who have congenital valve disease or valves damaged by rheumatic fever. (To help protect against contracting endocarditis, patients who already have valve disease are usually advised to receive antibiotics before any surgery or dental work that could lead to blood infections.)

Although rheumatic fever and these four other causes are most frequently at the root of valve disease, other cases may develop after heart attack or coronary artery disease.

Diagnosing Valve Disease

During the course of a thorough physical exam, a physician most often diagnoses that a person has heart valve disease by listening to the heart through a stethoscope. But the initial diagnosis may be followed by a chest X ray and electrocardiogram—and sometimes by echocardiography studies and diagnostic catheterization procedures.

Normal heart sounds come in pairs. Their sounds are often described as a continuous "lub-dub, lub-dub." The first "lub-dub" is the sound of the simultaneous shutting of the mitral and tricuspid valves, while the second is the closing of the aortic and pulmonary valves in quick succession. When there is a valve problem, however, a whooshing or murmuring sound is added to this normal "lub-dub"—indicating that blood is flowing through a defective valve. A physician's trained ear can even tell that a short, high-pitched murmur reveals stenosis (or narrowing), while a longer, lower-pitched murmur signals valvular regurgitation.

If your doctor detects a murmur, he or she may order a chest X ray to show if the heart is enlarged, or an electrocardiogram to provide information about the heart's electrical activity. Once valve disease is confirmed, your doctor may then turn to *echocardiography* for exact diagnosis.

Echocardiography bounces high-frequency sound waves off the heart to produce a picture of the thickness of the chamber walls, the valves' shapes and action, and the size of the valvular openings. And a sophisticated form of echocardiography called *Doppler echocardiography* can diagnose both stenosis and backflow, because it can determine how much blood is getting pushed through the valves.

If physicians need more information, or if you and your doctor are considering surgery, a *diagnostic cardiac catheterization* may also be recommended. In this procedure, a catheter, usually inserted in your groin area, delivers a dye to your heart chambers. Watching on a screen, physicians can see exactly what is happening in your heart as it happens. Thus, any narrowed valve, backflow, or blockage in your coronary arteries can be identified, and, if surgery is necessary, the appropriate procedure can be planned.

Treating Valve Disease

The treatment of heart valve disease ranges from using medications to reduce its symptoms to repairing or replacing a faulty valve through surgery.

Drugs don't cure heart valve disease, but they can minimize discomfort, decrease the heart's workload, and regulate the heart's rhythm. The single most commonly prescribed drugs for valve problems are digitalis-like medications, which increase the heart's pumping action and relieve some symptoms. Other prescribed drugs include diuretics, to lower the salt and fluid levels in the body; anticoagulants, to prevent blood clots; vasodilators, to enlarge blood vessels and lower blood pressure; and—the most recent—calcium channel blockers, which offer potential for delaying the need for heart valve surgery.

Balloon valvuloplasty is a procedure performed in the cardiac catheterization laboratory to widen a narrowed valve. A variation of the balloon angioplasty used on arteries, it involves inflating a tiny balloon on the tip of a catheter that has been inserted into the valve, to press back any deposits along the edge of the valve. When balloon valvuloplasty is the chosen treatment, it is most often used in narrowed tricuspid and pulmonary valves, sometimes in a narrowed mitral valve, but rarely in an aortic valve.

Surgery is the final and most invasive option for the treatment of valve disease. In surgery, valves may be either repaired or replaced. Repair may involve opening a narrowed valve, removing calcium deposits, or narrowing a valve that doesn't close fully. Repair may be used to treat congenital defects, and it has a good success record in cases of defective mitral valves.

Valve replacement is often used to treat aortic valve disease or any valve disease that's life-threatening. *Prosthetic* (or replacement) *valves* may be mechanical (made from plastics, carbon, and metal alloys) or biologic (made from human or animal tissue). Figure 21 shows illustrations of the three types of mechanical valves currently used (upper left, upper right, and lower left) and of a biologic valve (lower right).

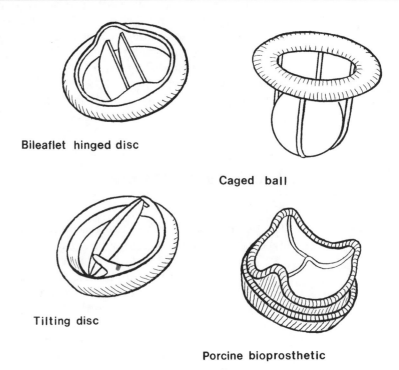

Bileaflet hinged disc

Caged ball

Tilting disc

Porcine bioprosthetic

FIGURE 21   *Four types of prosthetic heart valves.*

Mechanical valves are very reliable, some lasting 20 years or more before needing replacement. However, they may sometimes tend to cause blood clots, so patients with mechanical valves need to take anticoagulant drugs. Biologic valves don't last as long as mechanical ones: After about 10 years, many need to be replaced. But some biologic valves don't require the patient to take anticoagulants, so they may be a good choice for elderly patients or those whose medical conditions keep them from taking anticoagulants.

Preventing Valve Disease

You can't do as much to prevent heart valve disease as you can to prevent some other forms of heart disease, such as coronary artery disease. But you *can* maintain your best general health and eliminate from your life all the heart-health risk factors you possibly can.

One step you can take is to ensure that you and your children do not contract rheumatic fever. Since rheumatic fever comes from a bacterial infection such as strep throat, you need to have throat infections diagnosed early. And you need to be sure to complete the full 7-day course of antibiotics that your doctor prescribes for such an infection, to prevent rheumatic fever.

If you suspect that you have heart valve disease, be assured that many cases do not interfere with your leading a normal life. If you learn that you do have heart valve disease, remember that when it's diagnosed early, it's often effectively treated with drugs. But don't ignore the symptoms of heart valve disease. If you feel short of breath, have swelling in the ankles, or feel chest pain, consult your doctor. A thorough physical exam won't take much time—and it could save your life.

CHAPTER 29

Coronary Artery Disease, Angina, and Heart Attacks

Every year, about one and a quarter million Americans have heart attacks.

Some people who have a heart attack have previously experienced occasions of *angina pectoris* (*angina* = strangling pain, *pectoris* = chest). But the heart attack itself may come with or without warning. Some people experience such warning signs as shortness of breath, chest pain, sweating, or overall weariness. However, about one-third feel no noticeable signals.

Because most heart attacks stem from coronary artery disease, it's important to know what that disease is, how to prevent it, and what remedies are possible for those who develop it.

Coronary Artery Disease

Coronary artery disease (CAD) is a restriction of flow in the arteries supplying the heart with oxygen-rich blood. When this blockage merely *limits* the flow, the heart won't get enough nourishment—especially during physical exertion and high stress—and angina may occur. When the blockage completely *cuts off* the flow, a person will experience a heart attack.

Corona means crown, and the two main arteries that supply the heart with oxygen-rich blood are called coronary arteries because they surround the heart like a crown (see Figure 22). The right coronary artery branches

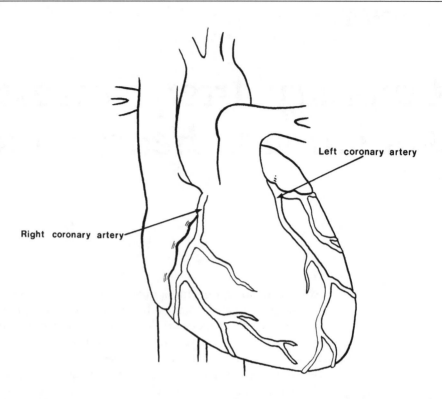

Left coronary artery

Right coronary artery

FIGURE 22　　　　*The coronary arteries surround the heart muscle and supply it with oxygen-rich blood.*

from the aorta and supplies blood to the bottom and right side of the heart. The left coronary artery, which consists of two main blood vessels, supplies the rest.

From the blood supplied by the coronary arteries, cells in the heart muscle take in their oxygen. They need more oxygen, of course, whenever the heart is called upon to work harder, like when you're climbing stairs, having sex, or exercising. Under these conditions, the coronary arteries expand. If, however, they can't deliver enough oxygenated blood, the heart experiences oxygen deprivation, called *myocardial ischemia.*

Healthy arteries have a smooth inner surface called the *endothelium.* But diseased arteries are partly blocked, hindering the flow of blood (see Figure 23). Arterial blockages are occasionally caused by a congenital defect, or may result from spasms in the muscle cells that expand and contract to control blood flow (see Figure 24). Most, however, are caused by atherosclerosis.

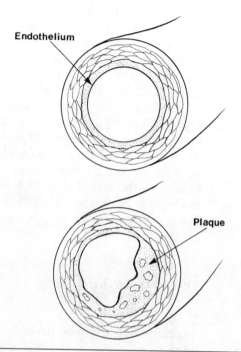

FIGURE 23   *Cross sections of two coronary arteries.*
The top one has a normal, smooth lining (endothelium). However, the bottom one has a buildup of atherosclerotic plaque on the endothelium, which narrows the opening available for blood flow.

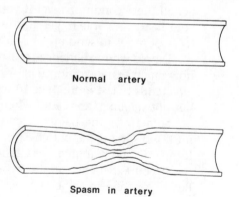

FIGURE 24   *Lengthwise sections of a normal artery and an artery with a spasm, which narrows the opening available for blood flow.*

Atherosclerosis is a buildup of fatty substances in and on the arterial wall. Blockage begins when substances such as cholesterol, carried in the blood, leave streaks on the artery's inner wall. If this wall is roughened or damaged, streaks form even more easily. This process can begin as early as during the late teens. However, most women are protected from atherosclerosis to some degree in early life by their hormones. (See chapter 11 for more details on women and coronary artery disease.)

Gradually, these fatty deposits accumulate, joined by fibrous tissue, various blood components, and calcium, and harden into plaque. When this happens, blood cannot flow smoothly through the artery.

Sometimes, the narrowed artery is suddenly and completely blocked by a blood clot, causing a heart attack. Or the existence of plaque may help the formation of clots: When plaque cracks, the body sends platelets to close the break; these platelets can then coagulate into a clot at the site of the break, completely blocking the artery.

What Is Angina?

Angina is not a disease itself, but rather a symptom of coronary artery disease.

The pain of angina is frequently felt as strong pressure in the middle of the chest. It may or may not radiate out to the shoulders, arms, or jaw. But the main way that it's distinguished from a heart attack is that it stops when you stop doing whatever brought it on.

Typically, angina is brought on by heightened physical activity, emotional stress, eating, or cold temperatures. Your heart must work harder under all these conditions, yet if your coronary arteries are partially blocked, your heart isn't able to get all the oxygenated blood it needs to do its job. Its response is to send up a cry for help in the form of chest pain.

People who experience recurring episodes of angina can often predict how much extra exertion will bring on pain. The pain associated with angina tends to last more than 10 seconds but less than 20 minutes, is steady but not stabbing, and fades when you rest and calm down.

Sometimes the pain of heartburn, inflammation, or arthritis can be mistaken for angina, but chest pain should never be ignored. For more information about angina, see chapter 24, "The Symptoms of Heart Disease."

If you experience angina, you of course need to consult your doctor. But there are also some changes you can make to your lifestyle that can reduce the severity of angina and the risks of developing coronary artery disease. You can avoid excess exertion, especially after meals, and reduce your stress level as much as possible. Your doctor will certainly recommend that you stop smoking if you currently do, may suggest changes in your diet to reduce your consumption of fat and cholesterol, and may start you on a program of regular aerobic exercise.

Diagnosing Coronary Artery Disease

The main symptom of coronary artery disease is angina—chest pain—but it's not always present. Sometimes the heart's oxygen deprivation (ischemia) causes no discomfort; in this case, people are said to have *silent ischemia*. This is the kind of ischemia most often experienced by people who have diabetes.

Diagnosing coronary artery disease involves your physician's taking your medical history, asking you about your symptoms, listening to your heart, and performing certain tests. These may start with a chest X ray and an *electrocardiogram (ECG)*.

A *baseline ECG* may be taken while you're sitting quietly. It will show your heart's activity and may reveal if your heart muscle isn't getting enough oxygen. An *exercise ECG*, also known as a *stress test*, will show how your heart responds to increasingly vigorous exercise. Your heart rate and blood pressure are monitored during this test as well. A drop in blood pressure during physical exertion may reveal coronary artery disease. The exercise ECG is accurate in identifying about three-fourths of the patients with coronary artery disease.

If further tests are needed, a physician may order *radioisotope scanning*, in which a harmless isotope is injected into your bloodstream, revealing information about blood flow. For example, an *exercise thallium test* is very accurate in revealing blockage. For people who cannot take an exercise test, a drug can be given that simulates exercise. Another diagnostic tool is *echocardiography*, a method that uses sound waves to produce an image of how the heart is functioning.

In some cases, such as when a patient with angina hasn't improved after lifestyle changes and medical treatment (see below), a cardiologist may want the patient to undergo *coronary angiography*. This diagnostic procedure takes place in the cardiac catheterization laboratory under mild sedation. Dye is injected to give physicians an X-ray "movie" of heart action and the flow of blood through valves and arteries. The number and severity of blockages can be seen, and decisions can be made about surgery or other treatment options.

More detailed information about the various diagnostic tests may be found in chapter 32, "Diagnosing Heart Diseases."

Treating Coronary Artery Disease

Drugs can relieve the chest pain and complications of coronary artery disease, but they cannot clear blocked arteries. So doctors focus on reducing symptoms and identifying those people who are at increased risk of death from heart disease.

Medications

Several medications, including nitrates, beta-blockers, and calcium channel blockers, help minimize chest pain.

Nitrates open the coronary arteries, improving blood flow to the heart, so the heart doesn't have to work so hard. The most recent means of administering nitrates are the skin patch, which allows a measured release of the drug into the body, and timed-release capsules, which are taken orally for prolonged effect.

Beta-blockers interrupt certain messages that the body sends to the heart. When your physical or emotional stress goes up, your body sends signals to your heart to work harder. Beta-blockers block the effect these signals have on the heart, so they reduce the amount of oxygen the heart demands.

One group of calcium channel blockers helps to keep arteries open and reduce blood pressure by relaxing the smooth muscle that surrounds the arteries in the body. The oxygen demand of the heart is also diminished by these drugs.

People with severe angina are often prescribed a combination of drugs. Aspirin may also be helpful, since it tends to lower the possibility of blood clots forming.

Angioplasty

In *percutaneous transluminal coronary angioplasty (PTCA),* sometimes simply called *angioplasty,* a balloon-tipped catheter is inserted into an artery and threaded through the arterial system until it reaches the blocked portion of a coronary artery (see Figure 25). Then a physician inflates the tiny balloon on the tip of the catheter. As the balloon expands, it presses against the plaque, flattening it and opening the passageway. The balloon is then deflated, the catheter is removed, and the result is improved blood flow.

Every year, about 250,000 Americans undergo PTCA, and most cases—about 90 percent—are successful at first. However, in about one-third of patients, the artery narrows again (a process called *restenosis*) within 6 months of the procedure. Many such patients choose to have the procedure repeated.

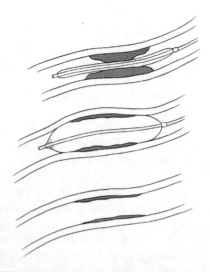

FIGURE 25

Lengthwise sections of an artery narrowed by atherosclerotic plaque and treated with balloon angioplasty.
The balloon has been inserted (top), inflated to flatten the plaque (middle), and removed to reveal a wider opening for blood flow (bottom).

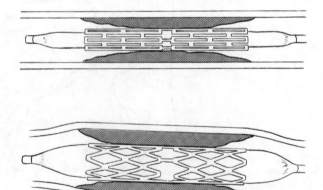

FIGURE 26

Lengthwise sections of an artery narrowed with atherosclerotic plaque and treated with angioplasty and a stent.
After the balloon and stent are inserted (top), the balloon is inflated, opening the stent (bottom). When the balloon is removed, the stent remains in place to maintain the wider opening.

A *stent*—a small wire-mesh device that acts as a brace—can also be inserted in a coronary artery to keep it open to blood flow (see Figure 26). When a stent is used, it usually accompanies PTCA, in which case its purpose is to maintain the opening that has been created by the expansion of the angioplasty balloon. Stents can also be used to close a tear in the wall of a blood vessel.

Two other variations on angioplasty are now in use: atherectomy and laser ablation.

Atherectomy makes use of a high-speed rotary drill (instead of a balloon) on the tip of the catheter. This diamond-tipped drill is positioned at the blockage, then spun up to 200,000 revolutions per minute to pare away plaque from the artery walls. Although the tiny pieces of plaque released into the bloodstream are too small to cause damage, these shavings are entrapped during the procedure and removed from the circulatory system.

Laser ablation is also sometimes used, although it is still considered somewhat experimental. In this procedure, the catheter's tip is equipped

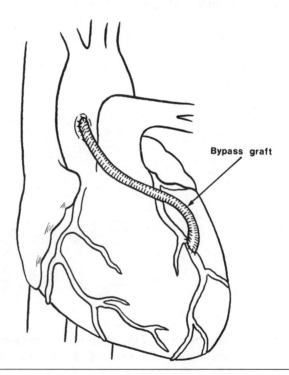

Bypass graft

FIGURE 27   *A bypass graft between the aorta and the left anterior descending coronary artery, which supplies oxygenated blood to the heart muscle.*

with a metal or fiber-optic probe. Carefully directed to the plaque in the artery, the laser uses light to "burn" away the plaque and open the vessel enough so that the balloon can further widen the opening.

Coronary Artery
Bypass Surgery

Coronary artery bypass surgery (CAB) has become a widely used and highly successful means of remedying a blocked coronary artery (see Figure 27). By grafting a healthy vein from the leg or artery from the chest wall, this procedure provides a new route around the blocked coronary artery to supply the heart muscle with oxygen-rich blood. Although research continues about the long-term effects of bypass surgery and about which patients benefit most, it is definitely appropriate in certain cases.

Patients with blockage of the main trunk of the left coronary artery and those with blockages in all three coronary arteries are clear candidates for bypass surgery. So are patients with severe angina that isn't relieved by drug therapy. In addition, those who cannot tolerate the medications prescribed for angina are often helped by surgery. Bypass surgery has been found to give full relief from angina to about 70 percent of people and partial relief to another 20 percent. (See chapter 33, "Heart Surgery," for more details about coronary artery bypass surgery.)

What Is a Heart Attack?

A heart attack occurs when the heart muscle fails to receive oxygen. The technical term is *acute myocardial infarction*, or *acute MI* (*myocardial* = heart muscle, and *infarction* = death of tissue from oxygen deprivation).

The outcome of the attack depends on several factors:

- Where the coronary blockage occurs. Blockage on the left—from the left main or left anterior descending arteries—is usually more dangerous.
- Whether heart rhythm is disturbed. If the blockage also causes irregular heartbeat (arrhythmia), it may cause sudden death. Either fast beating (tachycardia) or fluttering (ventricular fibrillation) may occur. Ventricular fibrillation prevents blood flow, which must be quickly restored through cardiopulmonary resuscitation (CPR) or shock therapy—defibrillation. (For more on CPR, see chapter 21.)
- Whether the heart is supplied by a collateral blood source. Sometimes a person's body responds to a gradual blockage by widening another vessel supplying the heart. If this is the fortunate case, the individual experiences less severe damage from the major blockage.

■ How soon medical care is available. In most cases, receiving medical attention within an hour of the attack's onset minimizes the amount of heart muscle tissue lost. Every minute counts, though, because the death of muscle cells is directly proportional to the length of time that passes before intervention. So if you or one of your family members or friends has a heart attack, that person needs to get medical care as quickly as possible.

Treating a Heart Attack

The goal of heart attack treatment is threefold: restoring blood flow to the heart muscle, reestablishing a regular heartbeat, and giving the heart time to recover.

Before acting, medical personnel make sure a person is having a heart attack, not experiencing symptoms of another condition. Experienced emergency care physicians and nurses can often tell that someone is having a heart attack just by looking at the person. They confirm their diagnosis by talking with the patient, checking heart rate and blood pressure, giving an electrocardiograph test, and taking a blood sample. The electrocardiograph aids in identifying which coronary artery is blocked, while the blood test detects enzymes that leak from damaged heart muscle cells.

During this time, the patient's symptoms are closely monitored. If the heartbeat is fluttering uncontrollably, the team may use an electrical-shock device, a *defibrillator,* to restore normal heart rhythm. If the heart has stopped beating altogether, emergency medical personnel will administer CPR to restore circulation.

As soon as the diagnosis of heart attack is confirmed, a physician will likely administer one or more drugs to the patient. A thrombolytic drug (usually TPA or streptokinase) will be given first to dissolve any blood clots blocking the coronary artery. This medication has been recognized as increasing survival chances when given as soon as possible after an attack.

Aspirin and either heparin, anticoagulants, or other blood-thinning agents may then be used as a follow-up to the thrombolytic agent. These reduce the chance that any blood clots will redevelop or increase in size. In addition, oxygen may be administered to increase the oxygen content of the blood still flowing through the heart, and morphine or other painkillers may be used to reduce discomfort. Beta-blockers, nitroglycerine, and rhythm-stabilizing drugs may also be part of the immediate treatment.

Most patients respond well to this initial drug treatment. They regain some of their heart function, and the rest of the body—which was deteriorating as a result of the heart's failure—stabilizes. Those patients whose hearts don't respond positively to drug therapy may need further emergency care: Balloon angioplasty, coronary artery bypass surgery, or a related procedure.

Whether a patient needs drug therapy or surgery to restore heart function and stabilize the heart, he or she may be hospitalized—for days or weeks. If physicians need to monitor a patient who has not yet undergone surgery, they may hospitalize the person in a unit equipped with continuous heart monitoring technology. When the patient's status is evaluated, one of three courses of action is chosen: The condition is treated medically with drugs, angioplasty is advised, or coronary artery bypass surgery is advised.

A patient who has had an emergency angioplasty or coronary artery bypass surgery will likely recover in an intensive care area devoted to heart patients—a coronary care unit. Follow-up testing that involves any and all of the methods originally used to diagnose heart disease may help evaluate the current state of the patient's heart.

The time it takes for full recovery—which is defined as a return to your normal activities—depends on how active you were before your heart attack, the severity of the attack, and your body's response to it. You'll recover more quickly if you avoid stress, temperature extremes, and conditions that place an added load on your heart. Take it easy, and follow your doctor's instructions.

Coping with a Heart Attack

Avoiding a heart attack, of course, is better than even the best ways of coping with one. So take all the steps you can to minimize your risk factors. But if you have heart disease or are at high risk for it, you need to know how to deal with a heart attack in case one occurs. You should:

- Recognize the warning signs of a heart attack.
- Know which hospitals near your home and office provide 24-hour emergency cardiac care.
- Learn the emergency procedures described in chapter 21.
- Remember that if you do have a heart attack, the more quickly you get medical aid, the better your chances will be for full recovery.

Although a heart attack is always serious, it need not be the end of life. Deaths from heart attack have been cut by over 25 percent during the past decade. Today, those who recover from a heart attack are able to return more fully to their past state of health than ever before.

CHAPTER 30

Diseases of the Peripheral Arteries and Veins

Your peripheral blood vessels are the ones distant from your heart; they are also the ones affected by *peripheral vascular disease (PVD)*. PVD may involve damage or blockage in either your arteries, which carry oxygen-rich blood to all body cells, or your veins, which carry oxygen-depleted blood back to your heart. The main forms that PVD takes include blood clots, inflammation, and the narrowing and blockage of blood vessels.

Diseases of the Arteries

Arterial Blockage   In the same way that coronary arteries can be narrowed and blocked by atherosclerotic plaque, the peripheral arteries can also be blocked.

Atherosclerosis is the buildup of deposits on the inner walls of the arteries, causing the vessels to thicken and lose flexibility. When enough plaque accumulates in an artery, the flow of blood through the area is slowed or even stopped.

A slowdown of blood flow may cause *ischemia*, which is oxygen deprivation in the cells. Atherosclerosis occurring in the coronary arteries can cause a heart attack, while the blockage of an artery to the brain can cause a stroke. In the peripheral arteries, blockage most often produces pain and cramping in the legs.

If leg cramps and pain develop when a person walks a certain distance, especially if it worsens with more strenuous exertion, the person is said to have *intermittent claudication*. Like the chest pain of angina, the leg pain of intermittent claudication tends to fade when the person stops the exertion. Exposure to cold temperatures and some medications (including beta-blockers) can also bring on the leg pain.

Exactly *where* a person feels pain depends on where the blockage occurs: The pain may occur in the calves, thighs, or buttocks. The severity of pain may also signal how severe the blockage is. In very serious cases, the toes may be bluish, the feet may feel cold, and the pulse in the legs may be weak. In rare cases, gangrene may set in and amputation may become necessary.

The risk factors for atherosclerosis in the peripheral arteries are the same as for the condition in the coronary arteries. People who smoke, are diabetic, or have high blood pressure or high blood cholesterol are at special risk. Therefore, any smoker with PVD will be advised to stop smoking. People with diabetes need to manage their diabetes carefully, and people who have poor circulation need to keep their feet warm and dry, and must take extra care to avoid injury.

How a Blockage Is Diagnosed

A physician makes a diagnosis of PVD by listening to a patient describe his or her symptoms, and by finding that the force of the pulse in the arteries of the feet is low. If confirmation is needed, *ultrasonography*—a method that uses sound waves to produce an image of blood flow—may be ordered. If the blockage seems serious enough to warrant surgery or angioplasty, diagnostic *arteriography* may be performed. This procedure involves mild sedation; a harmless dye is injected into the arteries, and cardiologists can then see the location and severity of the blockage of blood flow.

How a Blockage Is Treated

Most patients don't require surgery or angioplasty. Instead, their PVD is controlled by their losing weight (if they need to), their refraining from smoking (if they currently do so), and their sticking to a regular exercise program. Many people gradually increase the distance they can walk without pain, while others get relief from such forms of exercise as swimming or riding a stationary bicycle.

Balloon angioplasty is usually used only when the blockage is severe but found only in a short portion of the artery. A catheter with a balloon on its tip is threaded to the exact spot where the blockage is, then inflated to press the plaque against the walls of the artery and widen the opening for blood flow.

Surgery may be recommended in serious cases. A full cardiovascular examination would then need to be made, because coronary artery disease may be present with PVD. Surgery itself could take the form of bypass surgery (described in chapters 29 and 33) or *endarterectomy*, which is the opening and scraping out of the blocked vessel.

Aortic Aneurysm

An *aneurysm* is the bulging out of the wall of a weakened blood vessel. If the bulging becomes extreme and stretches the vessel wall beyond its limit, the vessel may rupture.

Because the aorta is the main artery carrying blood from the heart to the rest of the body, an aneurysm in this artery, called an *aortic aneurysm,* is especially serious. The bursting of this main artery can be fatal unless it's treated immediately.

An aortic aneurysm may be located in the abdominal area, below the renal arteries, or in the chest. It's usually caused by atherosclerosis, which weakens the wall of the vessel, although high blood pressure and/or congenital conditions sometimes also contribute to the problem.

There are three types of aortic aneurysms, classified by their shape (see Figure 28):

▶ 1. If the entire circumference of the aorta is involved, it's known as a *fusiform* aneurysm.

▶ 2. If only a portion of the circumference is affected, it's called a *saccular* aneurysm.

▶ 3. If the layers of the aortic wall separate or are torn, allowing blood to flow between the layers, it's called a *dissecting* aneurysm.

How Aneurysms Are Diagnosed

While some aneurysms cause no noticeable symptoms, others cause chest or back pain. If the aneurysm is in the chest, a person may also experience hoarseness, coughing, shortness of breath, and problems swallowing.

Often an aneurysm first shows up on a chest X ray. The size and location of the aneurysm can be estimated through echocardiography or through radiologic imaging—either magnetic resonance imaging (MRI) or computed tomography (CT) scanning. Patients who are found to have small aneurysms can be monitored and examined regularly, but those with large ones or dissecting ones need prompt treatment, because the rupture of an aneurysm can be fatal.

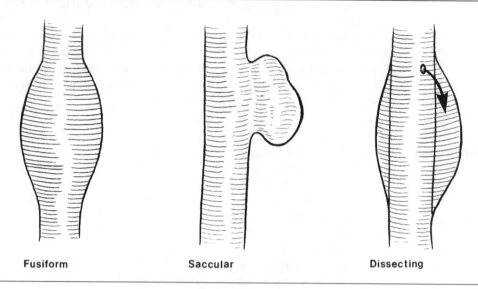

Fusiform	**Saccular**	**Dissecting**

FIGURE 28   *The three types of aortic aneurysms.*

How Aneurysms Are Treated

Aneurysms with a high danger of rupturing need to be repaired surgically. This is usually true of aneurysms that are expanding or are already very large. The operation entails replacing the damaged section with a synthetic graft.

Because an aneurysm, PVD, and coronary artery disease may all be present at the same time, physicians often recommend evaluating the entire cardiovascular system before repairing an aneurysm—unless, of course, there is a threat of imminent rupture. An angiogram can show the state of blood flow through the coronary arteries, and, if necessary, bypass surgery or angioplasty to remedy blocked coronary arteries can be performed *before* surgery to repair the aneurysm.

Other Problems in the Arteries

Two less frequent and less threatening disorders in the arteries are Buerger's disease and Raynaud's phenomenon.

Buerger's Disease

This is a smoking-related disease that causes inflammation of small and medium-sized arteries, and sometimes veins in the feet and legs. A rather rare disorder, it primarily affects male smokers aged 20 to 40.

Buerger's disease involves a severe constriction of the peripheral blood vessels. Although smoking causes some constriction of blood vessels in all those who smoke, those with this condition experience so much narrowing that *ischemia* (lack of oxygen) and *necrosis* (death of tissue) may result. Indeed, the most serious cases sometimes result in the amputation of fingers and toes. A person with Buerger's disease must, of course, stop smoking completely.

Raynaud's Phenomenon

This is another circulation disorder affecting the fingers and toes. Unlike Buerger's disease, which affects far more men than women, *Raynaud's phenomenon* is more common in women, by a ratio of five to one.

Raynaud's phenomenon involves severe constriction in the arteries of the fingers and toes when they're exposed to cold temperature, cigarettes, or emotional stress. A person with this condition may feel numbness and tingling, and may also notice a bluish discoloration of the skin followed by a reddening of the skin in affected areas.

Gradually warming the fingers and toes helps restore circulation. Those with the condition are advised to refrain from smoking, since smoking decreases circulation and constricts blood vessels. They are also urged to avoid cold temperatures and to be sure to wear warm gloves and socks when they can't avoid the cold. A number of medications to relieve the disorder are being tested; calcium channel blockers have been found to relieve symptoms in some cases.

Preventing Arterial Disease

The same factors that put you at risk for heart disease also increase your chances of developing arterial disease.

Cigarette smoking is by far the biggest and most avoidable risk factor for arterial disease. Of course, if you have diabetes or high blood pressure, it's more important than ever that you eliminate all the risks you can.

To decrease your risk factors, look back at Parts Two, Three, and Four of this handbook: Learn what your current risk factors are and what you can do to reduce or eliminate them.

Diseases of the Veins

Venous Blood Clots

A blood clot in the veins, called a *venous thrombus* (plural, *thrombi*), is a coagulated mass of blood. Nearly 6 million Americans have a blood clot in their veins—and the condition can be life-threatening.

The danger stems from the possibility that the clot may dislodge and travel to the lungs. There, it could form a blockage in a blood vessel in the lungs and completely block blood flow.

Blood clots in the veins are usually caused by reduced blood flow, which can lead the blood to coagulate, or by damage to a vein. There are also some genetic disorders that predispose a person to developing venous blood clots.

A reduced or slowed-down flow of blood to the legs and feet may contribute to clot formation. Sometimes blood flow becomes slower because of inactivity—perhaps being confined to bed, lengthy recuperation from a broken bone or an operation, or obesity leading to a sedentary life. Also, some people experience slower blood flow after sitting for hours in an automobile or plane. Other contributors to poor circulation to the legs include smoking, heart disease, diabetes, high blood pressure, inherited conditions, and certain tumors.

Clots in the veins near the skin's surface may cause inflammation and some pain, but they aren't considered as serious as clots in the deep veins, which are more likely to break loose and move to the lungs.

How Venous Blood Clots Are Diagnosed

Deep vein clots often cause pain and swelling, and a physician may be able to identify the condition just by pressing on a part of the leg. When necessary, however, the veins can be viewed by *ultrasonography*—a technique that uses sound waves to create an image on the screen—or with radioactive isotopes. Clots above the knee are sometimes identified by measuring blood flow with a blood pressure cuff around the leg.

Although this method is rarely used today, diagnosis may also be made by a *contrast venography exam,* which provides an X-ray image of the veins in the body. In this procedure, a dye is injected into the patient's feet while he or she is lying down. The patient is then moved into different positions so that physicians can see on a nearby X-ray screen the path of the blood flow through the veins.

How Venus Blood Clots Are Treated

Depending on the cause of the blood clot, it may be treated with blood-thinning or anticoagulant medications, or in some cases with clot-dissolving drugs. For patients who have already had a clot in the lungs and for those who can't take anticoagulants, a catheterization procedure may be performed to prevent further clots from moving to the lungs. A tiny umbrella-shaped filter is guided by a catheter to the vein that carries blood from the legs to the lungs. Permanently in place there, it prevents a clot from reaching the lungs.

People who experience a clot in the deep veins in their legs need to stay in bed with their legs elevated until the condition resolves—usually 3 to 5 days. Moist heat and medications can be used to reduce the swelling and pain. After the person is mobile again, he or she needs to wear elastic stockings below the knee and avoid standing for long periods.

Phlebitis

Phlebitis is an inflammation of a vein in the leg, usually a superficial vein. The area looks reddish and feels painful. The pain is treated with moist heat and aspirin or another nonsteroidal, anti-inflammatory medication.

The more dangerous form of phlebitis occurs in the deep veins of the legs. In these cases, the person usually feels greater pain and has a fever. This condition is more likely to result in clot formation and potential breaking off of the clot and embolization in the lungs.

Pulmonary Embolism

A *pulmonary embolus* is a blood clot that dislodges from where it formed in a vein and travels to the lungs, where it causes a blockage, or *pulmonary embolism*. There, because it blocks an artery, it needs prompt medical attention. Unfortunately, pulmonary embolism may have no warning symptoms, so it can cause sudden, unexpected death.

When symptoms are present, they usually include chest pain (especially upon inhaling), shortness of breath, coughing up blood, and occasionally dizziness and fainting. Even though some cases of pulmonary embolism resolve themselves, they often result in fluid in the lungs and injury to tissue.

How Pulmonary Embolism Is Diagnosed

Diagnosis usually begins with a test of the oxygen level in the blood in the arteries. A low oxygen level indicates that an embolus may be present. The diagnosis is usually confirmed by radioisotope scanning. Follow-up evaluation may include *pulmonary angiography*, in which dye is injected by catheter to reveal blood flow through the lungs.

How Pulmonary Embolism Is Treated

Surgery is needed in rare cases of pulmonary embolism, but most cases are treated with blood-thinning agents, anticoagulants, and clot-dissolving drugs.

Varicose Veins

Varicose veins are swollen, purple veins visible under the skin of the legs. Some women develop them during pregnancy as a result of hormonal changes and the extra pressure the fetus puts on the abdomen. Varicose veins can also be caused by being severely overweight or standing for long periods. A predisposition toward developing varicose veins can be inherited.

Varicose veins are caused by damage to superficial blood vessels, slow blood flow, or problems with the valves in the veins. Normal blood circulation in the legs is aided by valves that keep blood moving upward against the force of gravity. If these valves are weak or blood flow too slow, the blood may pool and cause veins to bulge. This may cause a tingling discomfort, but many who seek a remedy for varicose veins do so primarily because they find them unattractive.

How Varicose Veins Are Treated

Repair may involve injecting a salt solution that causes the veins to shrink. Surgical repair, a process called *stripping*, consists of tying the veins at certain intervals and removing the affected portion of vein. The body naturally responds by creating new circulatory pathways. People with varicose veins are advised to control their weight, avoid standing for long periods, and wear supportive—but not overly constrictive—stockings.

Preventing Peripheral Vascular Disease

Your best defense against peripheral vascular disease is the defense you've been reading about in every chapter of this book: Reduce your overall risk of developing heart disease. If you have diabetes, take care to manage it as well as possible. And if you have other risk factors for heart disease, make the changes you *can* make to give yourself the best chances for a long and healthy life.

CHAPTER 31

Heart Failure

The term *heart failure* may alarm you when you hear it for the first time.

Fortunately, this condition usually doesn't involve a complete work stoppage on the part of the heart. If it did, death would soon occur. Instead, heart failure describes a condition in which the heart isn't working efficiently *enough* to deliver all the oxygen-rich blood the body's cells need.

Sometimes you'll hear the term *congestive heart failure*, which means that there is also an accumulation of fluid (congestion) in the lungs and other body tissues.

About 3 million Americans have some degree of heart failure. Many of them, with treatment, continue to live normal lives, and some find that treatment can even reverse the severity of their condition.

There are four categories of heart failure. In increasing order of severity, they are:

- Class 1: The person may feel no recognizable symptoms and has no restrictions on exercise.
- Class 2: The person is comfortable at rest but feels discomfort during some physical activities.
- Class 3: The person is comfortable at rest but must severely restrict his or her physical activities.
- Class 4: The person may feel chest pain or other signs of a heart problem even at rest, and cannot engage in physical activity without discomfort.

Causes of Heart Failure

The most common cause of heart failure is coronary artery disease (discussed in detail in chapter 29). When the coronary arteries supplying blood to the heart muscle become blocked by plaque, the heart can't pump efficiently.

Coronary artery disease may lead to heart attack, but today more people are surviving heart attacks than in previous decades. Some of these survivors later develop heart failure, although other people with heart failure may never have had a heart attack.

Many problems associated with the heart and circulatory system take their toll over many years. Therefore, heart failure often shows up late in life. It also affects more women than men. High blood pressure, valve defects, heart rhythm problems, coronary artery disease, and heart muscle disease all make the heart work harder with less productivity. Drug abuse, congenital conditions, and alcoholism (which can lead to serious vitamin deficiencies) can also prevent the heart from operating efficiently and contribute to heart failure.

The body has a number of natural methods of protecting itself. In the case of heart failure, three main changes take place: (1) The heart pumps more often, trying to keep its weakened output at a normal level. (2) The heart chambers enlarge to try to pump out more blood. And (3) the kidneys retain more salt and water to increase blood volume. All these measures may, in the early stages of heart failure, keep the heart working at almost normal levels. But after years of enlarging and working harder, the heart eventually wears out.

Symptoms of Heart Failure

The right and left sides of the heart have their separate tasks to carry out. So, depending on the symptoms a person feels, a physician can tell which side of the heart isn't working efficiently.

Blood that has just picked up oxygen from the lungs flows into the left side of the heart—from there to be pumped throughout the body. If the left side isn't working well, blood and fluid will tend to back up in the lungs. So the person with heart failure on the left side will experience shortness of breath, fatigue, persistent coughing (especially at night), and may cough up bloody phlegm.

The right side of the heart receives oxygen-depleted blood returning to the heart from the body. Therefore, if the right side of the heart isn't performing adequately, a person will have slowed blood flow and a buildup of pressure in the veins. Fluids will be retained, and pressure will build in the liver, causing pain, and in the veins of the legs, causing swelling. Because the body has retained fluids, the person will feel a frequent need to urinate at night when he or she lies down and body fluid is more evenly distributed.

Fluid accumulation also makes the kidneys work harder, but sometimes they can't dispose of all the excess water and sodium. If the kidneys can't keep up, *kidney failure* will eventually occur. But this isn't necessarily a permanent condition: If the heart failure is treated, the functioning of the kidneys can return to normal.

Diagnosing Heart Failure

An experienced cardiologist can tell a great deal about the extent of heart failure by listening to a person's symptoms—and to the sounds in the person's chest.

With a stethoscope, a physician may hear the crackling sound of fluid in the lungs. The physician can also tell if fluid has leaked into the chest cavity by listening to a person's breathing or tapping on his or her chest. The distinct sounds of faulty valves or a very rapid heartbeat can also signal that a patient has heart failure. Breathing patterns are important because people with advanced heart failure may have altered breathing patterns.

The physician can feel an enlarged liver by pressing on the patient's abdomen and will notice if there is a bluish tint to the skin, especially in the fingers and toes. That blue tint, along with a possible coolness in the fingers and toes, is a sign that too little oxygen is reaching the extremities.

A chest X ray can reveal retention of fluid in the lungs. It can also show enlargement of the heart—a sign that one's heart has tried to compensate for its inefficiency by growing larger.

Modern diagnostic tools are also available to identify precisely the problems contributing to heart failure and the extent of the damage. These include electrocardiograms, echocardiograms, and such imaging techniques as *radionuclide angiocardiography* and *coronary angiography*. (See chapter 32, "Diagnosing Heart Diseases," for a discussion of the different types of diagnostic tools available.) Diagnosing the cause of heart failure can be tricky because often more than one type of heart condition is involved. Accurate diagnosis is important, however, because then treatment for reversible conditions can begin.

Types of Heart Failure

When your physician diagnoses heart failure, he or she will also explain what has been learned about its causes and what course of treatment should be considered. Some causes of heart failure are easier to treat than others.

The causes of heart failure that *usually* can be treated successfully are:

■ A persistently rapid heart rate.

■ A defect in one or more heart valves.

■ An abnormality in the heart's metabolism.

The causes of heart failure that *sometimes* can be treated successfully are:

■ Infections or inflammation of the heart or the surrounding sac (pericardium).

■ Prolonged, severe hypertension.

■ Poisoning of the heart muscle by alcohol or another toxin.

■ Very high deposits of iron in the heart muscle.

The causes of heart failure that *often* cannot be treated successfully are:

■ Severe intrinsic disease of the heart muscle tissue (cardiomyopathy).

■ Excessive protein deposits in the heart muscle tissue.

■ Enlargement of the heart chambers, with weakened pumping capacity.

■ Injury to the heart muscle from one or more heart attacks.

Treating Heart Failure

The first step your cardiologist will probably take after he or she finds that you have heart failure is to limit the amount of sodium or salt that you take in. Then he or she will prescribe one or more medications—depending on the factors causing your heart failure. These medications may work to lower your blood pressure, ease the load on your heart, and/or control your heart rhythm.

The following classes of drugs are often used to treat heart failure:

■ *Diuretics,* which help eliminate sodium and water from the kidneys.

■ *Digitalis,* which strengthens the heart's ability to pump.

- *Vasodilators,* which open the peripheral arteries. These drugs, including *ACE inhibitors,* lower the blood pressure and allow blood to move more easily through the vessels.
- *Calcium channel blockers,* which keep the vessels dilated and lower blood pressure.

In some cases, medications may also be prescribed to regulate the speed of the heartbeat or to reduce the likelihood of blood clot formation.

Certain heart conditions that contribute to heart failure can be corrected surgically. For example, a number of congenital heart defects can be corrected (see chapter 25); valves can be surgically repaired or replaced (see chapter 28); and blocked coronary arteries can be opened through angioplasty or remedied through coronary artery bypass surgery (see chapters 29 and 33).

A heart transplant is the treatment of last resort for heart failure. Currently, however, the need for donor hearts far exceeds the supply.

Preventing Heart Failure

Heart failure isn't the first heart condition a person typically experiences. Therefore, the best way to avoid heart failure is to practice healthy habits (a moderate diet, regular exercise) that reduce your chances of developing a heart problem of any type.

The second best way to avoid heart failure is to identify and treat early any of the risk factors that contribute to heart failure, such as high blood pressure or coronary artery disease. Reversing high blood pressure through dietary changes or drug therapy can head off more serious problems later. And remedying the plaque buildup of coronary artery disease through angioplasty or bypass surgery—and then following a course of healthy eating and lifestyle habits—will similarly reduce the likelihood of heart failure.

Heart failure is much more common in people over 70 than in younger people. Yet it is how we live our first 70 years that can make a difference in our chances of experiencing and recovering from heart failure. Although heart failure is frightening, it is not necessarily a death sentence. The sooner a diagnosis is made and treatment undertaken, the more likely it is that a person will regain his or her strength and health.

CHAPTER 32

Diagnosing Heart Diseases

The process of detecting and identifying heart diseases has become easier over the last 20 years. Diagnostic tests have become more sophisticated, and there are now many different types of tests available to help your doctor pinpoint the precise problem. For your doctor to take full advantage of these tests, though, it's important to begin with a thorough medical history and physical examination.

Your Medical History

A *medical history* is a review of your health status since birth, your family's health history, and your current lifestyle or habits. Information about your past illnesses, accidents, operations, time spent in the hospital, and allergies forms the foundation of an initial diagnosis. Other important pieces of information include your current symptoms, any medications you may be taking, and your family's history of strokes, heart disease, diabetes, or other illnesses. Finally, how you live day by day may also influence your doctor's appraisal of your condition.

When giving your history and explaining your present symptoms, you should describe them completely and in detail. For instance, chest pains, swelling of the ankles, and frequent urination at night are three separate symptoms, but together they reinforce a diagnosis of beginning heart failure. If you forget to mention a symptom, it's more difficult for your doctor to correctly diagnose your illness.

Your Physical Examination

A heart-related physical exam focuses on your heart rate, heart rhythm, blood pressure, your pulses in different places, signs of swelling, signs of vascular damage, and body sounds heard with the aid of a stethoscope. All these tests are painless and *noninvasive,* meaning that your doctor can perform them with instruments that don't enter the body or puncture the skin. In contrast, *invasive* testing uses instruments that must be inside your body to obtain information. A cardiovascular physical examination does *not* require invasive testing.

Blood pressure is taken using a *sphygmomanometer,* a simple pressure gauge. For details on how blood pressure is measured, see the section "Understanding Your Blood Pressure Reading" in chapter 8.

Although normal blood pressure varies with age and other factors (see Tables 11 and 12 in chapter 8), one standard is 120 over 80, or a diastolic pressure of 120 mm Hg and a systolic pressure of 80 mm Hg. However, ask your doctor to establish a satisfactory reading for you, as your standard may vary from this.

Blood pressure can also be used to determine whether there are blockages in the leg arteries or aorta. For example, three or even four cuffs may be placed on your leg. Blood pressure readings are then taken one at a time from your thigh to your ankle. A comparison of these readings can indicate atherosclerotic disease or blocked arteries.

A related test, called *plethysmography,* uses cuffs to measure changes in blood volume. This test can also help determine whether you have blocked arteries. Different types of plethysmography are used to diagnose the different types of blood vessel disease. These tests are usually performed in a special laboratory.

By feeling your pulse at various places on your body, your doctor can determine your heart rate, the regularity of your heart's rhythm, and any broad abnormalities in the flow of blood through your circulatory system.

Auscultation is the process of listening by means of a stethoscope to your heart sounds, the flow of blood through your vessels, and the noises created by your breathing. These sounds can tell your doctor a great deal about the condition of your heart, blood vessels, and lungs.

Your doctor may also use a light to check the blood vessels in your eyes, the only place on the body where blood vessels can be seen clearly. The condition of these vessels can indicate damage from high blood pressure or other disorders.

The findings of your initial physical examination may need to be confirmed by several other testing procedures.

Chest X Ray

When combined with auscultation, a chest X ray can provide a more exact diagnosis. Chest X rays use a small amount of radiation, and the X-ray procedure itself is painless. The X ray produces a shadowy image that a cardiologist can "read" to determine the size and shape of your heart, detect calcium deposits indicating heart disease or injury, and check the condition of your lungs.

Blood Tests

Chemical and microscopic analyses of the blood can be very revealing. For example, the presence of certain enzymes in the blood indicates damage to the heart muscle.

Drawing blood is a simple, almost painless process. Sometimes it involves only pricking the end of a finger or thumb with a special tool designed to release a single drop of blood. For tests that require more blood, a larger sample, but still only a few milliliters, can be taken from a vein by using a needle. In any case, there is no cause for concern about safety or severe pain.

Blood tests can be used to determine lipid levels (cholesterol and triglycerides), the presence of cardiac enzymes, the oxygen content of the blood, the amount of time the blood takes to clot, kidney and liver function, the possible presence of infection, and more. These tests can give your doctor a great deal of information about your current physical condition.

Electrocardiography

Electrocardiography (ECG) is the basic test of the heart's general condition. It is used specifically to determine possible heart failure and the presence of coronary artery disease. (This test was originally developed in the Netherlands, so the initials EKG, from the Dutch spelling for the procedure, are sometimes used. Both EKG and ECG refer to the same technique.)

An ECG records the heart's electrical activity. This recording, called an *electrocardiogram*, is made by a machine known as an *electrocardiograph*. The process is painless. Electrodes are placed on your body, and the machine detects the strength and patterns of your heart's electrical impulses. Your heart's electrical output is measured, but no electrical current is sent through your body. The recording reveals your heart rate and rhythm, damage to your heart, the occurrence of a heart attack, abnormalities in the structure of your heart, and whether your heart is receiving an adequate supply of oxygen.

An ECG given to a person who is sitting down is called a *baseline ECG*. An ECG given to person who is exercising is called a *stress test,* a *tolerance test,* or an *exercise ECG*. It is also possible, using a portable unit called a *Holter monitor,* to continue an ECG while a person goes through his or her normal daily routine. ECG readings may be transmitted over the telephone. This means that emergency medical personnel can administer the test in an ambulance on the way to a hospital and send the results to the hospital so that they're there for doctors to review before the patient arrives.

In combination with your medical history, physical examination, blood work, and chest X ray, an electrocardiogram completes your basic cardiovascular evaluation. If your doctor needs a more precise diagnosis, he or she can use a variety of more advanced diagnostic tests.

Echocardiography

Echocardiography uses sound waves to form an image of the heart. Echocardiography is used to detect valve and other heart problems, such as inflammation around the heart, congenital heart disease, and congestive heart failure. The procedure is painless and simple to perform. In routine echocardiography, a small instrument (a *transducer*) is placed on the skin of your chest above your heart. The transducer bounces the sound waves off your heart and translates the echoes it receives into a visual display of your heart.

Another form of this test, *transesophageal echocardiography (TEE),* can be used if additional information is required. In TEE, a small transducer is inserted into the mouth and down the esophagus (food pipe). This places the transducer very close to the heart, where it can produce more detailed images of the heart's structures.

Nuclear Scanning

In a sense, nuclear scanning of the heart is the reverse of an X ray. When making an X-ray image, radiation is sent through the body from an outside source. But in a nuclear scan, a small amount of radioactive material is injected into the bloodstream. The radiation coming from inside the body then makes it possible for a special camera to take pictures of the heart and its structures. This camera detects radiation in the same way that a Geiger counter does. The traces of radioactivity are tracked as they circulate through your body, producing an image that gives the cardiologist useful knowledge about your condition.

Radionuclide Ventriculography

To determine how well your heart's ventricles are working, a process called *radionuclide ventriculography* is used in one of two ways.

The *MUGA (MUltiGated Acquisition) scan* relies on a radioactive trace material that remains in the heart for several hours while images of the heart are recorded. In a *first-pass study,* on the other hand, the trace material does *not* remain in the body for as long a period. It is there only for a "first-pass." The MUGA scan evaluates the heart's overall function and can assess the damage done to heart tissue from a heart attack. The MUGA scan also accurately measures the amount of blood squeezed from the left ventricle with each stroke. This amount of blood, known to cardiologists as the *left ventricular ejection fraction*, is a prime indicator of your heart's health.

Perfusion Scan

In a *perfusion scan*, a radioactive material (usually thallium-201 or sestamibi) is injected into the bloodstream and then absorbed by the healthy heart muscle. Damaged heart muscle tissue or tissue not receiving an ample supply of blood absorbs less of the thallium or takes longer to absorb it, while scarred heart muscle tissue does not absorb thallium. Images of the thallium taken over time can show which parts of the heart muscle are not receiving enough (or any) oxygen-rich blood.

A perfusion scan may also be performed at the end of a stress test. This combination of tests is used in several ways: to determine whether blockages exist in the coronary arteries, to evaluate patients whose ECG is abnormal, and to estimate the probable success of angioplasty. If patients are too ill or weak to exercise, they may take a "mock" stress test, in which drugs are used to stimulate the blood flow and mimic the physical effects of exercise.

Single Photon Emission Computed Tomography (SPECT)

Single photon emission computed tomography (SPECT) is a nuclear scanning technique that provides a three-dimensional image of the heart. In this procedure, a person who has been given an injection of a radioactive material lies down on a special table. A camera is then rotated around the patient, so that pictures of the heart can be taken from different angles. This technique is useful for showing damaged heart muscle and decreased perfusion in the heart muscle.

Computed Tomography (CT or CAT) and Positron Emission Tomography (PET) Scanning

Computed tomography (CT or CAT scan) and *positron emission tomography (PET scan)* are nuclear imaging techniques that don't rely on an injected radioactive material. CT scanning generates images produced by a computer analysis of X-ray pictures made by rapidly rotating the X-ray source around the body. This process creates pictures of cross-sectional "slices" of the body. Positron emission tomography (PET) scanning is mostly used to determine which areas of the heart muscle are not receiving blood and have been damaged. It can also be used to measure blood flow in other areas of the body. PET scanning is expensive, however, and so is not widely used.

Magnetic Resonance Imaging (MRI)

Magnetic resonance imaging, or *MRI,* differs from the other scanning methods in that it uses magnetic fields and radio waves instead of X rays or injected radioactive material. MRI requires no injections. If you're undergoing an MRI, you'll lie down on a table that is then slid into a hollow magnet large enough to hold your entire body. Although this chamber may seem a little frightening, it's completely safe. If you have a pacemaker or hearing aid, however, be sure to tell your doctor before undergoing an MRI; the magnet may interfere with the proper functioning of these devices.

Among its many uses, MRI can detect heart tumors and help your doctor evaluate valve disease and congenital diseases of the heart.

Angiography

In *angiography*, a fine tube, or catheter, is inserted into a blood vessel in the groin or arm and guided into the heart. A special dye is injected from the catheter into the heart, allowing heart activity to be recorded by X ray in a kind of motion picture. In *coronary angiography,* this dye is injected into the coronary arteries. The images then let your cardiologist see any blockages that may be limiting blood flow to the heart muscle.

Because angiography is invasive—that is, an object is inserted through the skin into the body—there is some controversy about when it should be used. Nonetheless, angiography is currently the best way to determine how well the left ventricle is working, to locate any blockages in the coronary arteries, and to determine how much blockage exists. This test is especially useful to the surgeon who is going to replace blocked sections of the coronary arteries through a coronary bypass procedure (see chapter 33, "Heart Surgery") or to the cardiologist who will attempt to open a blocked coronary artery through balloon angioplasty (see chapter 29).

Electrophysiology Studies

An *electrophysiology (EP) study* is sometimes used when more information about the heart's electrical functions is needed to diagnose a problem.

Electrophysiology studies are generally conducted by inserting catheters tipped with electrodes through a vein into the right atrium and ventricle. When the catheters are in place, the electrodes sense the tiny electrical currents that the heart produces to make its chambers contract. The electrodes can also create a current of their own and cause the heart to contract. Electrophysiology studies can map or diagram the heart's own electrical pattern. And introducing a current into the heart can create an abnormal rhythm, which enables the cardiologist to examine certain arrhythmias more closely, to check whether certain medications are working, or to evaluate the heart's response to a pacemaker.

During an electrophysiology study, some people may faint, feel dizzy, or experience a hammering in the chest and a rapid heartbeat. In a few people, the heart may suddenly stop beating, so means of restarting the heart are always kept near at hand.

Your Cooperation Can Help in Your Diagnosis

Your doctor will only ask you to take the tests that he or she needs to make the right diagnosis—which is the first step toward relieving your symptoms and regaining your health. You can help your doctor help you by following any instructions that he or she gives before you take a test. For example, some tests require that you not eat for several hours before-hand. And remember to ask your doctor to discuss any test results with you.

CHAPTER 33

Heart Surgery

Today surgical correction of a number of heart problems is an everyday reality. In 1994 alone, more than 500,000 surgeries for coronary bypass or valve repair were performed in the United States. And despite the well-publicized shortage of donor organs, about 2,000 people benefitted from heart transplants.

Just decades ago, such surgery was a mere dream. Although surgeons during World War II had learned how to operate on the heart, they were limited in carrying out that knowledge. It was difficult to operate on a beating heart, and the heart couldn't be stopped for more than a few minutes without irreparable damage to the brain.

Two major advances in medicine made modern cardiac surgery possible: the heart-lung machine that took over the work of the heart, and cooling preservation techniques that allowed more time for surgical intervention without brain damage.

The Cardiopulmonary Bypass Machine

Known to most Americans as the *heart-lung machine, cardiopulmonary bypass technology* not only replaces the heart's pumping action but also supplies oxygenated blood that body cells need. With the heart's pumping action replaced by the heart-lung machine, the heart can be repaired more easily. For example, the heart can be opened to correct defects on the inside, and blocked coronary arteries can be bypassed to restore blood flow to the heart muscle.

Acting as both substitute heart and substitute lungs, the heart-lung machine carries blood from the patient's right atrium to a holding tank and then to a special chamber called an *oxygenator*. There, the blood travels through thin membranes that imitate the way the lungs allow blood to shed carbon dioxide and pick up oxygen. Finally, the oxygenated blood is filtered and sent to the patient's aorta, which then directs it throughout the body.

A modern heart-lung machine can maintain adequate blood flow and respiration for hours. Specially trained technicians called *perfusion technologists* ensure that this machine does its job properly during surgery. Still, surgeons strive to minimize the time a patient must depend on such artificial support.

Cooling Techniques

The second technological breakthrough permitted the heart to be stopped safely for an extended period. Damage to heart tissue is prevented by subjecting the heart to a cool temperature; this also results in a reduction in the heart's demand for oxygen.

Cooling is achieved in three ways. (1) Blood passing through the heart-lung machine is cooled, which in turn cools the whole body as blood reaches all body parts. (2) The heart itself is immersed in a cold saline bath. And (3) a solution of potassium is injected into the heart. The potassium has the effect of stopping the heart's electrical activity—its signal to pump. In this stilled, chilled condition, the heart is usually safe for about 2 to 4 hours.

Your Surgery Team

During open-heart surgery, a highly trained group of health professionals pool their knowledge and skills to act as a team. The members include:

- Your cardiovascular surgeon, who heads up the surgery team and performs key parts of the surgery him- or herself.
- Assisting surgeons, who act under the direction of your cardiovascular surgeon.

- The cardiovascular anesthesiologist, who administers and monitors appropriate levels of anesthesia and ventilator support.
- The perfusion technologist, who operates the heart-lung machine.
- Nurses specially trained to assist with cardiovascular cases.

Many different kinds of surgery are now performed on the heart or blood vessels, including coronary artery bypass surgery, valve repair or replacement surgery, surgery to correct arrhythmias, heart transplantation, repair of aneurysms, repair of congenital defects, and peripheral vascular bypass surgery.

Preparing for Your Surgery

Unless you have an emergency condition, your surgery will be scheduled for a day that is convenient for you and your surgeon, at a time when the hospital has an operating room available. The exact time may be a few days or several weeks after you and your doctor first discuss the surgery.

When your surgeon meets with you to discuss why your surgery is needed, he or she will have reviewed the findings from the diagnostic tests you have received or undergone. The surgeon should explain those test results, describe the operation and any risks involved, instruct you about preparing for your surgery, and give you a good estimate of the amount of improvement in your health (heart or vascular) that you can expect from the operation.

Be sure to express all your concerns and questions during this meeting. You deserve and should expect full explanations that are clear to you and any member of your family who accompanies you to the conference. This is a good time to ask questions about your activity level before the operation, how long recovery might take—and anything else you're wondering about. It's also a good time to review with your doctor the medications you're currently taking, in case some need to be changed or stopped before your surgery.

In addition to the information you'll receive from talking with your doctor, you can take advantage of other sources of information as well. Many hospitals hold informative sessions about open-heart surgery for patients and their families. Most will give you free literature or videotapes about the exact operation you're going to have and what you can expect during your hospitalization. Many doctors and hospitals also have specially trained nurses on staff to assist patients and their families in learning about and preparing for surgery.

As your surgery date approaches, several preparatory steps are common. You should report any changes in your health to your surgeon and doctor—especially if you experience fever, chills, coughing, or a runny nose during the week before your surgery. Such a respiratory illness could affect your recovery.

At the Hospital

You may be admitted to the hospital on the day before your surgery or, in some instances, early on the morning of your surgery. Even if you have recently had an electrocardiogram, blood tests, urinalysis, and chest X ray, you'll probably be given these again to make certain there's no change in your health status.

Anesthesia is safest on an empty stomach, so one standard instruction is that you have nothing to eat or drink after midnight the night before your surgery. You should also bathe the night before your surgery to reduce the amount of bacteria on your skin. Before your surgery, the area to be operated on will be washed, scrubbed with antiseptic, and—if necessary—shaved.

Before surgery, the anesthesiologist will visit with you, give you a short physical exam, and take your medical history again. You'll probably have to answer questions that you've answered before, but it's important that you give complete information, because that will help the anesthesiologist precisely monitor your anesthesia.

Nurses and others involved in your care may also ask several questions. These, too, may seem repetitious, but remember—the more your caregivers know about you, the better able they'll be to give you excellent care. Remember, too, that you and your family can ask all the questions you need to. The answers to some questions—such as where your family should wait, or when they'll hear a report on your progress—may be found in printed material that the hospital gives you, but you should always feel free to ask.

The Surgery Itself

Many types of surgery involve opening the heart's chambers—although coronary artery bypass is one type of heart surgery that doesn't. But whatever type of surgical procedure you're about to have, you'll find that the preliminary activities have much in common.

For example, you'll first be given a mild tranquilizer before being taken to the operating room. Electrodes will be placed on your back so that an ECG machine can show a continual reading of your heart's rhythm and electrical activity. After you receive a local anesthetic, intravenous (IV) lines will be inserted in a vein so that anesthesia can be administered as needed throughout your surgery. A Foley catheter will be inserted into your bladder to collect urine during your operation, and general anesthesia will then be administered.

When you're fully anesthetized, a tube will be inserted in your windpipe and connected to a respirator that will take over your breathing for you. Another tube will be inserted into your stomach to prevent fluid and air from collecting and causing distention and nausea, and an anticoagulant drug will be administered to prevent clotting. With all these preliminaries complete, the surgeon is now ready to open your chest.

From this point on, the surgical details will differ depending on the heart condition to be remedied. The sections that follow give brief overviews of several frequently performed surgeries.

Coronary Artery Bypass Surgery

The most common type of heart surgery, coronary artery bypass, involves grafting a segment of vein from the thigh or chest to circumvent or "bypass" a portion of a diseased coronary artery. (See chapter 29 for more details on coronary artery disease.) The blockage may be in the left main branch, which is crucial to supplying the heart with blood, or in the right coronary artery, which may not be quite as dangerous. Then again, multiple blockages in different coronary arteries may need to be bypassed. However, the number of bypasses (whether double, triple, or quadruple) doesn't necessarily indicate the severity of your heart condition.

Coronary artery bypass surgery is distinct from most other forms of heart surgery in that the chambers of the heart are not opened during the bypass procedure. The major goal of coronary artery bypass surgery is to give a new route for blood flow—in order that the heart muscle will receive the oxygen it needs to function.

Valve Repair or Replacement

Since valves regulate the flow of blood into and out of the ventricles, it's important that they open at the right time and that they close completely to prevent backflow. Two of the most common valve problems that require surgical repair are:

▶ 1. A rigid and partly blocked valve, which may need to be opened (or re-placed) to increase the flow of blood through it.

▶ 2. A valve that leaks, which may need to be tightened (or replaced).

Most often, valve repair is needed on the mitral or aortic valves—both on the left side, the harder working of the two sides of your heart. The *mitral* valve controls flow from the left atrium into the left ventricle, while the *aortic* valve controls flow from the left ventricle into the aorta and on throughout the body. (See chapter 28 for more details on diseases of the heart valves.)

Surgical repair of valve defects, especially mitral insufficiency, involves the surgeon's reconstructing the valve leaflets so that the valve will close properly. Surgical replacement can be carried out with artificial valves: either mechanical or biological devices. Mechanical valves usually last longer than biological ones, but the patient must take anticoagulant drugs the rest of his or her life.

Arrhythmias

Irregular heartbeats, whether they're too fast or too slow and whether or not they entail some other disturbance, are frequently treated first with medications. But in some cases, procedures performed in the catheterization laboratory or operating room may be required to deal effectively with the irregularity.

A wide range of pacing and rhythm-control devices can be implanted. For example, pacemakers are implanted in patients with various types of *bradycardia* (too slow a heartbeat). (See chapter 27 for more details on this and other types of arrhythmias.) And relatively small defibrillators can be implanted that detect a severe ventricular arrhythmia called *fibrillation* and deliver a shock to correct the condition.

Radio-frequency ablation is a means of using radio-frequency energy to eliminate electrical pathways that at times cause arrhythmias. When surgical ablation is chosen, the area causing the arrhythmia can be eliminated using computerized mapping techniques that precisely identify the incorrect paths. In another surgical technique called *maze surgery*, used occasionally in patients with severe atrial arrhythmias, surgeons make incisions in the atria that, when closed, create a new route—a maze—for the heart's electrical charge to move through efficiently.

Aneurysm Repair or Replacement

The weakening and bulging out of an area in the wall of the heart or an artery can often be repaired surgically before it causes death from heart failure or rupture. (See chapter 30 for more details on diseases of the peripheral arteries and veins.)

The aneurysm may be a *left ventricular aneurysm* or an *aortic aneurysm.* If the former develops after a heart attack, it signals that oxygen-deprivation has caused significant damage to the left ventricle. When arrhythmia or heart failure also develops, the surgeon may perform open-heart surgery to remove the part of the ventricular wall that has been damaged. Or the surgeon may use a prosthetic material to strengthen the weakened area.

Often, an aortic aneurysm is repaired with a section of prosthetic graft, frequently made of Dacron fabric.

Transplant

Heart transplantation is the treatment of last resort for patients with end-stage heart disease. Candidates for this drastic surgery have severe heart failure and little prospect of improvement without a replacement heart. Currently, 90 percent of heart transplant recipients are alive a year after their transplant, with a generally good quality of life.

The Texas Heart Institute has an outstanding record of success and innovation in the field of heart transplantation. Since the discovery and application of *cyclosporine,* a remarkable antirejection drug, in the early 1980s, approximately 600 patients have received heart transplants at the Texas Heart Institute. Nationwide, heart transplants are limited to about 2,000 each year due to a shortage of donor organs. The need is great to encourage more people to consider organ donation.

In some patients, surgeons can implant a mechanical device that helps the heart circulate blood while the patient waits for a donor heart. These mechanical circulatory devices, or heart-assist devices, are often referred to as "bridges" to transplantation, because they bridge the time gap from heart failure to heart transplantation. During this time period, most patients become healthier and better candidates for transplant. Some patients with electrical versions of these heart-assist devices can now wait for their transplant operations at home. When a suitable donor heart becomes available, the mechanical device is removed. In the future, such devices may be implanted permanently in some patients as an alternative to heart transplantation.

When a patient undergoes a heart transplant operation, the diseased heart is removed, and the donor heart is sewn into its place. In a very few instances, the patient's original heart will be left in place and the new heart connected to it. This is called a *heterotopic transplant.*

Potential rejection of the new heart is closely monitored in the days, months, and years following transplantation. This is done by taking a small piece of heart tissue, called a cardiac biopsy, during a catheterization procedure and analyzing the extent of rejection in this tissue sample. At the Texas Heart Institute, pathologists have developed a precise measuring tool to gauge the extent of rejection, using a scale from 1 to 10. Antirejection medications can be adjusted on the basis of the biopsy results.

Heart and Lung Transplants

In cases of patients whose lungs and hearts are both failing, the combination heart-lung transplant may be performed. Relatively rare in comparison to heart transplant, this surgery usually requires a longer recovery period. However, this procedure has been successful in many cases.

Recovering from Open-Heart Surgery

After your surgery is complete, you'll be moved to an intensive care unit (ICU). You'll probably stay there for 2 days or more, depending on your type of surgery and the severity of your condition.

While you're in the ICU, your blood pressure, temperature, and pulse will be continuously measured and monitored. Pressures in your heart chambers and the amount of blood flowing through your heart will likely be measured by a special tube, called a *Swan-Ganz catheter,* or by other similar methods. An ECG will constantly monitor your heart's rhythm and electrical activity. Any extra fluid or blood from around your heart will drain through a tube in your chest, and you'll be fed intravenously. You'll also be given medications to prevent complications, such as infection.

The ICU is a high-tech environment filled with highly trained staff. You'll receive frequent attention from physicians and nurses, you'll be monitored constantly, but you'll still feel the discomforts of recovering from surgery. Although the respirator tube that was placed in your windpipe will probably be taken out within 6 hours of your surgery, other tubes will stay in until you leave the ICU.

Every day will bring significant progress in your recovery. Depending on how quickly your condition stabilizes, your physician will move you to a less intensively monitored unit where you'll continue your recovery. Your cardiologist will generally monitor your condition during the remainder of your stay in the hospital after surgery. Throughout this time, it's important that you cough often to clear your lungs and keep your airways open. As your strength returns, your activities will gradually be increased, and you'll be put on a program of cardiac rehabilitation.

Cardiac Rehabilitation

Many physicians recommend that their heart surgery patients enroll in a structured program of cardiac rehabilitation. (See chapter 34 for details.) Whether sponsored by the hospital where you had your heart surgery or another organization, the program may include classes on heart-healthy nutrition, patient and family sessions about stress reduction, and an exercise plan carried out under the supervision of a physiologist experienced in cardiac care.

Enhancing Your Chances of Successful Recovery

You can do three things to increase your chances of successful recovery from heart surgery.

▶ **1.** *Talk with your cardiologist and surgeon.* Satisfy yourself that the surgery is necessary, and learn the answers to all your questions. Use this opportunity to deal with your fear. Remember, fears are natural, and talking about them will help relieve your anxiety.

▶ **2.** *Follow your doctor's instructions.* Also answer fully all the questions your doctor asks, because the information you give may affect how your doctor carries out his or her important role in your future health.

▶ **3.** *Know that your recovery depends as much on your attitude as on the physical benefits of the surgery.* You need to recover at your own pace and according to what's best for you—not according to someone else's timetable.

Open-heart surgery will probably seem frightening to you. Yet in many cases it is lifesaving. It can give you the opportunity to enjoy many more healthy and productive years.

CHAPTER 34

Recovering from Heart Surgery or Heart Disease

The process of recovering from heart disease or heart surgery is called *cardiac rehabilitation*. In the past, men and women recuperating from a heart attack or heart surgery were required to stay in bed as part of their convalescence. But those days spent in bed did nothing to help them regain their strength and stamina. As a result, many heart patients became invalids.

Experience and sound medical practice have changed the recovery process. Today, cardiac rehabilitation has two goals: to restore a person to as full and normal a life as possible, and to do so in the shortest time that his or her medical condition allows. A patient's rehabilitation program after heart disease or heart surgery is an essential part of his or her overall treatment.

Your Role in Cardiac Rehabilitation

How quickly and how well you recover from heart disease or heart surgery depends on several important factors that you can control (or at least influence): your mental attitude, your emotional reactions, your cardiovascular conditioning, your overall physical fitness and diet, and lifestyle changes that will decrease the risk of further heart-related problems. To give you the maximum benefit, your rehabilitation program should be designed especially for your needs.

Also, cardiac rehabilitation programs aren't just for people who have had a heart attack or heart operation. You can benefit from such programs if you have angina, a disease of the heart muscle, problems with your heart valves, or some other cardiovascular disease. In particular, anyone undergoing angioplasty to open a clogged coronary artery can enhance his or her chances of avoiding open-heart surgery by also following a recovery regimen.

Specialists, from your personal doctor and cardiologist to physical therapists and dietitians, are available to help you recover. Your friends and family are a part of your rehab team as well.

When Should Rehabilitation Begin?

Rehabilitation begins as soon as your condition has stabilized after a heart attack, other heart disease, or heart surgery. If your doctor doesn't suggest a formal plan, discuss your concerns and request a trial program. The sooner you begin, the more quickly you'll see results—and the more benefits you'll likely receive.

What Makes a Rehabilitation Program Successful?

A good cardiac rehabilitation program usually has five interrelated parts that work together to help you recover both physically and mentally. These parts correspond to the following five goals:

▶ 1. Understanding your condition.

▶ 2. Making the necessary emotional adjustments to your situation.

▶ 3. Learning how to live with your symptoms and limitations.

▶ 4. Improving your overall cardiovascular and physical fitness.

▶ 5. Living a heart-healthy life.

We'll now discuss each of these five components, and goals, of cardiac rehabilitation in detail.

Understanding Your Condition

If you have had a heart attack, you need to know what portion, if any, of your heart muscle has been irreversibly damaged. You also need to know what to do to prevent another one, and what is being done to treat the causes of your disease. If you have had a heart valve replaced, you need to know why it had to be replaced and how long the new valve can be expected to function. In essence, you need to understand your condition, what you can do to improve it, and the purpose of any treatment you're receiving, including a reason for each medication you're taking. The better you understand your condition, the easier it will be to speed your recovery.

Making the Necessary Emotional Adjustments to Your Situation

The emotional aspects of your recovery are also very important. If you have had a heart attack or have undergone open-heart surgery, the experience can elicit strong emotional reactions in you and your family and friends.

For most people, the first emotional reaction is denial. The feeling that "this can't be happening to me" then opens the door to self-doubt, because the event *is* happening to you. Facing your own mortality can also undermine your self-confidence, and when you lose confidence, you lose the ability to act. In addition, denial, along with shock and fear, often produces anger, which you may direct at both medical personnel and your family and friends.

The emotional impact of a heart attack or heart disease will also affect your family, friends, and coworkers, because they, too, will have serious questions about the future and fears about your condition. Role reversals, lifestyle changes, or even something as simple as new dietary requirements can produce stress and conflict in your family.

Doubts can multiply during the recovery period, when many patients begin to question whether they'll be able to continue working, whether they'll have another heart attack, and whether they can make the necessary changes in their lives. Anxiety and fear are common at this stage, for both you and your family. If you're recovering from heart surgery or heart disease, don't suppress your natural apprehension and worry. If you avoid all thoughts about your condition, you can't discuss it, and you may not hear about something that could relieve your fears and worries. Suppressing your feelings may also lead to problems in communicating with your family and friends. These problems can, in turn, produce depression, which creates another mental barrier to recovery.

You may also be abnormally aware of little aches and pains in your body. For a short time after a heart attack or surgery, or after a diagnosis of heart disease, many people think every muscle twitch or slight indigestion is the beginning of another heart crisis. However, you cannot recover successfully until you regain your mental equilibrium. Sometimes professional counseling is helpful; if you'd like to talk to a counselor, tell your doctor, who can recommend appropriate help.

The mental and emotional components of cardiac rehabilitation should begin while you're still in the hospital. When you're well enough, your doctor should explain what happened, why it happened, and what can be done about it. Straightforward, frank talk is important, because your understanding and acceptance are the first steps toward a good mental outlook. You can then use your past experiences to motivate yourself to lead a heart-healthier life.

Learning How to Live with Your Symptoms and Limitations

To feel as good as you can as soon as you can, you must do your part to control your symptoms and live within your limitations. Many people find it helpful to view their heart attack, heart disease, or surgery as a turning point in their life: Before the event, they lived one way, and afterward, they'll live another. The new way isn't better or worse than the old; it's just different.

Part of the new way of life entails following your doctor's instructions, understanding your condition, and paying attention to any symptoms you may experience. First, carefully follow all instructions about how and when to take your prescribed medications. Second, talk with your doctor about your condition and any side effects you might experience from the medications. And third, follow your doctor's recommendations about diet, smoking, and alcohol consumption. As your condition improves, your symptoms may change. If that happens, be sure to let your doctor know.

Physical limitations or restrictions can present another set of challenges. In most cases, any physical constraints will be minor and temporary. But if these restrictions will be long term, do your best to learn to live with them. Discuss them with your doctor, understand why they're being imposed, and work out the best arrangement to deal with them. Don't dwell on what you *can't* do; instead, concentrate on what you *can* do. And when you're feeling especially burdened by a physical limitation, try thinking about someone you know who's confronted with a physical challenge even greater than your own.

Improving Your Overall Cardiovascular and Physical Fitness

The key to leading an active life after a heart attack, heart disease, or surgery is improving your cardiovascular and physical conditioning. Improvement usually comes from following a regular exercise routine that will develop the capacity of your heart and lungs, increase your flexibility, and gradually strengthen your muscles. The routine should be designed specifically for you with the full approval of your doctor.

In addition to improving your strength and endurance, regular exercise can increase your sense of well-being, improve your self-image, and help control your weight. These benefits are particularly important for a person recovering from a heart problem. A fitness program helps many people recovering from a heart problem return to work, participate in family affairs, and resume their sex lives.

Almost anyone can benefit from an appropriate physical fitness plan; but if you're recovering from a heart attack or heart surgery, your benefits will be even greater.

Living a Heart-Healthy Life

After a heart attack or heart surgery, follow these general guidelines:

- Don't smoke, don't worry, and don't hurry.
- Eat a heart-smart diet.
- Start a fitness program and stick with it.

Following these guidelines will increase your chances of avoiding future problems, improve your overall health, and contribute to a positive outlook on life. You'll find easy-to-follow programs for each of these guidelines described in Part Five of this handbook.

Note: Don't forget to consult your doctor before starting any exercise program, especially after heart surgery.

Recovery and Sex

A major concern of many people recovering from a heart problem is returning to a satisfactory sex life. The demand placed on the heart during sex is about the same as that of climbing a couple of flights of stairs or taking a brisk walk, and most people are up to that degree of physical exertion a few weeks after a heart attack or heart surgery. The *physical* ability to engage in sex, though, is often not the problem.

Many experts believe that your mental or emotional state strongly affects your ability to enjoy sex. If you have had a heart attack or heart surgery, you may be worried about dying, the physical demands of sex, or other similar concerns. It isn't surprising, then, that sexual difficulties and reduced sexual desire are common among those recovering from heart disease. It's also common for your partner to have fears and concerns about resuming sexual activities. In time, however, most people are able to return to their usual sex life.

Because some medications reduce or inhibit sexual desire, you may want to ask your doctor whether those are possible side effects of your medications. Of course, if you should experience chest pains, an irregular heart rate, or a greater than normal shortness of breath during sex, stop!

If you have questions about resuming your sexual activities, talk to your doctor. Your concerns and questions are appropriate: Your doctor won't be embarrassed—and you shouldn't be either.

The Importance of a Positive Attitude

Your recovery will probably be aided the most by a positive attitude. Heart attack patients who become depressed have a lower survival rate and a higher chance of experiencing another heart attack than patients who maintain a positive attitude.

The contribution of a positive attitude to good health is recognized but difficult to measure. Generally, though, a person who wants to recover will have a better chance of doing so.

The Importance of Gradual Change

One of the keys to recovery is *gradual* change. That is, you should:

- *Gradually* change your way of life in order to become more heart-healthy.
- *Gradually* change your diet to lower your consumption of fats, sugar, and salt.
- *Gradually* make an exercise program part of your daily routine.
- *Gradually* examine attitudes or fears that hinder your progress.

In essence, think in terms of *gradual improvement*. The habits of a lifetime cannot be corrected overnight. However, your heart problem may provide you with extra incentive to change your lifestyle.

Resources for More Information

Aging

Eldercare Locater
1112 16th Street NW, Suite 100
Washington, DC 20036
800–677–1116

> Information regarding home-delivered meals, transportation, legal assistance, housing options, adult day care, home health services, and senior centers in locations near you.

National Council on Aging
409 Third Street SW, Suite 200
Washington, DC 20024
800–424–9046

> Information and publications about various topics including family caregivers, senior employment, and long-term care facilities.

National Institutes on Aging
PO Box 8057
Gaithersburg, MD 20898–8057
800–222–2225

> Provides health information on all aspects of aging, including diseases and disorders, safety, nutrition, and care. Services available Monday through Friday, 8:30 A.M. to 5 P.M., Eastern Time.

Children of Aging Parents
1609 Woodbourne Road, Suite 302A
Levittown, PA 19057–1151
800–CAPS294 or 800–227–7294

> A national clearinghouse of information for caregivers of the elderly. Provides listing of resources available in individual states and sometimes by county. Services available Monday through Friday, 9 A.M. to 3 P.M., Eastern Time.

Alcohol

800-ALCOHOL

> This hotline is available 24 hours a day, seven days a week, to offer counseling and assistance in finding local treatment centers.

Al-Anon Family Group Headquarters
Alateen
PO Box 862
Midtown Station
New York, NY 10018–0862
800–356–9996

> Information and support for families affected by alcoholism.

Alcoholics Anonymous, Inc.
General Services Office
PO Box 459
Grand Central Station
New York, NY 10163
212–870–3400

> Sobriety support for anyone who has a problem with alcohol.

Cancer

AMC Cancer Research Center
1600 Pierce Street
Denver, CO 80214
800–525–3777

> Information about new and ongoing cancer research.

Cancer Care, Inc.
National Cancer Institute
1180 Avenue of the Americas

New York, NY 10036
212–221–3300

> Information about the physical and emotional effects of cancer on patients and their families.

Cancer Information Service
800–4–CANCER (800–422–6237)

> Information about cancers, treatment options, and local resources; provided by the National Cancer Institute.

National Cancer Institute
Office of Cancer Communications
Building 31, Room 10A16
Bethesda, MD 20892
301–496–5583

> Information about cancers, treatment options, and local resources. For questions about cancer, call the toll-free number operated by the National Cancer Institute: 800–4–CANCER (800–422–6237).

Cardiovascular Health

American Heart Association
National Center
7272 Greenview Avenue
Dallas, TX 75231–4596
800–242–8721 or 800–AHA–USA1

> Information and publications about the prevention, diagnosis, and treatment of cardiovascular diseases.

Heart Information Service
Texas Heart Institute
PO Box 20345
Houston, TX 77225–0345
800–292–2221

> Information about the prevention, diagnosis, and treatment of cardiovascular diseases in children and adults. Call Monday through Friday, 8 A.M. to 5 P.M., Central Time.

National Heart, Lung, and Blood Institute
Information Center
PO Box 30105
Bethesda, MD 20824–0105
301–251–1222

> Information about cholesterol, high blood pressure, smoking, asthma, and heart attacks.

National Marfan Foundation
382 Main Street
Port Washington, NY 11050
800–8–MARFAN (800–862–7326) or 516–883–8712

> Information for individuals affected by the Marfan Syndrome and support for family members.

Sudden Arrhythmia Death Syndrome Foundation
PO Box 58767
Salt Lake City, UT 84158
800–786–7723

> Information about Long Q-T Syndrome and other arrhythmias.

Diabetes

American Diabetes Association, Inc.
1660 Duke Street
Alexandria, VA 22314
800–232–3472

> Information about the disease, treatment options, and ongoing research.

Juvenile Diabetes Foundation International
1200 Wall Street, 19th Floor
New York, NY 10005
800–533–2873

> Information about the disease, treatment options, and ongoing research.

National Diabetes Information Clearinghouse
One Information Way
Bethesda, MD 20892–3560
301–654–3327

> Information about various educational materials. Maintains a meeting registry that includes regional, national, and international meetings and conferences.

Drugs

National Clearinghouse for Alcohol and Drug Information
6000 Executive Boulevard
PO Box 2345

Rockville, MD 20852
800–729–6686

Provides information and fact sheets about drug and alcohol usage.

National Institute on Drug Abuse
800–662–4357

Provides information and referral to a treatment center.

Fitness

American College of Obstetricians and Gynecologists
409 12th Street SW
Washington, DC 20024–2188

Write and request a copy of technical bulletin no. 189, "Exercise During Pregnancy and the Postpartum Period."

American College of Sports Medicine
PO Box 1440
Indianapolis, IN 46206–1440

Send a self-addressed, stamped envelope to receive general information about fitness and exercise.

American Running and Fitness Association
4405 East West Highway, Suite 405
Bethesda, MD 20814
800–776–2732

Information and educational materials that explain the symptoms and treatment of stress fractures, shin splints, and more. Call Monday through Friday, 9 A.M. to 5 P.M., Eastern Time.

National Youth Sports Foundation for the Prevention of Athletic Injuries
10 Meredith Circle
Needham, MA 02192
617–449–2499

Information and educational materials promoting the safety and well-being of children and adolescents participating in sports.

President's Council on Physical Fitness and Sports
701 Pennsylvania Avenue NW
Washington, DC 20004
202–272–3421

Information on walking, jogging, and exercise and weight-control fitness for Americans of all ages.

General Health Services and Information

Centers for Disease Control and Prevention
1600 Clifton Road NE
Mail Stop D25
Atlanta, GA 30333
404–332–4555

> Recorded messages on a variety of health topics, including vaccines, precautions for international travel, and infectious diseases such as the flu.

National Insurance Helpline
1001 Pennsylvania Avenue NW
Washington, DC 20004
800–942–4242

> Information about how to shop for health and life insurance. No company recommendations or price comparisons provided. Call Monday through Friday, 8 A.M. to 8 P.M., Eastern Time.

National Consumers League
1701 K Street NW, Suite 1200
Washington, DC 20006
202–835-3323

> Call for a consumer's guide to hospice care, a 34-page booklet providing basic information, which sells for $4.

National Health Information Center
PO Box 1133
Washington, DC 20013–1133
800–336–4797

> Information about disease prevention and health services; provides toll-free numbers of organizations and health services.

National Library of Medicine
8600 Rockville Pike
Bethesda, MD 20894
800–272–4787

> Sends health hotline's directory and provides other health-related services.

Nutrition

Meat and Poultry Hotline
U.S. Department of Agriculture/FSIS

2925 South 14th Street and Independence Avenue
Washington, DC 20205
800–535–4555

> Information about the safety, labeling, storage, preparation, and nutritional value of meat and poultry. Dietitians available to answer questions. Call Monday through Friday, 10 A.M. to 4 P.M., Eastern Time.

National Center for Nutrition and Dietetics (NCND)
216 West Jackson Boulevard, Suite 800
Chicago, IL 60606–6995
800–366–1655

> Information about food, diet, and nutrition. Call Monday through Friday, 9 A.M. to 4 P.M., Central Time. Recorded messages available 24 hours daily.

National Cholesterol Education Program
NHLBI Information Center
PO Box 30105
Bethesda, MD 20824–0105
301–251–1222

> Distributes literature about how to select and prepare low-cholesterol foods for children, including "Cholesterol in Children—Healthy Eating Is a Family Affair" and "Eating with Your Heart in Mind." Spanish versions available.

Nutrition Information Service
University of Alabama at Birmingham
1675 University Boulevard, Room 449
Birmingham, AL 35294–3360
800–231–3438

> Information about peak-performance eating, including topics such as fluid intake, vitamin and mineral supplements, and carbohydrate loading. Call Monday through Friday, 9 A.M. to 4 P.M., Central Time.

Seafood Hotline
U.S. Food and Drug Administration
800–332–4010

> Information about the purchasing, handling, storing, preparation, and nutritional value of fish and seafood. Call Monday through Friday, noon to 4 P.M., Eastern Time.

The Superintendent of Documents
Consumer Information Center
Department 159-Y
Pueblo, CO 81009

> Copies of the Food Guide Pyramid booklet are available by sending a $1.00 check or money order to this address.

Organ Donation and Transplantation

American Organ Transplant Association
PO Box 277
Missouri City, TX 77459
713–261–2682

> Information for transplant patients and their families.

LifeGift Organ Donation Center
5615 Kirby, Suite 900
Houston, TX 77005
800–633–6562 or 713–523–4458 in Houston

> Information and support for people who are awaiting transplant and potential donors; a not-for-profit, federally certified organization.

United Network for Organ Sharing (UNOS)
1100 Boulders Parkway, Suite 500
Richmond, VA 23225
804–330–8504

> A federally supported organization helping medical personnel match people who are awaiting transplant with potential donors.

Prescription Drug Information

FDA Bulletin Board (computer modem access only)
800–222–0185
301–443–7318 (for technical assistance)

> Free access to the Food and Drug Administation's computer bulletin-board system via modem. Lists FDA recalls, newly approved drugs and devices, and provides AIDS updates.

Pharmaceutical Manufacturers Association
1100 15th Street NW
Washington, DC 20005
800–862–4110

> Information about various prescription drugs and ongoing research.

Smoking

American Cancer Society
National Office
1599 Clifton Road NE

Atlanta, GA 30329
800–ACS–2345

Information about smoking-cessation groups. Ask about "Fresh Start," the quit-smoking program, and its brochure, "Seven-Day Plan to Help You Stop Smoking Cigarettes."

American Heart Association
National Center
7320 Greenville Avenue
Dallas, TX 75231
800–AHA–USA1

Distributes stop-smoking literature, including "Calling It Quits."

American Lung Association
1740 Broadway, 14th Floor
New York, NY 10019–4374
800–586–4872 or 800–LUNG–USA

Distributes literature, including "Freedom from Smoking in 20 Days" and "A Lifetime of Freedom from Smoking."

Stroke

Courage Stroke Network
3915 Golden Valley Road
Golden Valley, MN 55422
800–553–6321

Referral to the nearest Stroke Club or guidance on forming your own. Stroke Clubs are primarily independent, although some are affiliated with local chapters of the Easter Seal Society or the American Heart Association.

National Aphasia Association
PO Box 1887
Murray Hill Station
New York, NY 10156–0611
800–922–4622

Information and support for the long-term needs of aphasic patients and their families.

National Institute of Neurological Disorders and Stroke
NINDS Information Office
Building 31, Room 8A06
Bethesda, MD 20892
301–496–5751

General information about stroke and various neurological disorders.

National Stroke Association
300 East Hampden Avenue, Suite 200
Englewood, CO 80110–2622
800–787–6537

Sends literature on stroke, its causes, prevention, and recovery. Provides referrals for individuals seeking information on physicians, treatments, rehabilitation, and community care programs. Services available Monday through Friday, 8 A.M. to 4:30 P.M., Mountain Time.

Glossary

Abdominal aorta. The portion of the aorta in the abdomen.

Ablation. Elimination or removal.

Alveoli. Air sacs in the lungs where oxygen and carbon dioxide are exchanged.

Aneurysm. A saclike protrusion from a blood vessel or the heart, resulting from a weakening of the vessel wall or heart muscle.

Angina or angina pectoris. Chest pain that occurs when diseased blood vessels restrict blood flow to the heart.

Angiography. An X-ray technique that makes use of a dye injected into the coronary arteries to study blood circulation through those vessels. The test allows physicians to measure the degrees of obstruction to blood flow. (Circulation through an artery is not seriously reduced until the inside diameter of the vessel is more than 75 percent obstructed.)

Angioplasty. A nonsurgical technique for treating diseased arteries by temporarily inserting into an artery a catheter with a tiny balloon at its tip. The balloon is then inflated briefly to reduce blockage in the artery.

Angiotensin-converting enzyme (ACE) inhibitor. A drug that lowers blood pressure by interfering with the breakdown of a proteinlike substance involved in blood pressure regulation.

Annulus. The ring around a heart valve where the valve leaflet merges with the heart muscle.

Anticoagulant. Any drug that keeps blood from clotting; a blood thinner.

Antihypertensive. Any drug or other therapy that lowers blood pressure.

Aorta. The largest artery in the body and the initial blood-supply vessel from the heart.

Aortic valve. The valve that regulates blood flow from the heart into the aorta.

Aphasia. The inability to speak, write, or understand spoken or written language because of brain injury or disease.

Arrhythmia (or dysrhythmia). An abnormal heartbeat.

Arterioles. Small, muscular branches of arteries. When they contract, they increase resistance to blood flow, and blood pressure in the arteries increases.

Arteriosclerosis. A disease process, commonly called hardening of the arteries, which includes a variety of conditions that cause artery walls to thicken and lose elasticity.

Arteritis. Inflammation of the arteries.

Artery. A vessel that carries oxygen-rich blood to the body.

Ascending aorta. The first portion of the aorta, emerging from the heart's left ventricle.

Atherectomy. A nonsurgical technique for treating diseased arteries with a rotating device that cuts or shaves away obstructing material inside the artery.

Atherosclerosis. A disease process that leads to the accumulation of a waxy substance, called plaque, inside blood vessels.

Atria. The two upper or holding chambers of the heart.

Atrial septal defect. See *Septal defect.*

Atrioventricular block. An interruption or disturbance of the electrical signal between the heart's atria (upper two chambers) and ventricles (lower two chambers).

Atrioventricular (AV) node. A group of cells located between the atria (upper two chambers) and the ventricles (lower two chambers) that regulates the electrical current (heart rhythm) that passes through it to the ventricles.

Atrium (right and left). Either one of the heart's two upper chambers.

Beta-blocker. An antihypertensive drug that limits the activity of epinephrine, a hormone that increases blood pressure.

Biopsy. The process by which a small sample of tissue is taken for examination.

Blalock-Taussig procedure. The insertion of a palliative shunt between the subclavian and pulmonary arteries, used to increase the supply of oxygenated blood in blue babies (see below).

Blood clot. A jellylike mass of blood tissue formed by clotting factors in the blood. Clots stop the flow of blood from an injury; they can also form inside an artery whose walls are damaged by atherosclerotic buildup and can cause a heart attack or stroke.

Blood pressure. The force or pressure exerted by the heart in pumping blood; the pressure of blood in the arteries.

Blue babies. Babies who have a blue tinge to their skin (cyanosis) resulting from insufficient oxygen in the arterial blood. This condition often indicates a heart defect.

Bradycardia. Abnormally slow heartbeat.

Bundle-branch block. A condition in which portions of the heart's conduction system are defective and unable to conduct the electrical signal normally, causing arrhythmias.

Calcium channel blocker (or calcium blocker). A drug that lowers blood pressure by regulating calcium-related electrical activity in the heart.

Capillaries. Microscropically small blood vessels between arteries and veins that distribute oxygenated blood to the body's tissues.

Cardiac. Pertaining to the heart.

Cardiac arrest. The stopping of the heartbeat, usually because of interference with the electrical signal (often associated with coronary heart disease).

Cardiac catheterization. A procedure that involves inserting a fine, hollow tube (catheter) into an artery, usually in the groin area, and passing that tube into the heart. Often used in conjunction with angiography and other procedures, cardiac catheterization has become a prime tool for visualizing the heart and blood vessels and diagnosing and treating heart disease.

Cardiac enzymes. Complex substances capable of speeding up certain biochemical processes in the cardiac muscle. Abnormal levels of these enzymes indicate that a heart attack has occurred.

Cardiac output. The amount of blood the heart pumps through the circulatory system in one minute.

Cardiology. The study of the heart and its function in health and disease.

Cardiomyopathy. A disease of the heart muscle that leads to generalized deterioration of the muscle and its pumping ability.

Cardiopulmonary bypass technology. The process by which a machine is used to do the work of the heart and lungs so that the heart can be stopped during surgery.

Cardiovascular (CV). Pertaining to the heart and blood vessels. The cardiovascular system consists of the heart and all the blood vessels that circulate blood throughout the body.

Cardioversion. A technique of applying an electrical shock to the chest in an attempt to convert an abnormal heartbeat to a normal one.

Carotid artery. A major artery (right and left) in the neck supplying blood to the brain.

Cerebral embolism. A blood clot formed in one part of the body and then carried by the bloodstream to the brain, where it blocks an artery.

Cerebral hemorrhage. Bleeding within the brain resulting from a ruptured blood vessel, aneurysm, or a head injury.

Cerebral thrombosis. Formation of a blood clot in an artery that supplies part of the brain.

Cerebrovascular. Pertaining to the blood vessels of the brain.

Cerebrovascular accident. Also called cerebral vascular accident, apoplexy, or stroke. An impeded blood supply to some part of the brain, resulting in injury to brain tissue.

Cerebrovascular occlusion. The obstruction or closing of a blood vessel in the brain.

Cholesterol. A fatty substance that occurs naturally in the body, in animal fats, and in dairy products, and that is transported in the blood. Limited quantities are essential to the normal development of cell membranes.

Cineangiography. The technique of taking moving pictures to show the passage of an opaque dye through blood vessels, which allows physicians to diagnose diseases of the heart and blood vessels.

Circulatory system. Pertaining to the heart, blood vessels, and the circulation of blood.

Claudication. A tiredness or pain in the arms and legs caused by an inadequate supply of oxygen to the muscles, usually due to narrowed arteries.

Collateral circulation. Blood flow through small, nearby vessels in response to blockage of a main blood vessel.

Computed tomography (CT or CAT scan). An X-ray technique that uses a computer to create cross-sectional images of the body.

Conduction system. Special muscle fibers that conduct electrical impulses throughout the muscle of the heart.

Congenital. Refers to conditions existing at birth.

Congenital heart defects. Malformation of the heart or of its major blood vessels present at birth.

Congestive heart failure. A condition in which the heart cannot pump all the blood returning to it, leading to a backup of blood in vessels and the accumulation of fluid in body tissues, including the lungs.

Coronary arteries. Two arteries arising from the aorta that arch down over the top of the heart and divide into branches. They provide blood to the heart muscle.

Coronary artery bypass (CAB). Surgical rerouting of blood around a diseased vessel that supplies the heart by grafting either a piece of vein from the leg or the artery from under the breastbone.

Coronary artery disease (CAD). A narrowing of the inside diameter of arteries that supply the heart with blood. The condition arises from the accumulation of plaque and greatly increases a person's risk of having a heart attack.

Coronary heart disease. Disease of the heart caused by atherosclerotic narrowing of the coronary arteries and likely to produce angina pectoris or heart attack; a general term.

Coronary occlusion. An obstruction of one of the coronary arteries that hinders blood flow to some part of the heart muscle.

Coronary thrombosis. Formation of a clot in one of the arteries that carry blood to the heart muscle. Also called coronary occlusion.

Cyanosis. Blueness of skin caused by insufficient oxygen in the blood.

Cyanotic heart disease. A birth defect of the heart that causes oxygen-depleted (blue) blood to circulate to the body without first passing through the lungs.

Death rate, age-adjusted. A death rate that has been standardized for age so that different populations can be compared or the same population can be compared over time.

Deep-vein thrombosis. A blood clot in the deep vein in the calf.

Defibrillator. An electronic device that helps reestablish normal contraction rhythms in a malfunctioning heart.

Diabetes (diabetes mellitus). A disease in which the body doesn't produce or properly use insulin, which is needed to convert sugar and starch into the energy needed in daily life.

Diastolic blood pressure. The lowest blood pressure measured in the arteries, it occurs when the heart muscle is relaxed between beats.

Diuretic. A drug that lowers blood pressure by stimulating fluid loss; promotes urine production.

Doppler ultrasound. A technology that uses sound waves to assess blood flow within the heart and blood vessels and to identify leaking valves.

Ductus arteriosus. See *Patent ductus arteriosus.*

Dysarthria. The imperfect articulation of speech resulting from muscular problems caused by damage to the brain or nervous system.

Dyspnea. A shortness of breath.

Echocardiography. A method of studying the heart's structure and function by analyzing sound waves bounced off the heart and recorded by an electronic sensor placed on the chest. A computer processes the information to produce a two- or three-dimensional moving picture that shows how the heart and heart valves are functioning.

Edema. Swelling caused by fluid accumulation in body tissues.

Ejection fraction. A measurement of what portion of blood is pumped out of a filled ventricle. The normal rate is 50 percent or more.

Electrocardiogram (ECG or EKG). A test in which several electronic sensors are placed on the body to monitor electrical activity associated with the heartbeat.

Electroencephalogram (EEG). A graphic record of the electrical impulses produced by the brain.

Electrophysiological study (EPS). A test that uses cardiac catheterization to study patients who have arrhythmias (abnormal heartbeats). An electrical current stimulates the heart in an effort to provoke an arrhythmia, which is immediately treated with medication. EPS is used primarily to identify the origin of arrhythmias and to test the effectiveness of drugs used to treat them.

Embolus. Also called embolism; a blood clot that forms in a blood vessel in one part of the body and travels to another part.

Endarterectomy. Surgical removal of plaque deposits or blood clots in an artery.

Endocarditis. A bacterial infection of the heart's inner lining (endothelium).

Endocardium. The smooth membrane covering the inside surfaces of the heart.

Endothelium. The smooth inner lining of many body structures, including the heart (endocardium) and blood vessels.

Enlarged heart. A state in which the heart is larger than normal due to heredity, long-term heavy exercise, or diseases and disorders such as obesity, high blood pressure, and coronary artery disease.

Enzyme. A complex chemical capable of speeding up specific biochemical processes in the body.

Epicardium. The thin membrane covering the outside surface of the heart muscle.

Estrogen. A female hormone produced by the ovaries that may protect women against heart disease. Estrogen is not produced after menopause.

Exercise stress test. A fairly common test for diagnosing coronary artery disease, especially in patients who have symptoms of heart disease. The test helps physicians assess blood flow through coronary arteries in response to exercise, usually walking, at varied speeds and for various lengths of time on a treadmill. A stress test may include use of electrocardiography, echocardiography, and injected radioactive substances. Also called exercise test, stress test, or treadmill test.

Familial hypercholesterolemia. A genetic predisposition to dangerously high cholesterol levels.

Fatty acids. Chemical components of triglycerides (fats).

Fibrillation. Rapid, uncoordinated contractions of individual heart muscle fibers. The heart chamber involved can't contract all at once and pumps blood ineffectively, if at all.

Flutter. The rapid, ineffective contractions of any heart chamber. A flutter is considered to be more coordinated than fibrillation.

Gated blood pool scan. An analysis of how blood pools in the heart during rest and exercise. The test makes use of a radioactive substance injected into the blood to tag or label red blood cells. The test provides an estimate of the heart's overall ability to pump and its ability to compensate for one or more blocked arteries. Also called a MUGA scan.

Heart attack. Death of, or damage to, part of the heart muscle due to an insufficient blood supply.

Heart block. General term for conditions in which the electrical impulse that activates the heart muscle cells is delayed or interrupted somewhere along its path.

Heart failure. See congestive heart failure.

Heart-lung machine. An apparatus that oxygenates and pumps blood to and from the body during open-heart surgery.

Heredity. The genetic transmission of a particular quality or trait from parent to offspring.

High blood pressure. A chronic increase in blood pressure above its normal range.

High-density lipoprotein (HDL). A component of cholesterol, HDL helps protect against heart disease by promoting cholesterol breakdown and removal from the blood; hence, its nickname "good cholesterol."

Holter monitor. A portable device for recording heartbeats over a period of 24 hours or more.

Hypertension. High blood pressure.

Hypertrophic obstructive cardiomyopathy (HOCM). An overgrown heart muscle that creates a bulge into the ventricle and impedes blood flow.

Hypoglycemia. Low levels of glucose in the blood.

Hypotension. Abnormally low blood pressure.

Hypoxia. Less than normal content of oxygen in the organs and tissues of the body.

Immunosuppressive medications. Any drug that suppresses the body's immune system. These medications are used to minimize the chances that the body will reject a newly transplanted organ such as a heart.

Impedance plethysmography. A noninvasive diagnostic test used to evaluate blood flow through the leg.

Infarct. The area of heart tissue permanently damaged by an inadequate supply of oxygen.

Inferior vena cava. The large vein returning blood from the legs and abdomen to the heart.

Inotropic medications. Any drug that increases the strength of the heart's contraction.

Intravascular echocardiography. A marriage of echocardiography and cardiac catheterization. A miniature echo device on the tip of a catheter is used to generate images from inside the heart and blood vessels.

Ischemia. Decreased blood flow to an organ, usually due to constriction or obstruction of an artery.

Ischemic heart disease. Also called coronary artery disease and coronary heart disease, this term is applied to heart ailments caused by narrowing of the coronary arteries, and therefore characterized by a decreased blood supply to the heart.

Jugular veins. The veins that carry blood back from the head to the heart.

Lesion. An injury or wound. An atherosclerotic lesion is an injury to an artery due to hardening of the arteries.

Lipid. Triglyceride, cholesterol, or other fatty substances insoluble in blood.

Lipoprotein. A lipid surrounded by a protein; the protein makes the lipid soluble in blood.

Low-density lipoprotein (LDL). The body's primary cholesterol-carrying molecule. High blood levels of LDL increase a person's risk of heart disease by promoting cholesterol attachment and accumulation in blood vessels; hence, the nickname "bad cholesterol."

Lumen. The hollow area within a tube, such as a blood vessel.

Magnetic resonance imaging (MRI). A technique that produces images of the heart and other body structures by measuring the response of certain elements in the body (such as hydrogen) to a magnetic field. When stimulated by radio waves, the elements emit distinctive signals in a magnetic field. MRI can produce detailed pictures of the heart and its various structures without the need to inject a dye.

Mitral valve. The structure that controls blood flow between the heart's left atrium (upper chamber) and left ventricle (lower chamber).

Mitral valve prolapse (MVP). A condition that occurs when the leaflets of the mitral valve between the left atrium (upper chamber) and left ventricle (lower chamber) bulge into the ventricle and permit backflow of blood into the atrium. The condition is often associated with progressive mitral regurgitation.

Monounsaturated fat. A type of fat found in many foods but predominantly in avocados and canola, olive, and peanut oil. Monounsaturated fat tends to lower LDL cholesterol levels, and some studies suggest that it may do so without also lowering HDL cholesterol levels.

Mortality. The total number of deaths from a given disease in a population during an interval of time, usually a year.

Murmur. Noises superimposed on normal heart sounds. They are caused by congenital defects or damaged heart valves that do not close properly and allow blood to leak back into the chamber from which it has come.

Myocardial infarction. The damage or death of an area of the heart muscle (myocardium) resulting from a blocked blood supply to the area. The affected tissue dies, injuring the heart. Symptoms include prolonged, intense chest pain and a decrease in blood pressure that often causes shock.

Myocardial ischemia. Deficient blood flow to part of the heart muscle.

Myocardium. The muscular wall of the heart. It contracts to pump blood out of the heart and then relaxes as the heart refills with returning blood.

Necrosis. Referring to the death of tissue within a certain area.

Nitroglycerin. A drug that helps relax and dilate arteries, often used to treat cardiac chest pain (angina).

Noninvasive procedures. Any diagnostic or treatment procedure in which no instrument enters the body.

Obesity. The condition of being significantly overweight. The term is usually applied to the condition of being 30 percent or more over one's healthy body weight. Obesity puts a strain on the heart and can increase the chance of developing high blood pressure and diabetes.

Occluded artery. An artery in which the blood flow has been impaired by a blockage.

Open-heart surgery. An operation in which the chest and heart are opened surgically while the bloodstream is diverted through a heart-lung (cardiopulmonary bypass) machine.

Pacemaker. A surgically implanted electronic device that helps regulate the heartbeat.

Palpitation. An uncomfortable sensation within the chest caused by an irregular heartbeat.

Patent ductus arteriosus (PDA). A congenital defect in which the opening between the aorta and the pulmonary artery does not close after birth.

Percutaneous transluminal coronary angioplasty (PTCA). See *Angioplasty.*

Pericardiocentesis. A diagnostic procedure using a needle to withdraw fluid from the sac or membrane surrounding the heart (pericardium).

Pericarditis. Inflammation of the outer membrane surrounding the heart. Rheumatic fever, tuberculosis, and many other agents are its possible causes.

Pericardium. The outer fibrous sac that surrounds the heart.

Plaque. A deposit of fatty (and other) substances in the inner lining of an artery wall; it is characteristic of atherosclerosis.

Platelets. One of the three types of cells found in blood; they aid in the clotting of the blood.

Polyunsaturated fat. The major fat constituent in most vegetable oils, including corn, safflower, sunflower, and soybean oils, which are all liquid at room temperature. Polyunsaturated fat actually tends to lower LDL cholesterol levels but may also reduce HDL cholesterol levels.

Positron emission tomography (PET). A test that uses positron emitting substances to assess information about the metabolism of elements that can be used to indicate whether heart muscle is alive and functioning. A ring of radiosensitive detectors positioned around the chest reconstructs a two- or three-dimensional image of the heart.

Prevalence. The total number of cases of a given disease that exist in a population at a specific time.

Pulmonary. Referring to the lungs and respiratory system.

Pulmonary valve. The heart valve between the right ventricle and the pulmonary artery. It controls blood flow from the heart into the lungs.

Pulmonary vein. The blood vessel that carries newly oxygenated blood from the lungs back to the left atrium of the heart.

Radionuclide ventriculography. A diagnostic test used to determine the size and shape of the heart's pumping chambers (the ventricles).

Regurgitation. Backward flow of blood through a defective heart valve.

Renal. Pertaining to the kidneys.

Rheumatic fever. A disease, usually occurring in childhood, that may follow a streptococcal infection. Symptoms may include fever, sore or swollen joints, skin rash, involuntary muscle twitching, and development of nodules under the skin. If the infection involves the heart, scars may form on heart valves, and the heart's outer lining may be damaged.

Risk factor. An element or condition involving a certain hazard or danger. When referring to heart and blood vessels, a risk factor is associated with an increased chance of developing cardiovascular disease, including stroke.

Rubella. Commonly known as German measles. A viral disease generally lasting 3 to 5 days. Signs include a rash and swollen lymph nodes. If contracted while pregnant, particularly in the first trimester, it can cause serious birth defects.

Saturated fat. Type of fat found in foods of animal origin and a few of vegetable origin; they are usually solid at room temperature. Abundant in meat and dairy products, saturated fat tends to increase LDL cholesterol levels, and it may raise the risk of certain types of cancer.

Septal defect. A hole in the wall of the heart separating the atria, or in the wall of the heart separating the ventricles.

Septum. The muscular wall dividing a chamber on the left side of the heart from the chamber on the right.

Shock. A condition in which body function is impaired because the volume of fluid circulating through the body is insufficient to maintain normal metabolism. This may be caused by blood loss or by a disturbance in the function of the circulatory system.

Shunt. A connector that allows blood to flow between two locations.

Sick sinus syndrome. The failure of the sinus node to regulate the heart's rhythm.

Silent ischemia. Episodes of cardiac ischemia that are not accompanied by chest pain.

Sinoatrial (SA) node. The natural pacemaker of the heart; also called the sinus node. The SA node is a group of specialized cells in the top of the right atrium which produces the electrical impulses that travel down to eventually reach the ventricular muscle, causing the heart to contract.

Sodium. A mineral essential to life found in nearly all plant and animal tissue. Table salt (sodium chloride) is nearly half sodium.

Sphygmomanometer. An instrument used to measure blood pressure.

Stenosis. The narrowing or constriction of an opening, such as a blood vessel or heart valve.

Stent. A device made of expandable, metal mesh that is placed (by using a balloon on the tip of a catheter) at the site of a narrowing artery. The stent is then expanded and left in place to keep the artery open.

Sternum. The breastbone.

Stethoscope. An instrument for listening to sounds within the body.

Streptococcal infection (strep infection). An infection, usually in the throat, resulting from the presence of streptococcus bacteria.

Streptokinase. A clot-dissolving drug used to treat heart attack patients.

Stress. Bodily or mental tension resulting from physical, chemical, or emotional factors. Stress can refer to physical exertion as well as mental anxiety.

Stroke. A sudden disruption of blood flow to the brain, caused either by a clot or a leak in a blood vessel.

Subarachnoid hemorrhage. Bleeding from a blood vessel on the surface of the brain into the space between the brain and the skull.

Sudden death. Death that occurs unexpectedly and instantaneously or shortly after the onset of symptoms. The most common underlying reason for patients dying suddenly is cardiovascular disease—in particular, coronary heart disease.

Superior vena cava. The large vein that returns blood from the head and arms to the heart.

Syncope. A temporary, insufficient blood supply to the brain which causes a loss of consciousness. Usually caused by a serious arrhythmia.

Systolic blood pressure. The highest blood pressure measured in the arteries. It occurs when the heart contracts with each heartbeat.

Tachycardia. Accelerated beating of the heart. Paroxysmal tachycardia is a particular form of rapid heart action, occurring in seizures that may last from a few seconds to several days.

Tachypnea. Rapid breathing.

Thallium-201 stress test. An X-ray study that follows the path of radioactive potassium carried by the blood into heart muscle. Damaged or dead muscle can be defined, as can the extent of narrowing in an artery.

Thrombolysis. The breaking up of a blood clot.

Thrombolytic therapy. A drug that dissolves blood clots.

Thrombosis. A blood clot that forms inside the blood vessel or cavity of the heart.

Thrombus. A blood clot.

Tissue plasminogen activator (TPA). A clot-dissolving drug used to treat heart attack patients.

Transesophageal echocardiography (TEE). A diagnostic test that analyzes sound waves bounced off the heart. The sound waves are sent through a tubelike device inserted in the mouth and passed down the esophagus (food pipe), which ends near the heart. This technique is useful in studying patients whose heart and blood vessels, for various reasons, are difficult to assess with standard echocardiography.

Trans **fat.** Created when hydrogen is forced through an ordinary vegetable oil (hydrogenation), converting some polyunsaturates to monounsaturates, and some monounsaturates to saturates. *Trans* fat, like saturated fat, tends to raise LDL cholesterol levels, but, unlike saturated fat, tends to lower HDL cholesterol levels at the same time.

Transient ischemic attack (TIA). A temporary, strokelike event that lasts for only a short time and is caused by a temporarily blocked blood vessel.

Transplantation. Replacing a defective organ with one from a donor.

Tricuspid valve. The structure that controls blood flow from the heart's right atrium (upper chamber) into the right ventricle (lower chamber).

Triglyceride. The chemical term for fat; normally stored as an energy source in fat tissue. High triglyceride levels may thicken the blood and make a person more susceptible to clot formation. High triglyceride levels tend to accompany high cholesterol levels and other risk factors for heart disease such as obesity.

Ultrasound. High-frequency sound vibrations, not audible to the human ear, used in medical diagnosis.

Valvuloplasty. The reshaping of a heart valve through surgical or catheterization techniques.

Varicose vein. Any vein that is abnormally dilated.

Vascular. Pertaining to the blood vessels.

Vasodilators. Any medication that dilates (widens) the arteries.

Vasopressors. Any medication that elevates blood pressure.

Vein. Any one of a series of blood vessels of the vascular system that carries blood from various parts of the body back to the heart; returns oxygen-depleted blood to the heart.

Ventricle (right and left). One of the two lower chambers of the heart.

Ventricular fibrillation (VF). A condition in which the ventricles contract in a rapid, unsynchronized fashion. When fibrillation occurs, the ventricles cannot pump blood throughout the body.

Ventricular tachycardia. An arrhythmia (abnormal heartbeat) in the ventricle characterized by a very fast heartbeat.

Vertigo. A feeling of dizziness or spinning.

Wolff-Parkinson-White syndrome. A condition in which an extra electrical pathway connects the atria (two upper chambers) and the ventricles (two lower chambers). It may cause a rapid heartbeat.

X ray. Form of radiation used to create a picture of internal body structures on film.

Selected References

Chapter 1

Thompson GR, Wilson PW. Coronary risk factors and their assessment. London: Science Press, 1992.

Chapter 2

The American College of Obstetricians and Gynecologists. Exercise during pregnancy and the postpartum period. Washington, DC: ACOG, 1994; ACOG Technical Bulletin No. 189.

The American College of Obstetricians and Gynecologists. Women and exercise. Washington, DC: ACOG, 1992; ACOG Technical Bulletin No. 173.

American Heart Association and National Heart, Lung, and Blood Institute. Exercise and your heart: A guide to physical activity. Dallas, TX: American Heart Association, 1993.

Blair SN, Kohl HW 3d, Paffenbarger RS Jr, et al. Physical fitness and all-cause mortality: A prospective study of healthy men and women. Journal of the American Medical Association 1989; 262:2395–401.

Centers for Disease Control and Prevention. Prevalence of sedentary lifestyle—behavioral risk factor surveillance system, United States, 1991. Morbidity and Mortality Weekly Report 1993; 42(29):576–9.

Mittleman MA, Machure M, Tofler GH, et al. Triggering of acute myocardial infarction by heavy physical exertion. Protection against triggering by regular exertion. Determinants of Myocardial Infarction Onset Study Investigators. New England Journal of Medicine 1993; 329(23): 1677–83.

Sandvik L, Erikssen J, Thaulow E, et al. Physical fitness as a predictor of mortality among healthy middle-aged Norwegian men. New England Journal of Medicine 1993; 328(8):533–7.

Schmied LA, Steinberg H, Moss T, Sykes EA. Aerobic exercise and Type A behaviour. Journal of Sports Sciences 1994; 12:433–45.

Sol N, Foster C, eds. ACSM's health/fitness facility standards and guidelines / American College of Sports Medicine. Champaign, IL: Human Kinetic Books, 1992.

Vaitkevicius PV, Fleg JL, Engel JH, et al. Effects of age and aerobic capacity on arterial stiffness in healthy adults. Circulation 1993; 88[part 1]: 1456–62.

Weyerer S, Kupfer B. Physical exercise and psychological health. Sports Medicine 1994; 17:108–16.

Chapter 3

Boeing H, Frentzel-Beyme R, Berger M, et al. Case-control study on stomach cancer in Germany. International Journal of Cancer 1991; 47:858–64.

Bolton-Smith C, Woodward M, Tunstall-Pedoe H. The Scottish Heart Health Study. Dietary intake by food frequency questionnaire and odds ratios for coronary heart disease risk. II. The antioxidant vitamins and fibre. European Journal of Clinical Nutrition 1992; 46:85–93.

Cooley DA, Moore CE. Eat smart for a healthy heart cookbook. Hauppage, NY: Barron's, 1987.

Enstrom JE, Kanin LE, Klein MA. Vitamin C intake and mortality among a sample of the United States population. Epidemiology 1992; 3:194–202.

Hemila H. Does vitamin C alleviate the symptoms of the common cold? A review of current evidence. Scandinavian Journal of Infectious Diseases 1994; 26:1–6.

Hemila H. Vitamin C and the common cold. British Journal of Nutrition 1992; 67:3–16.

Hennekens CH. Antioxidant vitamins and cancer. American Journal of Medicine 1994; 97:25–45; discussion 22S–8S.

Human Nutrition Information Service. The food guide pyramid. Washington, DC: U.S. Department of Agriculture, 1992; Home and Garden Bulletin No. 252.

Lalanne E. Eating right for a new you: Peak nutrition for fitness after fifty. New York: Plume/Penguin, 1992.

La Vecchia C, D'Avanzo B, Negri E, et al. Attributable risks for stomach cancer in northern Italy. International Journal of Cancer 1995; 60: 748–52.

Love JM, Gudas LJ. Vitamin A, differentiation and cancer. Current Opinion in Cell Biology 1994; 6:825–31.

McKenney JM, Proctor JD, Harris S, et al. A comparison of the efficacy and toxic effects of sustained- vs immediate-release niacin in hyper-cholesterolemic patients. Journal of the American Medical Association 1994; 271:672–7.

Mera SL. Diet and disease. British Journal of Biomedical Science 1994; 51:189–206.

National Research Council, National Academy of Sciences. Recommended dietary allowances, 10th ed. Washington, DC: National Academy Press, 1989.

Porrini M, Simonetti P, Testolin G, et al. Relation between diet composition and coronary heart disease risk factors. Journal of Epidemiology and Community Health 1991; 45:148–51.

Public Health Service. Nutrition and your health: Dietary guidelines for Americans. Washington, DC: U.S. Department of Agriculture, U.S. Department of Health and Human Services, 1990; Home and Garden Bulletin No. 232.

Public Health Service. The Surgeon General's report of nutrition and health / U.S. Department of Health and Human Services; introduction by Marion Nestle. New York: Warner Books, 1989.

Richardson LA. Diets and weight loss. Harrisonburg, VA: Banta, 1993.

Singh RB, Ghosh S, Niaz AM, et al. Epidemiologic study of diet and coronary risk factors in relation to central obesity and insulin levels in rural and urban population of north India. International Journal of Cardiology 1995; 47:245–55.

Singh RB, Rastogi SS, Sircar AR, et al. Dietary strategies for risk-factor modification to prevent cardiovascular diseases. Nutrition 1991; 7:210–4.

Willett WC. Diet and health: What should we eat? Science 1994; 264:532–7.

Willett WC, Ascherio A. Trans fatty acids: Are the effects only marginal? American Journal of Public Health 1994; 84:722–4.

Woodard DA, Limacher MC. The impact of diet on coronary heart disease. Medical Clinics of North America 1993; 77:849–62.

Chapter 4

National Task Force on the Prevention and Treatment of Obesity. Weight cycling. Journal of the American Medical Association 1994; 272(15): 1196–202.

Public Health Service. Nutrition and your health: Dietary guideline for Americans. Washington, DC: U.S. Department of Agriculture, U.S. Department of Health and Human Services, 1990; Home and Garden Bulletin No. 232.

Public Health Service. The Surgeon General's report of nutrition and health / U.S. Department of Health and Human Services; introduction by Marion Nestle. New York: Warner Books, 1989.

Chapter 5

American Heart Association. Heart and stroke facts: 1994 statistical supplement. Dallas, TX: American Heart Association, 1993.

Centers for Disease Control and Prevention. Cigarette smoking—attributable mortality and years of potential life lost—United States, 1990. Morbidity and Mortality Weekly Report 1993; 42(33):645–9.

Heart disease: Women at risk. Consumer Reports 1993 May; 300–4.

Shiu M. Refusing to treat smokers is unethical and a dangerous precedent. British Medical Journal 1993; 306(6884):1048–9.

Chapter 6

American Heart Association. Rationale of the Diet-Heart Statement of the American Heart Association. Publication #71–0030. Dallas, TX: American Heart Association, 1995.

Gaziano JM, Buring JE, Breslow JL, et al. Moderate alcohol intake, increased levels of high-density lipoprotein and its subfractions, and decreased risk of myocardial infarction. New England Journal of Medicine 1993; 329(25):1829–34.

Institute for Health Policy, Brandeis University, for The Robert Wood Johnson Foundation. Substance abuse: The nation's number one health problem. Princeton, NJ: The Robert Wood Johnson Foundation, 1993.

Chapter 7

Eliot RS, Iles RL, Kumar N, Morales-Ballejo H. Emotions and coronary heart disease. Heart Disease and Stroke 1994; 3:361–4.

Thompson GR, Wilson PW. Coronary risk factors and their assessment. London: Science Press, 1992.

Chapter 8

American Heart Association. Heart and stroke facts: 1995 statistical supplement. Dallas, TX: American Heart Association, 1995.

Caulfield M, Lavender P, Farrall M, et al. Linkage of the angiotensinogen gene to essential hypertension. New England Journal of Medicine 1994; 330:1629–33.

Clark LT. Improving compliance and increasing control of hypertension: Needs of special hypertensive populations. American Heart Journal 1991; 121:664–9.

Hollenberg NK. Hypertension and the kidney: Determinants of the response to antihypertensive therapy and their implications. American Heart Journal 1993; 125(2 Pt 2):604–8.

National Institutes of Health. Fifth report of the Joint National Committee on Detection, Evaluation, and Treatment of High Blood Pressure. Archives of Internal Medicine 1993; 153:154–83.

Chapter 9

Castelli WP. Epidemiology of triglycerides: A view from Framingham. American Journal of Cardiology 1992; 70(19):3H–9H.

Grundy SM. Etiologies and treatment of hyperlipidemia. In: Willerson JT, ed. Treatment of heart diseases. New York: Raven Press, 1992:4.3–4.79.

Hoeg JM, Klimov AN. Cholesterol and atherosclerosis: "The new is the old rediscovered" (editorial). American Journal of Cardiology 1993; 72: 1071–2.

Kannel WB, Wilson PW. Efficacy of lipid profiles in prediction of coronary disease. American Heart Journal 1992; 124:768–74.

Kinosian B, Glick H, Garland G. Cholesterol and coronary heart disease: Predicting risks by levels and ratios. Annals of Internal Medicine 1994; 121:641–7.

Stamler J, Wentworth D, Neaton JD. Is the relationship between serum cholesterol and risk of premature death from coronary heart disease continuous and graded? Findings in 356,222 primary screenees of the Multiple Risk Factor Intervention Trial. Journal of the American Medical Association 1986; 256(20):2823–8.

Summary of the second report of the National Cholesterol Education Program (NCEP) Expert Panel on Detection, Evaluation, and Treatment of High Blood Pressure Cholesterol in Adults (Adult Treatment Panel II). Journal of the American Medical Association 1993; 269(23):3015–23.

Chapter 10

The Diabetes Control and Complications Trial Research Group. The effect of intensive treatment of diabetes on the development and progression of long-term complications in insulin-dependent diabetes mellitus. New England Journal of Medicine 1993; 329(14):977–86.

King H, Rewers M. Global estimates for prevalence of diabetes mellitus and impaired glucose tolerance in adults. WHO Ad Hoc Diabetes Reporting Group. Diabetes Care 1993;16(1):157–77.

National Institute of Diabetes and Digestive and Kidney Diseases. Diabetes overview: National diabetes information clearinghouse. Washington, DC: Public Health Service, U.S. Department of Health and Human Services, National Institutes of Health; 1994. NIH Publication No. 94–3235.

Public Health Service. Diabetes in adults. Washington, DC: U.S. Department of Health and Human Services, National Institutes of Health; 1990. NIH Publication No. 90–2904.

Chapter 11

American Heart Association. Heart and stroke facts: 1995 statistical supplement. Dallas, TX: American Heart Association, 1994.

Ayanian JZ, Epstein AM. Differences in the use of procedures between women and men hospitalized for coronary heart disease. New England Journal of Medicine 1991; 325:221–5.

Barrett-Connor EL, Cohn BA, Wingard DL, Edelstein SL. Why is diabetes mellitus a stronger risk factor for fatal ischemic heart disease in women than in men? The Rancho Bernardo Study. Journal of the American Medical Association 1991; 265(5):627–31.

Croft P, Hannaford PC. Risk factors for acute myocardial infarction in women: Evidence from the Royal College of General Practitioners' oral contraception study. British Medical Journal 1989; 298(6667):165–8.

Hannan EL, Bernard HR, Kilburn HC Jr, O'Donnell JF. Gender differences in mortality rates for coronary artery bypass surgery. American Heart Journal 1992; 123(4 Pt 1):866–72.

Karlson BW, Herlitz J, Hartford M. Prognosis in myocardial infarction in relation to gender. American Heart Journal 1994; 128(3):477–83.

Kawachi I, Colditz GA, Stampfer MJ, et al. Smoking cessation and time course of decreased risks of coronary heart disease in middle-aged women. Archives of Internal Medicine 1994; 154(2):169–75.

Kelsey SF, James M, Holubkov AL, et al. Results of percutaneous transluminal coronary angioplasty in women: 1985–1986 National Heart, Lung, and

Blood Institute's Coronary Angioplasty Registry. Circulation 1993; 87:720–7.

Manson JE. Postmenopausal hormone therapy and atherosclerotic disease. American Heart Journal 1994; 128(6 Pt 2):1337–43.

National Center for Health Statistics. Provisional number of deaths for the 10 leading causes of death by age, race, and sex: United States, 1992. Monthly Vital Statistics Report 1993; 41(13).

Ness RB, Harris T, Cobb J, et al. Number of pregnancies and the subsequent risk of cardiovascular disease. New England Journal of Medicine 1993; 328:1528–33.

Romm PA, Green CE, Reagan K, Rackley CE. Relation of serum lipoprotein cholesterol levels to presence and severity of angiographic coronary artery disease. American Journal of Cardiology 1991; 67:479–83.

Steingart RM, Packer M, Hamm P. Sex differences in the management of coronary artery disease. New England Journal of Medicine 1991; 325:226–30.

Wilkinson P, Laji K, Ranjadayalan K, et al. Acute myocardial infarction in women: Survival analysis in first six months. British Medical Journal 1994; 309(6954):566–9.

Chapter 12

American Heart Association. Heart and stroke facts: 1995 statistical supplement. Dallas, TX: American Heart Association, 1994.

Blair SN, Kohl HW 3rd, Barlow CE, et al. Changes in physical fitness and all-cause mortality: A prospective study of healthy and unhealthy men. Journal of the American Medical Association 1995; 273:1093–8.

Burris JF. Practical considerations in treating the elderly hypertensive patient. American Journal of Medicine 1991; 90(4B):28S–31S.

Finucane FF, Madans JH, Bush TL, et al. Decreased risk of stroke among postmenopausal hormone users. Results from a national cohort. Archives of Internal Medicine 1993; 153:73–9.

Hall WD. Hypertension in the elderly with a special focus on treatment with angiotensin-converting enzyme inhibitors and calcium antagonists. American Journal of Cardiology 1992; 69:33E–42E.

Johnson K, Kligman EW. Preventive nutrition: Disease-specific dietary interventions for older adults. Geriatrics 1992; 47:39–40, 45–9.

Kris-Etherton PM, Krummel D. Role of nutrition in the prevention and treatment of coronary heart disease in women. Journal of the American Dietetic Association 1993; 93:987–93.

Montague TJ, Ikuta RM, Wong RY, et al. Comparison of risks and patterns of practice in patients older and younger than 70 years with acute myocardial infarction in a two-year period (1987–1989). American Journal of Cardiology 1991; 68:843–7.

O'Malley K, Cox JP, O'Brien E. Choice of drug treatment for elderly hypertensive patients. American Journal of Medicine 1991; 90(3A):27S-33S.

Paffenbarger RS Jr, Hyde RT, Wing AL, et al. The association of changes in physical-activity level and other lifestyle characteristics with mortality among men. New England Journal of Medicine 1993; 328:538–45.

Ryan C. Hypertension in the elderly patient. American Heart Journal 1991; 122(4 Pt 2):1225–7.

Sempos CT, Cleeman JI, Carroll MD, et al. Prevalence of high blood cholesterol among U.S. adults. An update based on guidelines from the second report of the National Cholesterol Education Program Adult Treatment Panel. Journal of the American Medical Association 1993; 269:3009–14.

Sherman SE, D'Agostino RB, Cobb JL, Kannel WB. Does exercise reduce mortality rates in the elderly? Experience from the Framingham Heart Study. American Heart Journal 1994; 128:965–72.

Chapter 13

American Heart Association. Heart and stroke facts: 1995 statistical supplement. Dallas, TX: American Heart Association, 1994.

Centers for Disease Control and Prevention. Current cigarette smoking by persons 18 years of age and over, according to sex, race, and age: United States, selected years 1965–92. National Center for Health Statistics, 1993.

Levy RA. Ethnic and racial differences in response to medicines: Preserving individualized therapy in managed pharmaceutical programs. Pharmaceutical Medicine 1993; 7:139.

Luft FC, Miller JZ, Grim CE, et al. Salt sensitivity and resistance of blood pressure. Age and race as factors in physiological responses. Hypertension 1991; 17(1 Suppl):1102–8.

National Center for Health Statistics. The advance report of final mortality statistics, 1988. Public Health Service, U.S. Department of Health and Human Services, 1990.

Public Health Service. Healthy people 2000: National health promotion and disease prevention objectives—full report, with commentary. Washington, DC: U.S. Department of Health and Human Services, 1991; DHHS Publication No. (PHS)91–50212.

Sorlie PD, Backlund E, Johnson NJ, Rogot E. Mortality by Hispanic status in the United States. Journal of the American Medical Association 1993; 270(20):2464–8.

Whittle J, Conigliaro J, Good CB, Lofgren RP. Racial differences in the use of invasive cardiovascular procedures in Department of Veterans Affairs medical system. New England Journal of Medicine 1993; 329(9): 621–7.

Chapter 14

Castro-Beiras A, Muniz J, Fernandez-Fuertes I. Family history as an independent risk factor for ischaemic heart disease in a low incidence area (Galicia, Spain). European Heart Journal 1993; 14:1445–50.

Marenberg ME, Risch N, Berkman LF, et al. Genetic susceptibility to death from coronary heart disease in a study of twins. New England Journal of Medicine 1994; 330:1041–6.

Sol N, Foster C, editors. ACSM's health/fitness facility standards and guidelines / American College of Sports Medicine. Champaign, IL: Human Kinetic Books, 1992.

Chapter 15

American Heart Association and National Heart, Lung, and Blood Institute. Exercise and your heart: A guide to physical activity. Dallas, TX: American Heart Association, 1993.

Dishman RK. Compliance/adherence in health related exercise. Health Psychology 1982; 1:237–67.

Fletcher GF, Froelicher VF, Hartley LH, et al. Exercise standards: A statement for health professionals from the American Heart Association. Circulation 1990; 82:2286–322.

Morris CK, Myers J, Froelicher VF, et al. Nomogram based on metabolic equivalents and age for assessing aerobic exercise capacity in men. Journal of the American College of Cardiology 1993; 22(1):175–82.

Pate RR, Pratt M, Blair SN, et al. Physical activity and public health: A recommendation from the Centers for Disease Control and Prevention and the American College of Sports Medicine. Journal of the American Medical Association 1995; 273(5):402–7.

Public Health Service. Healthy People 2000: National health promotion and disease prevention objectives—full report, with commentary. Washington, DC: U.S. Department of Health and Human Service, 1991; DHHS Publication No. (PHS)91–50212.

Sallis JF, Haskell WL, Fortmann SP, et al. Predictors of adoption and maintenance of physical exercise in a community sample. Preventive Medicine 1986; 15:331–41.

Chapter 16

American Heart Association. Heart and stroke facts: 1995 statistical supplement. Dallas, TX: American Heart Association, 1994.

American Heart Association and National Heart, Lung, and Blood Institute. Exercise and your heart: A guide to physical activity. Dallas, TX: American Heart Association, 1993.

Dishman RK. Compliance/adherence in health related exercise. Health Psychology 1982; 1:237–67.

Fletcher GF, Froelicher VF, Hartley LH, et al. Exercise standards: A statement for health professionals from the American Heart Association. Circulation 1990; 82:2286–322.

Morris CK, Myers J, Froelicher VF, et al. Nomogram based on metabolic equivalents and age for assessing aerobic exercise capacity in men. Journal of the American College of Cardiology 1993; 22(1):175–82.

Public Health Service. Healthy People 2000: National health promotion and disease prevention objectives—full report, with commentary. Washington, DC: U.S. Department of Health and Human Services, 1991; DHHS Publication No. (PHS)91–50212.

Sallis JF, Haskell WL, Fortmann SP, et al. Predictors of adoption and maintenance of physical exercise in a community sample. Preventive Medicine 1986; 15:331.

Shephard RJ. Nutritional benefits of exercise. Journal of Sports Medicine and Physical Fitness 1989; 29:83–90.

Chapter 17

Centers for Disease Control and Prevention. Cigarette smoking—attributable mortality and years of potential life lost—United States, 1990. Morbidity and Mortality Weekly Report 1993; 42(33):645–9.

Chapter 18

Eliot RS. From stress to strength: How to lighten your load and save your life. New York: Bantam, 1993.

Chapter 19

Cooley DA, Moore CE. Eat smart for a healthy heart cookbook. Hauppage, NY: Barron's, 1987.

Moran V. Get the fat out: 501 ways to cut the fat in any diet. New York: Crown, 1994.

Winston M, ed. American Heart Association cookbook. 5th ed. New York: Times Books, 1991.

Chapter 21

Chandra NC, Hazinski MF, Stapleton E, eds. Instructor's manual for basic life support. Dallas, TX: American Heart Association, 1994.

Hazinski MF, Chameides L. Instructor's manual for pediatric basic life support. Dallas, TX: American Heart Association, 1994.

Chapters 23 to 34

American Academy of Pediatrics Committee on Sports Medicine. Recommendations for participation in competitive sports. Pediatrics 1988; 81:737–9.

The American College of Cardiology and the American College of Sports Medicine. Recommendations for determining eligibility for competition in athletes with cardiovascular abnormalities. Journal of the American College of Cardiology 1994; 24:845–99.

Angelini P. Balloon catheter coronary angioplasty. Mount Kisco, New York: Futura, 1987.

Cooley DA. Surgical treatment of aortic aneurysms. Philadelphia: W.B. Saunders, 1986.

Cooley DA. Techniques in cardiac surgery. Philadelphia: W.B. Saunders, 1984.

Frazier OH, Macris MP, Radovancevic B. Support and replacement of the failing heart. Philadelphia: Lippincott, 1995.

Garson A, Bricker JT, McNamara DG. The science and practice of pediatric cardiology. Philadelphia: Lea & Febiger, 1990.

Gillette PC, Garson A. Pediatric arrhythmias: Electrophysiology and pacing. Philadelphia: W.B. Saunders, 1990.

Hallman GL, Cooley DA, Gutgesell HP. Surgical treatment of congenital heart disease, 3rd ed. Philadelphia: Lea & Febiger, 1987.

Kirklin JW, Barratt-Boyes BG. Cardiac surgery, 2nd ed. New York: Churchill Livingstone, 1993.

Leachman DR, Leachman RD. Coronary and peripheral angiography and angioplasty. Philadelphia: Lippincott, 1989.

McCaffrey FM, Braden DS, Strong WB. Sudden cardiac death in young athletes: A review. American Journal of Diseases of Children 1991; 145: 177–83.

Mullins CE, Mayer DC. Congenital heart disease: A diagrammatic atlas. New York: Wiley-Liss, 1988.

Netter FH. The Ciba collection of medical illustrations, volume 5, the heart. West Caldwell, NJ: Ciba Pharmaceutical Company, 1978.

Schlant RC, Alexander RW, eds. Hurst's the heart: Arteries and veins, 8th ed. New York: McGraw-Hill, 1994.

Willerson JT, ed. Treatment of heart disease. New York: Gower Medical Publishing, 1992.

Willerson JT, Cohn JN, eds. Cardiovascular medicine. New York: Churchill Livingstone, 1995.

Index